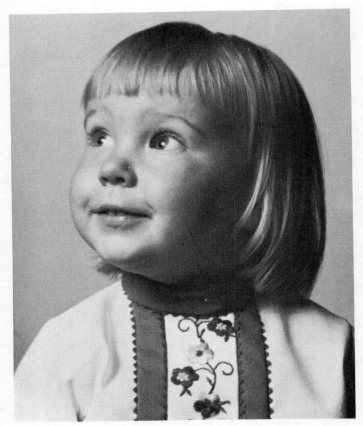

Heredity colors the eyes; environment puts the light in them.

PEDIATRICS
FOR
PRACTICAL NURSES
2nd Edition

Eleanor Dumont Thompson, R.N.

Formerly Pediatric Clinical Instructor, Practical Nurse
Students, Mary Hitchcock Memorial Hospital, Hanover,
N.H. Formerly Instructor of Pediatrics, Nursing Instructor,
and Instructor, Body Structure and Function, Hanover
School of Practical Nursing, Hanover, N.H.

W. B. SAUNDERS COMPANY
Philadelphia • London • Toronto

W. B. Saunders Company: West Washington Square
Philadelphia, Pa.   19105

12 Dyott Street
London, WC1A   1DB

833 Oxford Street
Toronto 18, Ontario

Pediatrics for Practical Nurses   ISBN 0-7216-8841-1

Print No.:   9   8   7   6   5   4

TO
JULIE

PREFACE TO THE SECOND EDITION

Since the original publication of this text, many exciting advances have developed in the field of pediatrics. In this second edition I have tried to incorporate the newer trends, while bearing in mind the role and responsibilities of the practical nursing student. The organization of the book around specific areas of growth and development from the prenatal period to adolescence has been maintained. I have completely reorganized Chapter Six, Disorders of the Newborn, so that the congenital anomalies are now grouped together for more uniformity of thought.

I have given more emphasis to the emotional aspects of illness and to the practical nurse's role in providing emotional support to the child and his family. The value of play and the contributions of the student in this area have been covered more fully.

Current programs for child care on a local, national, and international level are discussed. Modern methods of detection and treatment of such conditions as erythroblastosis fetalis, Down's syndrome, and congenital heart defects are discussed, and the nursing care is given in detail. The section on mental retardation has been greatly expanded. New illustrations and diagrams help to clarify the material and to make it more interesting to the student. A glossary has been added as a study guide.

At the suggestions of many educators in the field of practical nursing throughout the United States and Canada, I have added a discussion of the following disease conditions to the text: bronchitis, congenital heart defects, cystic fibrosis, dislocation of the hip, acute glomerulonephritis, lead poisoning, asthma, phenylketonuria, aspirin poisoning, thalassemia, kwashiorkor, atelectasis, Wilms' tumor, esophageal stricture, drug abuse, battered child syndrome, and the child with emotional disturbance.

ELEANOR DUMONT THOMPSON

ACKNOWLEDGMENTS

Many professional persons have willingly reviewed and/or offered the use of their facilities so that the revision of this book could be made possible. My sincere thanks are extended to the following:

Robert A. Joy, M.D., Manchester, N.H. Fellow of the American Academy of Pediatrics. Mrs. Georgina T. Westover, R.N., B.S., Instructor, Sacred Heart Hospital, School of Nursing, Manchester, N.H., Former Coordinator, Exeter School of Practical Nursing, Exeter, N.H. Sister Nora Therese Barrett, R.N., B.S., Director, St. Vincent Hospital, School of Practical Nursing, Montclair, N.J. Mrs. Ruth M. Greenspan, B.S., R.N., Associate Director St. Barnabas Medical Center, School of Practical Nursing, Livingston, N.J. Miss Gloria Harris, R.N., B.S., Senior Instructor, St. Vincent Hospital, School of Practical Nursing, Montclair, N.J.

I have also retained many pertinent suggestions and illustrations made possible by contributors to the first edition. My appreciation is extended to Mr. Lawrence DeBonis, photographer, and to all the parents who allowed their children to be photographed or who submitted pictures for use in the text.

I am grateful to the staff of the W. B. Saunders Company for their assistance, and to the publishers, companies, and other disciplines who granted permission to reproduce photographs and other materials.

In conclusion, I would like to acknowledge the cooperation of the members of my family, my husband Carl, our nine year old daughter Justine and our three year old newcomer to this edition, Julie. I also appreciate the confidence shown by so many in the first edition which provided the stimulus for the updating of this text.

ELEANOR DUMONT THOMPSON

PREFACE TO THE FIRST EDITION

In recent years, practical nurse programs have developed rapidly. The practical nurse is recognized as a valuable team member, and the scope of her activities has broadened. *Pediatrics for Practical Nurses* was written to help meet the needs of the student in the area of child care. The number of hours spent in pediatric study is necessarily limited in a course of practical nursing. I feel, therefore, that the student and graduate should own a comprehensive textbook in this particular area.

This book is organized around specific areas of growth and development from the prenatal period to adolescence. The practical nurse working on the children's ward cares for patients who are in the process of growth. Once she has considered the needs of the well child of a particular age, she advances to the disease conditions and their effect on the patient. The disease conditions were selected for their prevalence and for the variety of nursing procedures required in their treatment. A certain amount of intended repetition emphasizes specific points, e.g., charting and preventing infection.

Information on nutrition, immunizations, safety, and agencies concerned with child care has been included to create an awareness of the necessity of preventive pediatrics. Nursing care and procedures associated with the child in the home and hospital are presented. I have tried to give the student a better understanding of the effects of illness and hospitalization on the child and his family, as well as to develop an appreciation of her role and contributions in this particular area.

Each chapter is introduced by a suggested vocabulary. Vocabulary deficiencies or improper spelling may create great difficulties in learning and teaching. The selected words are commonly used in charting and

refer to the material about to be covered. Suggestions for study are
included at the end of each chapter to help the student to review and
correlate the material presented.

ELEANOR DUMONT THOMPSON

CONTENTS

Chapter 1

INTRODUCTION

VOCABULARY

Attention	*Humanity*
Charter	*Mortality*
Conference	*Opportunity*
Contribute	*Participate*
Cripple	*Poverty*
Depression	*Welfare*

Pediatrics is defined as the branch of medicine that deals with the child and his development and care, and the diseases of children and their treatment. The word is derived from the Greek *pais, paidos* child + *iatreia* cure. A medical doctor who specializes in pediatrics is called a *pediatrician.* Pediatric nursing as a specialty paralleled the establishment of departments of pediatrics in medical schools, the founding of children's hospitals, and the development of separate units for children in foundling homes and general hospitals.

THE CHILDREN'S BUREAU

Lillian Wald, a nurse who was interested in the welfare of children, is credited with suggesting the establishment of a federal children's bureau. She felt that if a nation could have a bureau dedicated to its farm crops, it should certainly have one to look after its "child crop." She and Florence Kelley, an ardent foe of child labor, were jointly responsible for the far-reaching conception of a children's bureau. The time was 1903.* It took several years before the bill was given the needed support by the first While House Conference on Children and Youth (see p. 4). The act directed the Children's Bureau "to investigate and report upon all matters pertaining to the welfare of children and child life among all classes of people."

Once the Children's Bureau was established, it focused its attention on the problems of infant mortality. This study was followed by one that dealt with maternal mortality. These investigations gave great impetus to

---

*Bradbury and Oettinger, pp. 1, 2.

drives for improvement in maternal and child health. Another early effort was made in the area of birth registration. This study eventually led to birth registrations in all states.

In the 1930's the Children's Bureau began to investigate the effects of the economic depression on children. It found that the health and nutrition of children throughout the nation was declining because of the great increase in poverty. As a result of the research done in this area, hot lunch programs were established in many schools.

During the depression, many adolescents found home life unbearable because of unemployment. Great numbers of adolescents wandered throughout the country in search for work. Since there was none to be found, they were not welcome in most communities. In 1933, the chief of the bureau made suggestions that were instrumental in the establishment of the Civilian Conservation Corps. These work camps provided opportunities for training in a wholesome environment and they proved very successful.

Throughout the 1920's and 1930's the Children's Bureau had been observing the conditions under which children were forced to work. The observations were appalling. A description of 13 and 14 year old children working in coal mines was particularly vivid.

Black coal dust is everywhere, covering the windows and filling the air and lungs of the workers. The slate is sharp so that slate pickers often cut or bruise their hands; the coal is carried down the chute in water and this means sore and swollen hands for the pickers. The first few weeks after the boy begins work his fingers bleed almost continuously, and are called "red tops" by the other boys.*

In one community, 64 per cent of the children under 16 years of age worked regularly standing in cold, damp and drafty sheds, doing wet, dirty, and sometimes unsanitary and dangerous work.* School attendance was sporadic. A child was considered well educated if he finished eighth grade.

These studies paved the way to a constitutional amendment that controls child labor. The *Fair Labor Standards Act* passed in 1938 established a general minimum working age of 16, a minimum working age of 18 for jobs considered hazardous. More importantly, this act paved the way for the establishment of national minimum standards for child labor, and provided a means for enforcement.†

In 1935, President Franklin D. Roosevelt signed the Social Security Act. Provisions for children were included in this act. A system was established whereby the states would be given financial assistance from the federal government for the development of child health programs and services for crippled children and child welfare, particularly in rural

---

*Bradbury and Oettinger, p. 40.
† Bradbury and Oettinger, p. 52.

areas. As larger yearly appropriations from the government have been made available, these programs have broadened.

During World War II the Children's Bureau had to adapt its program to meet the problems that faced the child and his family. The absence of fathers and the need for mothers to be employed in war plants created a new crisis.

Between 1946 and 1956, further advances were made in programs for maternal and child health, medical care for crippled children, and child welfare. Studies were reviewed, and further research was directed toward juvenile delinquency, mental retardation, adoption, and the emotional health of children.

In Miami, Florida, the immigration of Cuban citizens and unattached children presented a challenging problem. At the end of January 1962, there were 2450 unaccompanied Cuban children in foster care— 964 in the Miami area and 1486 in 67 communities in 30 states. The vast majority of these children were under the care of Catholic agencies. The Florida State Department of Public Welfare agreed to be the agent for the Department of Health, Education, and Welfare in planning for these children and in using federal funds for their care.*

Project Head Start, sponsored by the Office of Economic Opportunity, has proven itself an effective educational instrument. Deprived preschoolers have increased their academic skills and readiness for school through this program. Follow Through, another new program, will do just as its name implies by carrying over to the kindergarten and first grade the work which was begun in Head Start. Through this latter program, it is hoped that the initial gains made by a child will not be lost.

The members of the current Children's Bureau find themselves wrestling with some rather unique problems. Special emphasis is being given to mentally retarded children, juvenile delinquents, abused and neglected children, children of working mothers, refugees, and children of migrant agricultural workers. The Children's Bureau works actively with international organizations, two of which are the United Nations International Children's Emergency Fund (UNICEF) and the World Health Organization (WHO). Through these and other groups the health and welfare of children in undeveloped countries are being improved.

Unfortunately, only the bare highlights of the many accomplishments of the Children's Bureau can be reviewed in a pediatric text. Of course, this work was not accomplished alone, but was and is a team effort on the part of many federal, state, and local organizations, both public and private. The Children's Bureau wants every citizen to be a part of its campaign. This is evidenced by the great number of publications it distributes in an effort to educate the people of our country to

*Bradbury and Oettinger, p. 120.

the needs of its children.* All of us in the health field can contribute to this vast effort. The practical nurse who practices her vocation dedicatedly makes a significant contribution to humanity, for history shows us that the great accomplishments made in our country are, after all, the results of a job well done by each individual.

WHITE HOUSE CONFERENCES

The First White House Conference on Children and Youth was called by President Theodore Roosevelt in 1909. A similar conference now gathers every 10 years. As a result of the first meeting, the United States Children's Bureau was founded.

In the White House Conference on Child Health and Protection (1930), the famous *Children's Charter* was drawn up. This is considered to be one of the most important documents in child-care history. It lists 19 statements relative to needs of children in the areas of education, health, welfare, and protection. This declaration has been widely distributed throughout the world.

Preparations for the 1970 White House Conference on Children and Youth are now in progress, with approximately six million Americans becoming involved in its planning. President Nixon has appointed Stephen Hess as its National Chairman. This conference will be divided into two sessions—a Children's Conference (ages 0–13) which will be held December 13–18, 1970 and a Youth Conference to follow in June, 1971. The Children's Conference will stress the emergence of identity in the child. He will be seen as a person with feelings, needs, and potential. The president has asked the Youth Conference to search for a national youth policy to enable the United States to provide a coherent policy on matters pertaining to youth, e.g., military service, voting, education, government service, and so forth. Briefly three basic goals of the Youth Conference are: involvement of youth in our society, especially in the governmental process; accenting the quality of life, i.e., the good that is accomplished by youth rather than the negative, more publicized actions of youth; and establishing communications between the young people and government. Today's youth, when contrasted with those described by the 1960 Conference, are not apathetic; they are active and concerned with the country's problems.

CHANGING ATTITUDES IN CHILD CARE

The diseases of children have not always been studied as a separate entity. At one time children were placed in adult units, and there were no pediatricians. Emphasis was placed on the disease instead of the

*A list of publications may be obtained by writing to the Superintendent of Documents, U.S. Government Printing Office, Washington, D.C. 20402.

individual. This fortunately has changed. The child is no longer considered a "miniature adult." We understand him better and treat his mind as well as his body. We learn as much about our patient and his disease as we can, so that we can give him personal attention. As the practical nurse student advances through her pediatric experience, she will see for herself how each child responds differently to the problems of hospitalization.

Many advances in medical and surgical techniques have been made through the years. For instance, children with heart problems are now treated by a pediatric cardiologist. Much of the complex surgery required by the newborn with a congenital defect is provided by the pediatric surgeon. Emotional problems are managed by pediatric psychiatrists. Many hospital laboratories are better equipped to test pediatric specimens. The medical profession and allied agencies work as a team for the total well-being of the patient. Children with defects previously thought to be incompatible with life are taken to special diagnostic and treatment centers where they receive expert attention.

THE PUBLIC HEALTH DEPARTMENT

The public health department assumes a great deal of responsibility or the prevention of disease and death during childhood. This is done on a national, state, and local level. The water, milk, and food supplies of communities are inspected. Maintenance of proper sewerage and garbage disposal is enforced. Epidemics are investigated, and when necessary persons capable of transmitting diseases are isolated. The public health department is also concerned with the inspection of housing. It has recently directed its attention to the pressing needs of the American Indian and natives of Alaska for better health services.

Laws requiring the licensing of physicians and pharmacists indirectly affect the health of the child and the general public. Protection is also afforded by the Pure Food and Drug Act which controls medicines, poisons, and the purity of foods. Programs for disaster relief, care and rehabilitation of handicapped children, foster child care, family counseling, family day care, protective services for abused or neglected children, and education of the public are maintained and supported by governmental and private agencies. State licensing bureaus control the regulation of motor vehicles. This and the protection given the public through law enforcement agencies is of increasing importance since automobile accidents rank among the leading causes of injury and death of children.

STUDY QUESTIONS

1. Define the following: pediatrics, pediatrician, Children's Charter, Fair Labor Standards Act, UNICEF.

2. How often does the White House Conference on Children and Youth meet?
3. Where is the United States Children's Bureau Located?
4. How will the 1970 White House Conference differ from the previous conferences?

BIBLIOGRAPHY

Blake, F. G., and Wright, F. H.: Essentials of Pediatric Nursing. 7th Ed. Philadelphia, J. B. Lippincott Co., 1963.
Bradbury, D., and Oettinger, K.: Five Decades of Action for Children. Washington, D.C., Children's Bureau, Department of Health, Education, and Welfare, 1962.
Closing the "Generation Gap" — Search for a National Policy. Interview with Nixon's Adviser on Youth. U.S. News & World Report, pp. 56-59, Feb. 1970.
Dorland's Illustrated Medical Dictionary. 24th Ed. Philadelphia, W. B. Saunders Co. 1965.
Hess, Stephen: The White House Conference on Children: A Progress Report. Government Printing Office, 1970.
Marlow, D.: Textbook of Pediatric Nursing. 3rd Ed. Philadelphia, W. B. Saunders Co., 1969.
The White House: President's Statement on the Appointment of Stephen Hess As National Chairman of the White House Conference on Children and Youth. Government Printing Office, 1969.
United States Department of Health, Education, and Welfare: It's Your Children's Bureau. Government Printing Office, 1964.

Chapter 2

THE PRENATAL PERIOD

VOCABULARY

Ailment	*Pregnant*
Delivery	*Protein*
Discuss	*Public*
Disturb	*Health*
Encourage	*Toxemia*
Influence	*Trauma*
Midwife	

No discussion of pediatrics is complete unless one considers the influences of the prenatal period upon the baby and expectant mother. Ideally, preparation for parenthood is an extension of knowledge received throughout childhood. In our culture we believe that young men and women should be free to select their marital partners. Few couples give any thought to the advisability of the union in regard to their hereditary backgrounds and the effect that these might have on their offspring. Some states require a physical examination before a marriage license is issued, but the majority require merely a blood test for syphilis.

Young couples preparing for marriage should be encouraged to seek advice from their doctor and others in the field of marriage counseling. It is wise for the prospective bride to have a premarital pelvic examination so that any minor ailments may be corrected. It is equally advantageous for a woman to have a complete physical examination prior to conception. This will reassure her that she is in good health or will provide an opportunity for the doctor to detect and deal with disorders that would be more hazardous to treat during pregnancy. Physical and emotional preparation for marriage is essential because it is such an important and responsible career.

PRENATAL HEALTH SUPERVISION

A physical examination and certain laboratory tests are performed on the expectant mother early in pregnancy. The results of these tests indicate what treatment, if any, is necessary to improve the health of the

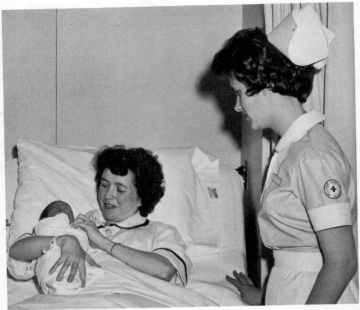

Figure 1. Pediatric nursing is an extension of maternity nursing. The fields are interdependent. (Courtesy of Saint Vincent Hospital School of Practical Nursing, Montclair, N. J.)

expectant mother and to protect the fetus. For instance, while treating the patient for such diseases as tuberculosis, diabetes, anemia, or heart and kidney disorders, the doctor will also be preventing the baby from the possibility of premature birth, toxemias, or anoxia. When the doctor measures and examines the pelvis, he becomes aware of some of the difficulties which could result and makes adequate plans for the delivery to minimize trauma to both mother and child. If a mother is known to be Rh negative, the physician makes special preparations for the handling of a baby with erythroblastosis fetalis. Widespread premarital blood tests are responsible for the decrease in congenital forms of syphilis.

An expectant mother may be vaccinated against polio to protect her from the more serious form of the disease, which may occur during pregnancy. It will also protect the baby from acquiring the disease from her during the prenatal and postnatal period. The nurse warns the expectant mother of the danger of contracting German measles during the first three months of pregnancy, because of the possibility of congenital malformation of the fetus. This hazard will lessen as more of the population become vaccinated against rubella. Likewise, the nurse teaches the pregnant woman the importance of including sufficient protein and vitamins in her diet to guard against premature birth and other complications.

The period of birth and the first and second days following birth are the most dangerous times in the life of the child. One can easily see why it is so necessary for an expectant mother to receive the best medical care possible in a hospital with adequate resources. A prospective mother may obtain the services of an obstetrician or she may prefer to see her family doctor. Clinics may be sponsored by a hospital, private agency, or the maternal and child health division of the department of health. The death rate of infants in the United States is not low enough. It falls behind several other countries in this respect. The main reasons

1st Month—Length 2.5-4 mm. (0.1-0.16 inches) (smaller than a BB shot). Rudiments of eyes, ears and nose appear. First traces of all organs become differentiated.

6th Month—Length 28-34 cm. (11.1-13.4 inches). Weight 650 Gm. (1.4 pounds). Skin wrinkles. Eyebrows and eyelashes appear. If born, fetus never survives.

2nd Month—Length 2.5 cm. (1 inch). Fetus markedly bent. Extremities rudimentary. Head disproportionately large, because of development of brain. External genitalia appear, but sex cannot be differentiated.

7th Month—Length 35-38 cm. (13.8-15.0 inches). Weight 1200 Gm. (2.6 pounds). Skin red and covered with vernix. Pupillary membranes disappear from eyes. If born, fetus breathes, cries, moves but usually dies.

3rd Month—Length 7-9 cm. (2.8-3.6 inches). Weight 5-20 Gm. (77-308 grains). Fingers and toes distinct, with soft nails.

8th Month—Length 38-43 cm. (15.0-17.0 inches). Weight 1600-1900 Gm. (3.5-4.2 pounds). Appearance of "little old man." If born, may live with proper care.

4th Month—Length 10-17 cm. (3.9-6.7 inches). Weight 55-120 Gm. (1.9-4.2 ounces). Sex can be definitely differentiated. Downy hair (lanugo) appears on head.

9th Month—Length 42-48 cm. (16.6-18.9 inches). Weight 1700-2600 Gm. (3.7-5.7 pounds). Face loses wrinkled appearance due to subcutaneous fat deposit. If born, good chance to survive.

5th Month—Length 18-27 cm. (7.1-10.6 inches). Weight 280-300 Gm. (9.9-10.6 ounces). Lanugo over entire body with small amount on head. Fetal movements usually felt by mother. Heart sounds perceptible.

10th Month—Length 48-52 cm. (18.9-20.5 inches). Weight 3000-3600 Gm. (6.6-7.9 pounds). Skin smooth, without lanugo (except about shoulders), covered with vernix. Scalp hair usually dark. Fingers and toes with well developed nails projecting beyond their tips. Eyes uniformly slate colored; impossible to predict final hue.

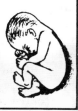

Figure 2. Changes in the fetus during the 10 lunar months of gestation. (From Schering Corporation.)

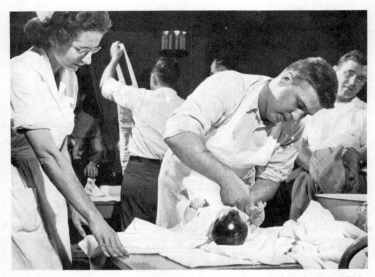

Figure 3.   What a help this will be for a busy mother, and bath time will be fun for father and baby. (From Davis, M. E., and Rubin, R.: DeLee's Obstetrics for Nurses. 17th Ed., 1962.)

for our failure to have a lower death rate are premature birth and inadequate prenatal care. This is particularly evident in the poor sections of large cities and rural areas. The need for accessible clinics for these citizens is great. Relatively few babies are delivered in the home. The midwife of yesterday has virtually disappeared. The registered nurse midwife available in some parts of the country must have advanced training in order to qualify for membership in the American College of Nurse Midwifery. She may deliver a baby in the home providing that there are no foreseeable complications. She works closely with an obstetrician and calls upon him if she feels that it is necessary.

A great deal of emphasis today is placed on the education of prospective parents. The trend is to revert to the more natural aspects of birth and child care. Natural childbirth, breast feeding, rooming-in, and demand feeding schedules are gaining popularity. Classes for expectant parents are sponsored by hospitals and other interested agencies, and include such topics as the structure and function of the reproductive system, prenatal care, labor and delivery, and care of the newborn. Parents who understand what is going to happen are less afraid. They receive the information enthusiastically since their interest is at its peak. These classes include lectures, demonstrations, and question and answer sessions. The principles and attitudes discussed help parents to become more receptive to further knowledge in the care and guidance of the child following birth.

The expectant mother must receive special attention. She needs an opportunity to talk to an understanding person about her feelings concerning her unborn child. The doctor may refer a mother who is very upset to a psychiatrist. Prompt treatment of emotional problems often prevents a disturbed mother-child relationship after the child has been born.

STUDY QUESTIONS

1. What are the advantages of physical examinations before marriage and conceptions?
2. List several hereditary diseases.
3. Mrs. Abbott, pregnant with her first child, has just returned from the doctor's office. She asks you why the doctor asked her so many questions about her past life. What would you reply?
4. What facilities are available in your community for the unwed mother?
5. Review the nutritional requirements of the expectant mother. (Consult your nutrition text.) How do the requirements differ from that of a nonpregnant woman?
6. What do you consider good prenatal care?
7. How can you contribute to the education of prospective parents?

BIBLIOGRAPHY

Blake, F. G., and Wright, F. H.: Essentials of Pediatric Nursing. Philadelphia, J. B. Lippincott Co., 1963.

Davis, M., and Rubin, R.: DeLee's Obstetrics for Nurses. 18th Ed. Philadelphia, W. B. Saunders Co., 1966.

Marlow, D. R.: Textbook of Pediatric Nursing. 3rd Ed. Philadelphia, W. B. Saunders Co., 1969.

Smith, C. S.: Maternal-Child Nursing. Philadelphia, W. B. Saunders Co., 1963.

Chapter 3

THE CHILD, THE HOSPITAL, THE PRACTICAL NURSE

VOCABULARY

Admitted	*Medication*
Ambulatory	*Specimen*
Cheerful	*Strapped*
Crying	*Stretcher*
Fearful	*Urine*
Lumbar puncture	*Wheel chair*

THE CHILDREN'S WARD

The student practical nurse may find her first day on the children's ward confusing because it is noisy and cluttered—it differs in many respects from adult divisions. The student's uniform will undoubtedly become crushed and crumpled within minutes. The pediatric ward or hospital is designed to meet the needs of children and their parents. A cheerful, casual atmosphere helps to bridge the gap between home and hospital, and is in keeping with the child's emotional as well as physical needs. Two newer trends are for patients to wear their own clothing while they are hospitalized and for the nurses to wear pastel uniforms or colorful smocks. Colored bedspreads and wagons or strollers for transportation are also more homelike.

The physical structure of the division includes furniture of the proper height for the child, soundproof ceilings, and color schemes with eye appeal. There is a special treatment room for the doctor to examine the patient. In this way the other children do not become disturbed by the proceedings. Some hospitals have a schoolroom. When this is not available, it is necessary for the teacher to visit each child individually in his room. Today's modern general hospitals have separate waiting rooms for children. This is more relaxing for parents, since they don't have to worry about their child disturbing adult patients, and it is less frightening to the child.

Most pediatric departments include a playroom in their structural

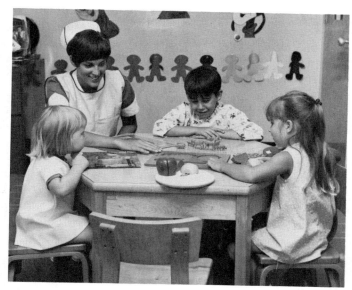

Figure 4. Children are no longer considered "miniature adults." Student practical nurse wears colorful smock over uniform. (Courtesy of St. Barnabas Medical Center, School of Practical Nursing, Livingston, N.J.)

plan. (See Fig. 4.) It is generally large and light in color. Bulletin boards and blackboards are within reach of the patients. Mobiles may be suspended from the ceiling. Some playrooms are equipped with an aquarium of fish and blossoming plants since children love living things. A variety of toys suitable for different age groups is available. This room may be under the supervision of a play lady or nursery school teacher. Parents usually enjoy taking their children to the playroom and observing the various activities. The practical nurse assisting should allow each child freedom to develop independently, and should avoid excessive demands or partiality. Further discussion on the value of play to the child is found on page 229.

Some children are not able to be taken to the playroom because of their physical condition. In such cases the nurse should provide a comfortable chair for the patient's mother so that she will be able to cuddle or read to him according to his needs and state of health.

Mealtimes on the children's ward differ from those on adult divisions. Patients whose conditions permit may be served together around small tables. This provides a homelike setting and offers the child a satisfying social experience.

The daily routine differs widely from adult wards, for obvious reasons. Although rigid schedules should be discouraged, children benefit from a certain amount of routine. Meals, rest, and play are carried out at approximately the same time each day. Continuity in nursing care whereby the same nurse cares for the child daily promotes further security for the child. Visiting hours on the pediatric unit are usually very liberal, for the child receives security from seeing his parents. They are encouraged to come as often as possible. Chairs which convert into beds for "rooming-in" facilities are now available.

SAFETY

The practical nurse must be especially conscious of safety measures on the children's ward. *Accidents are a major cause of death among infants and children.* By demonstrating her concern about safety regulations, the nurse not only reduces unnecessary accidents, but sets a good example for the parents of children who are placed in her care. Although the physical layout of each institution cannot be altered by personnel, there are many simple safety measures that can be carried out by the entire hospital team. The following is a list of measures applicable to the children's unit:

Do

1. Keep cribsides up at all times when the patient is unattended in bed.
2. Close safety pins at once and put them out of the child's reach.
3. Wash your hands before and after caring for each patient.
4. Fasten gates to children's rooms when leaving.
5. Check wheel chairs and stretchers before placing patients in them.
6. Place fans out of reach of the patient.
7. Inspect toys for sharp edges and removable parts.
8. Apply restraints correctly to prevent constriction of a part.
9. Keep medications and solutions out of reach of the child.
10. Lock the medication cabinet when not in use.
11. Identify the patient properly before giving medications.
12. Place electrical heating plates away from the patient's bed. Remain in the room while the unit is on.
13. Cap hot water bottles tightly. The water temperature should not be over 115° F.
14. Check thermometers for breakage before inserting, and remain with the patient while taking the temperature.
15. Prevent cross-infection. Diapers, toys, and materials that belong in one patient's unit should not be borrowed for another patient's use.
16. Take proper precautions when oxygen is in use.
17. Locate fire exits and extinguishers on your unit, and learn how to use them properly. Become familiar with your hospital fire manual.
18. Handle infants and small children carefully.

Do Not

1. Prop nursing bottles or force feedings on small children. There is danger of choking which may cause lung disease or sudden death.
2. Allow ambulatory patients to use wheel chairs or stretchers as toys.
3. Remove dressings or bandages unless specifically instructed.

4. Leave medications at the bedside.
5. Give oily medications to a crying child (because of the danger of choking).

Many other safety measures must be carried out as each student becomes more familiar with the hazards of her individual unit. The nurse must use her eyes to see with, not just to look at, and then must take the necessary precautions.

THE CHILD'S REACTION TO HOSPITALIZATION

The child's reaction to hospitalization depends on many factors such as his age, the amount of preparation he has been given, the security of his home life, and whether or not he has ever been in a hospital before. Many children cannot grasp what is going to happen to them even though they have been well prepared. At a time when the child needs his parents most he is separated from them, placed in the hands of strangers, and even fed different foods. Add to this a totally new environment and tummy ache, and you have the picture of one unhappy child. Each child reacts differently to hospitalization. One may be demanding and exhibit temper tantrums whole another becomes withdrawn. The

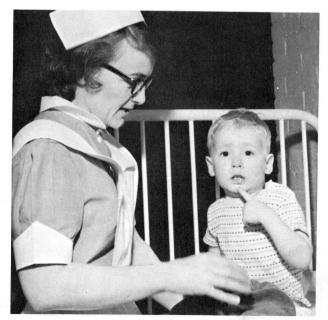

Figure 5. The nurse just came . . . will mother leave? Will she come back. . . .? Can I get to her? Does she still love me? (Courtesy of Moore General Hospital, School of Practical Nursing, Grasmere, N.H.)

"good" child on the ward may be going through greater torment than the one who cries and shows his resentment outwardly. The best prepared nurse cannot do for a child what his own mother can do.*

The child sees the nurse as someone who cares for him physically as his mother would and also as someone who is a source of security and comfort. He realizes that she sometimes administers strange treatments which can be painful. Soon he discovers her relationship with his parents and the doctor and that she is a liaison between hospital and home. Older children view the nurse as a health teacher and model to imitate. The patient learns to know "his" nurses if the changeover of nurses caring for him is kept at a minimum.

PARENTS' FEELINGS

The parents of the hospitalized youngster need to have interest directed toward them as well as the child. If they are frightened and tense the child will soon sense it. Some of the main reasons for their apprehension are:

Guilt Feelings. Parents sometimes feel that they are to blame for the child's illness. For example, they may have neglected to have the baby immunized or may have exposed him unknowingly to the disease. The practical nurse indicates by her manner that she does not blame the parents for the child's condition, even though she may sometimes feel otherwise.

Fear of the Unknown. They do not understand the ways of a hospital. The disease itself may be relatively rare. Poor communications may also result in unneccessary fears. The practical nurse can try to explain the use of some of the equipment she is using in simple terms. She should listen attentively and try to straighten out misconceptions. Very often parents are "left in the dark" about some of the most simple routines of the hospital merely because everyone just presumes that they have already been informed.

Fear of Improper Care. The public realizes that many hospitals are crowded and understaffed. Parents may also lack confidence in the doctor. Rooming-in may resolve this problem. The practical nurse should also attend to the needs of the child promptly and cheerfully which should indicate to the parents that he will be in good hands. Extended visiting hours for pediatric units are also beneficial.

Fear of Financial Burden. Hospital and doctor bills are expensive, particularly in long-term cases. The social service worker may be of help in such instances.

Fear That the Child Will Suffer. This may be due to the nature of the child's illness, or it may be fear of painful treatments or emotional

---

*Blake, p. 16.

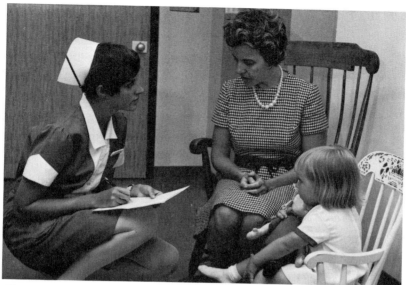

Figure 6. Establishing rapport with mother and patient is an important part of the admission procedure. (Courtesy of St. Barnabas Medical Center, School of Practical Nursing, Livingston, N.J.)

deprivation. Parents need reassurance that their child will receive medication for pain whenever necessary. It is also helpful to mention that although a lot of hospital equipment looks foreboding, very often their use presents little or no discomfort, i.e., x-rays, electrocardiograms, cast cutters, etc. Also, if a procedure is known to be painful, patients are frequently anesthetized or given analgesics beforehand.

Fear That Others in the Family May Contract the Disease. Parents may worry that the disease, e.g., eczema, is infectious, when actually there is no such problem. Reassurance by the nurse or doctor is indicated.

Fear That Their Child Will Transfer His Affection to Hospital Personnel. This is more noticeable when the mother is unable to assist with the child's care. The practical nurse should allow parents to assist with or administer the routine care of their child whenever possible.

The nurse must realize that parents are not themselves when they have such burdensome worries. Sometimes even the most mature adult may ask questions that seem illogical. It is not uncommon for mothers to cry. If the practical nurse could know the life history of each parent who enters the hospital with a sick child, she would be in a better position to understand his behavior and accept him as an individual. Behavior is not only a response to the current situation, but often involves attitudes resulting from early childhood experiences. Do not be too quick to pass judgment on individuals whose behavior may seem demanding or unreasonable. *An understanding of people and their problems is essential for the successful pediatric nurse.*

ADMISSION

As a member of the nursing team, the practical nurse is often called upon to admit the new patient. As well as knowing how to do the procedure skillfully, she must be prepared to meet the emotional needs of those involved. The impression she gives, whether good or bad, will definitely affect her patient's adjustment. When the inexperienced student admits her first patient, she may be nervous and frightened. After completing the procedure, she should stop for just a moment and recall her anxieties. Does she realize that the parents and child she has just left are equally as upset? She will never have to do that procedure for the first time again, but almost every admission will bring her in contact with a mother and child undergoing an experience that is unfamiliar to them. Empathy in dealing with the fears of the child and his parents makes the admission procedure stimulating rather than merely a task to be completed.

A child must be prepared for hospitalization. If possible, a tour of the pediatric ward by the parents and child before admission is advisable, and will enable the parents to meet the personnel who will be caring for their child. Recalling your original tour of the hospital may help you to understand the anxieties of the small patient. Your reaction depended on how familiar you were with such institutions. A child does not have this advantage to cushion his impressions.

Between the ages of one and three the child is very worried about being separated from his parents. After three he may become more fearful about what is going to happen to him. The parents should try and be as matter-of-fact about this new experience as possible. Unless he has been hospitalized before, the child tries to imagine what will happen to him. It is not necessary to go into much detail, since the child's imagination is great and giving information that is beyond his understanding may create unnecessary fears. It would seem logical to dwell on the more pleasant aspects, but not to the extent of saying that hospitalization will involve no discomforts. For example, one might mention that his meals will be served on a tray, that he may take a bath from a basin at his bedside, and that he will be with other children. The fact that he may have a buzzer to call the nurse if necessary may add to his security. The parents may also plan with the child what favorite toy or book he is going to bring. Perhaps more important than explaining certain occurrences is listening to how he feels and encouraging questions. Prepare him a few days but not weeks in advance. Never lure him to the hospital pretending it's some place else. In emergency situations there is little time for such preparation. The entire medical team must try to give added emotional support to the child in such cases.

Prepare the equipment for the admission procedure in advance. This will save time and will make you feel more secure. Once the smaller details are attended to concentrate on the approach to the patient and his family. The initial greeting should show warmth and friendliness. Smile and introduce yourself.

Some hospitals allow the patient to be taken to the playroom for a short time before going to his room. When the mother tells you the child's name, associate it with someone you know who has the same name. This will help you to remember it. It creates a much warmer feeling to speak of "John" or "Susy" than "your little boy [or girl]."

When the child and his parents are taken to the child's room, introduce them to the other children present. Explain the admission procedure carefully. Avoid discussing information the child will not understand in front of him. The mother is encouraged to do as much for her child as possible, e.g., remove his clothes. Try not to appear rushed. A matter-of-fact attitude must be maintained regardless of the patient's condition. A soft voice and quiet approach is less frightening to the child. If you look anxious, it will merely create unnecessary worry for everyone concerned. A nurse may look troubled when her apprehension has nothing to do with the patient involved. Take one step at a time. Calmness is catching. The mother is seated comfortably. The nurse remains available to answer questions that might arise. When there is a good relationship between mother and nurse, the child benefits from a higher level of care.

PHYSICAL EXAMINATION OF THE PATIENT

Taking the Pulse and Respiration

When the practical nurse takes the pulse, she feels the wave of blood as it is forced through the artery. The pulse rate varies considerably in different children of the same age and size. The pulse rate of the newborn is high (120 to 150 beats per minute) as is the respiratory rate (35 to 50 times per minute). Both pulse and respiratory rate gradually slow down with age until the adult values are reached.

The nurse takes the pulse of the older child the same as she would for an adult. She may find taking the pulse of the infant more difficult at first. The most common site is the radial pulse (at the thumb side of the wrist just above the radial artery). It is taken while the infant is at rest. The temporal pulse may also be taken. This usually does not disturb the sleeping infant. Actually, the pulse may be taken in any area where a large artery lies close to the skin, especially if the artery runs across a bone and has very little soft tissue about it. The following are the most common sites: radial, temporal (just in front of the ear), mandibular (on the lower jawbone), carotid (on each side of the front of the neck), and femoral (in the groin).* The doctor may also order apical

*Thompson and LeBaron, p. 691.

CHILD'S NAME_____BIRTH DATE _____

We want to make your child as comfortable and happy as possible. If we know about his or her nick-name, favorite friends, pets, food preferences and, above all, normal pattern of living, we can help your child feel more at home. Won't you please help us by telling us about your child.

Nickname _____

Parent's name _____

Address and phone number _____

Child's religion _____ Baptized ?_____

Names and ages of your other children_____

Does your child need help with dressing_____ Washing face_____ Combing hair_____ Brushing teeth_____

Has your child been in a hospital before _____

Does the child know why he or she is being admitted to the hospital _____

Does your child seem to make friends with unfamiliar grownups easily_____

_____

SCHOOL

Does your child attend nursery school _____ Grade school _____

Name of school _____ Grade_____

Name of best friend(s) _____

Name of favorite teacher _____

List any special interests (hobbies, favorite book, favorite TV, radio programs, etc.) _____

_____

Is there anything else about your child that you feel we should know to make his or her hospital stay as pleasant as

possible? _____

_____

To reorder, specify SIMILAC Form No. 330.23A

Figure 7. The parents of the newly admitted child are requested to fill in an information sheet such as that shown above. This is of value to the nurse and other personnel in determining the care of the individual patient. It also involves the parents in planning the care of their child. (Habit and Care Sheet. Ross Laboratories—Similac, form No. 330.23A.)

CHILD'S NAME _____ BIRTH DATE _____

EATING HABITS

Is your child breast fed _____ Uses bottle _____ Spoon _____ Cup _____ Feeds self alone _____

Feeds self with help _____ If on a schedule, at what hours _____

What is his present formula _____

What fruit juices does your child drink _____ From bottle _____ From cup _____

Is your child allergic to any foods _____

What foods does your child especially like _____

or dislike _____

Are there any other feeding routines or aids that we should know about _____

ELIMINATION

Is your child toilet trained for bowel movement _____ For urination _____

For how long _____ Does your child wear diapers _____ Does your child use a toilet chair or toilet _____

What is word used for urination _____ Bowel movement _____

Is child taken to toilet at night _____ If so, at what time _____

SLEEPING HABITS

Is your child a heavy sleeper _____ When is bedtime _____ Are naps taken _____

If so, at what time _____ Does your child sleep alone _____ Crib _____

Bed with sides _____ Adult bed _____ Does your child climb out of bed _____

Describe any special bedtime routine, e.g., having prayers heard, taking teddy bear or doll to bed, etc. _____

_____

_____

PLAY

Has your child a favorite toy _____ Did you bring it along _____

Any favorite games _____

Is the child used to playing alone _____ With other children _____ With grownups _____

Does your child have a pet at home _____ What is it _____ What is its name _____

COPYRIGHT 1958 ROSS LABORATORIES LITHO IN U.S.A.   390-330-030.23A

Figure 7. (Continued).

pulses in which the nurse counts the infant's heartbeats with a stethoscope placed over the heart. The rate, force, and rhythm, or qualities, of the pulse are very important, since the pulse indicates the condition of the heart and circulation. The pulse should be taken for one full minute to determine these qualities.

The act of breathing consists of an exchange of gases. It is the continual process of drawing in and then expelling air from the lungs. During inspiration, oxygen is taken into the blood; during expiration carbon dioxide is forced from the lungs. Respiration is controlled and regulated by the respiratory center located in the medulla and pons of the brain, and by the proportion of carbon dioxide in the blood.

The child's respirations are taken as for the adult. The practical nurse notes for one minute the number of times the chest or abdomen rises and falls. The rate and character of respirations are important in determining the patient's general condition. The pulse and respiration rates are recorded in even numbers on the graphic chart.

The following terms are commonly used in describing respirations: shallow breathing, dyspnea (difficult breathing), orthopnea (the patient has to sit up in order to breathe). Cyanosis is a bluish color of the skin and mucous membranes caused by an inadequate amount of oxygen in the hemoglobin of the blood.

Blood Pressure

Blood pressure is defined as the pressure of the blood on the walls of the arteries. The procedure for measuring the blood pressure of children is the same as for adults. A stethoscope and sphygmomanometer are used. Blood pressure cuffs vary in size for children, so the practical nurse must choose one that is suited to the size of her patient. It is difficult to determine the blood pressure of infants, and the procedure is often inaccurate. On admission, blood pressure is required only for the older child. The exact age may vary somewhat with the institution. One hospital suggests that the child be at least eight years old. The nurse explains to the patient what she is about to do.

Blood pressure is lower in children than in adults (see Table 12–1, p. 251). The 7 to 10 year old may have a systolic range of 75 to 120 mm. Hg and a diastolic range of 40 to 75 mm.Hg. If a patient needs to have his blood pressure taken throughout his stay in the hospital, the nurse observes the previous readings before she charts her current one. If she notices a great difference, she rechecks the blood pressure. Unusual readings are charted and reported to the nurse in charge. Many factors account for variations in blood pressure. Included are sex, age, exercise, pain, and emotion. A blood pressure taken when a child is frightened or crying will not be accurate.

Taking the Temperature

For the smaller pediatric patient, a rectal temperature is taken unless contraindicated. It is accurate and safe and the child cannot bite and break the thermometer. It should be taken last because it may make the child cry, which influences pulse rate, respiratory rate, and blood pressure.

Place the patient in a comfortable position either on his side with knees slightly flexed or on his stomach. It is difficult to take the toddler's temperature when he is lying on his back since the feet are in a good kicking position. After inserting the thermometer into the rectum, shift your grip from the end of it, placing the palm of your hand across the buttocks, and hold the thermometer lightly, between two fingers. This prevents the child from twisting and injuring himself and gives a better hold on him. Hold the thermometer in place for three to five minutes.

A mother will sometimes show interest in how to read a thermometer. The student should take advantage of this teaching opportunity. The thermometer is most easily read when the sharp edge of its triangular shape is pointed toward the nurse. In this position the degree marks are above and the numbers below the mercury. It is then rolled very slightly until the band of mercury appears.

Remember that a healthy body temperature does not remain constant. Slight variations from the assumed 98.6° F. may be considered normal. The rectal temperature is approximately one degree higher than the oral temperature. If a great variation from normal is dis-

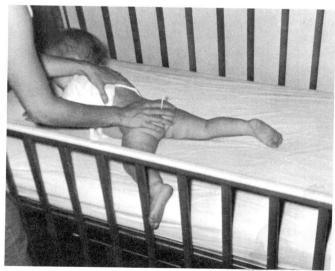

Figure 8. The nurse will prevent injury to the child from the thermometer if she holds it in place as shown.

covered, retake the temperature, being sure that the mercury in the thermometer is shaken down properly. If the same reading is obtained, report it immediately to the team leader or head nurse and enter it on the chart. It is not uncommon for infants and young children to have convulsions from a high fever which would only produce chills in an adult.

Weight

Weight must be recorded accurately on admission. The weight of a patient provides a means of determining his progress and also is necessary to determine the dosage of certain medications. The way in which the nurse weighs the child depends on his age.

The infant is weighed completely naked in a warm room. A fresh diaper or scale paper is placed on the scale. This prevents cross-contamination, the spread of germs from one infant to another. The scale is balanced to compensate for the weight of the diaper. There are various ways of balancing scales; the nurse should request specific instruction for the particular scale used. The infant is placed gently on the scale. The nurse's left hand is held slightly above the infant to make sure that he does not fall. The nurse regulates the weights with her right hand. The scale should be read when the infant is lying still. If the mother is present, she may distract the patient by speaking softly to him. Once the exact weight is determined, the infant is removed from the scale, wrapped in a blanket, and given to his mother to soothe. Record the weight immediately on a piece of paper. The scale paper is disposed of in the proper receptacle. The unsoiled diaper is returned to the patient's unit.

The older child is weighed in the same manner as an adult. A paper towel is placed on the scale for the patient to stand on. The patient is generally weighed in a hospital gown. The shoes are removed. If the child is unable to stand on the scales it may be necessary for the nurse to hold the child and read the combined weights. She then weighs herself and subtracts her weight from the combined weight to obtain that of the patient. Occasionally, a child is weighed who is wearing a cast. The nurse records this as, for example, weight 34 pounds with cast on right arm.

The undressed child is observed for such objective symptoms as skin coloring, abrasions, rash, swelling, facial expressions (fear, pain, fatigue), discharge from nose or ears, dyspnea, conditions of joints, odor of breath, condition of teeth, coughing, or other unusual abnormalities or markings.

Height

The older child has his height taken when he is weighed. The infant must be measured while lying on a flat surface beside a metal tape measure or yardstick. The knees should be pressed flat on the table. Measure from the top of the head to the heels and record.

Collection of Urine Specimens

A urine specimen is obtained from the newly admitted patient. Certain general principles should be observed regarding the collection of specimens:

1. Explain the procedure to the patient.
2. Use a clean container.
3. An uncontaminated specimen requires catheterization and is obtained from the pediatric patient by a registered nurse or doctor.
4. Label all specimens clearly and attach the proper laboratory slip.
5. Record in nurses' notes.

Additional measures must be taken to obtain a specimen from an infant or small child who is unable to urinate voluntarily:

1. Cleanse the genitals and dry them before applying and after removing receptacle.
2. When removing adhesive tape, pull the skin away from the tape, not the tape from the skin. This will lessen the irritation.

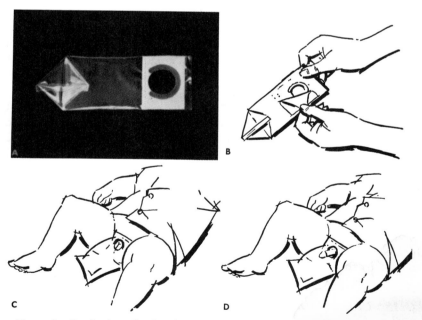

Figure 9. Sterilon's pediatric urine collector for use with both sexes. *A*, Urine collector bag. *B*, Removing paper backing exposing adhesive surface. *C*, On the female, the round opening in the bag is placed so as to cover the upper half of the external genitalia. *D*, On the male, the penis is projected through the round opening in the bag. (Courtesy Sterilon Corporation, Buffalo, New York.)

3. Babies frequently void during feedings and temperature taking. Keep a clean, padded receptable at the bedside (a soap dish may be adequate).
4. Restrain the child if necessary, using the type of restraint suitable for the child's age, e.g., jacket or extremity restraint.
5. At least 15 cc. of urine is required for proper testing.

ADMISSION OF A CHILD WITH A CONTAGIOUS DISEASE

Any patient who is suspected of having a contagious disease must be isolated until a definite diagnosis has been established. A pediatric hospital will have an isolation ward for this purpose. The smaller children's division of a general hospital may not have these facilities. The nurse admitting the patient must take certain precautions. The purpose of medical aseptic technique is to prevent the spread of the disease to the nurse and others. Proper *handwashing* cannot be overemphasized.

The patient is placed in a private room. All unnecessary furnishings are removed before his arrival. Place an ample supply of paper towels and soap near the sink. Attach a paper bag to the bed for the patient to use as a wastebasket. Equipment for daily patient care is placed in the unit. This includes: thermometer, bath equipment, bedpan, urinal, tissues, and linen. Such equipment remains there until the patient is discharged and will then be terminally disinfected. Linen is changed daily. An ample supply of gowns, masks, and newspapers saves much time and energy. A clean area is prepared according to hospital procedure. The floor is always considered contaminated. Anything that touches the floor must be discarded. Toys are tied to the bed with a short tape, and must be washable.

The practical nurse may be asked to assist the doctor during the physical examination. In taking the blood pressure, the patient's arm and bed are protected by a clean gown or sheet to prevent contamination of the sphygomomanometer. When a flashlight, otoscope, or opthalmoscope are used they are protected by a paper towel. Any part that comes in direct contact with the patient must be disinfected. All the specimens that leave the room are marked "precaution" and placed in a clean outer container according to hospital procedure. Trays necessary for general ward use are not brought into the patient's room. Remove the necessary articles, place them on a smaller metal or paper tray, and carry it to the bedside. Further information is presented on page 262.

LUMBAR PUNCTURE

The practical nurse is sometimes requested to assist the physician with a lumbar puncture which is also referred to as a "spinal tap." It is done to obtain spinal fluid for examination or to reduce pressure within

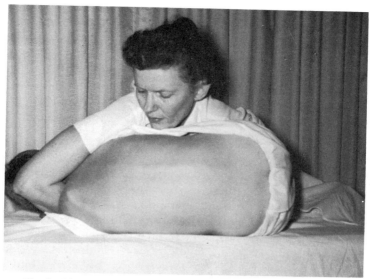

Figure 10. Positioning the child for a lumbar puncture. The nurse holds the head and legs of the patient in the crook of her elbows and clasps her hands together in front of the patient. She leans forward slightly, placing some of her weight on the body of the child.

the brain in such conditions as hydrocephalus or meningitis. Disposable lumbar puncture sets are now available.

Normal spinal fluid is clear like water. The pressure ranges from 60 to 180 mm. Hg. It is somewhat lower in infants. The procedure for children is essentially the same as for adults. The main difference lies in the patient's ability to cooperate with positioning. The nurse explains to the child that he must lie quietly and that she will help him to do this. The way in which the child is held can directly affect the success of the procedure. The patient lies on his side with his back parallel to the side of the treatment table. His knees are flexed and his head is brought down close to the flexed knees. The nurse can keep the child in this position if she places his head in the crook of one arm and his knees in the crook of her other arm. She then clasps her own hands together at the front of the child and leans forward, gently placing her chest against the patient. (See Fig. 10.)

Once the child is positioned, the doctor prepares the lower back using sterile technique. The solutions generally used for this are alcohol and iodine. They are poured by a second nurse. A vial of 1 per cent Novocain is also necessary unless this is provided in the sterile setup. The top of the vial is cleansed with an alcohol sponge. Once the area has been locally anesthetized, the doctor inserts a special hollow needle into the patient's lower back. He collects the spinal fluid in two or three test tubes. When the procedure is completed, a sterile Bandaid is placed over the injection site and the child is comforted. Specimens are labeled and

taken to the laboratory with the appropriate requisition form. The
doctor may prefer to do this himself. Children do not usually suffer
from headaches and may play quietly after the procedure unless ordered otherwise. The nurse charts the date and time of the lumbar
puncture, and the name of the attending physician. She also charts the
amount of fluid obtained; its character, e.g., cloudly or bloody; whether
or not specimens were sent to the laboratory; and the reaction of the
patient to the procedure. She cleans and restocks the treatment room.

MEDICATIONS

The student practical nurse learns how to administer medications.
She is supervised by her instructor during her training period. Whether
she will be allowed to dispense medications following graduation depends on the policy of the hospital in which she is employed.*

The responsibility of giving medications to children is a serious one.
The practical nurse must realize her limitations in this area. Children are
smaller than adults and their medications have to be adapted to their
size and age. For instance, a student nurse who takes one adult aspirin
receives 5 grains. A mother who gives her three year old child one baby
aspirin is administering 1¼ grains, which is only one-fourth the 5 grain
tablet taken by the nurse. Infants require even less. The doctor determines the dosage of medication for each child on an *individual* basis by
weight or age;

Weight: Clark's Rule

$$\frac{\text{weight of child in pounds}}{150} \times \text{average adult dose} = \text{child's dose}$$

Age: Young's Rule

$$\frac{\text{age of child}}{\text{age of child} + 12} \times \text{average adult dose} = \text{child's dose}$$

Since there is no set dosage to rely on, the possibility for error is
increased. Besides knowing the correct amount and route of a drug, the
nurse must also be aware of the toxic side effects that might occur.
Children react more quickly and violently to medication. Their reactions
are not as predictable as they are in adult patients. The entire area of
pediatric drug therapy is currently under close scrutiny. *The nurse must
always know what medications her patient is receiving regardless of whether or
not she administers them personally.* Medications should not be placed in a

---

*See the Index for specific medications. They are presented under the disease condi-
tions for which they are used.

bottle of water or milk. They may be partially refused and the nurse would not be positive about the amount of the drug consumed.

Intramuscular Injections. This procedure is essentially the same for children as for adults. Whenever possible, a second nurse should assist to distract the child and restrain him when necessary. The nurse must be thoroughly familiar with the technique and she must use good equipment. The needle should be sharp. A 1½ inch long, No. 22 gauge needle is used for the older child; a 1 inch long, No. 22 gauge needle is used for the infant.* *The contents of an ampule are not intended to be a single dose for a child except for a few clearly stated cases.* The injection site is varied. The nurse selects an area with enough muscle tissue to prevent injecting the medication into subcutaneous tissue. The usual sites for injection are the buttocks and the thighs. Some authorities discourage the use of the buttocks in infants and small children because of the danger of injuring the sciatic nerve.

The nurse should anticipate some protest from children in regard to injections. The child's first injection is particularly important, since it establishes the pattern for his future acceptance of shots. Injections are more of a threat to toddlers and preschool children who are too little to understand the necessity for them. The nurse should not be offended or become indignant when the child acts hostile to her. He needs to vent his anger. She should remain with him until he has calmed down and can focus his attention on more pleasant things. The nurse should not reject or show disapproval of the uncooperative child.

Rectal Medications. Some drugs come in the form of suppositories, e.g., aspirin, glycerin. Children's suppositories are long and thin in comparison to the cone-shaped types administered to adults. The nurse wearing a rubber glove or finger cot inserts the lubricated suppository well beyond the anal sphincter about one-half as far as the forefinger will reach. The nurse applies pressure to the anus by gently holding the buttocks together until the patient's desire to expel the suppository subsides.

STUDY QUESTIONS

1. What is the purpose of the playroom?
2. Observe a patient being admitted. How could the nurse have carried out her functions more effectively?
3. Define systolic and diastolic blood pressure. What is hypertension?
4. Nine year old Chris Jones has just been admitted to the ward with a severe laceration of the leg. You are assigned to take his blood pressure. How would you explain this to Chris?
5. What is meant by an apical pulse?

*Blake, and Wright, p. 122.

6. Compile a list of safety measures that would be effective on the children's ward in your hospital. Underline those measures that apply to the practical nurse.
7. List several ways in which children show their insecurities.
8. Of what value are visiting hours to the child, the parents, the practical nurse?
9. Discuss how you would obtain a urine specimen from a four month old baby.
10. Mrs. Lang, the head nurse, has just told you to prepare Room 101 for a new admission who is suspected of having tuberculosis. The patient is four years old. How would you do this?
11. What is the role of the practical nurse in assisting with a lumbar puncture?
12. What special precautions must be taken when giving medications to children? How and where are medications charted in your hospital?

BIBLIOGRAPHY

Benz, G. S.: Pediatric Nursing. 5th Ed. St. Louis, C. V. Mosby Co., 1964.
Blake, F.: The Child, His Parents and the Nurse. Philadelphia, J. B. Lippincott Co., 1954.
Blake, F., and Wright, F. H.: Essentials of Pediatric Nursing. 7th Ed. Philadelphia, J. B. Lippincott Co., 1963.
Brigley, C.: Pediatrics for the Practical Nurse. New York, Delmar Publishers, Inc., 1965.
Broadribb, V.: Foundations of Pediatric Nursing. Philadelphia, J. B. Lippincott Co., 1967.
Culver, V. M.: Modern Bedside Nursing. 7th Ed. Philadelphia, W. B. Saunders Co. 1969.
Hemmendinger, M.: "Rx: Admit parents at all times." Child Study, 34(No. 1):3, 1956.
Jones, J. D., and Stedman, D.: Emotional Stresses. Baby Talk Magazine. July 1969, pp. 11-15.
Leifer, G.: Principles and Techniques in Pediatric Nursing. Philadelphia, W. B. Saunders Co., 1965.
Marlow, D.: Textbook of Pediatric Nursing. 3rd Ed. Philadelphia, W. B. Saunders Co., 1969.
Mason, M.: Basic Medical-Surgical Nursing. 2nd Ed. New York, The Macmillan Co., 1967.
Nelson, W. E. (Editor): Textbook of Pediatrics. 9th Ed. Philadelphia, W. B. Saunders Co., 1968.
Price, A.: The Art, Science and Spirit of Nursing. 3rd Ed. Philadelphia, W. B. Saunders Co., 1965.
Rapeir, D., Koch, M., Moran, L., Geronsin, J., Cady, E., and Jensen, D.: Practical Nursing. 3rd Ed. St. Louis, The C. V. Mosby Co., 1968.
Spock, B.: Baby and Child Care. Rev. Ed. New York, Duell, Sloan and Pearce, Inc., 1968.
Thompson, E., and LeBaron, M.: Simplified Nursing. 7th Ed. Philadelphia, J. B. Lippincott Co., 1960.
Verville, E.: Behavior Problems of Children. Philadelphia, W. B. Saunders Co., 1967.

Chapter 4

THE NEWBORN

VOCABULARY

Buttock	*Moro reflex*
Circumcision	*Mucus*
Fontanel	*Physiological*
Formula	*Regurgitated*
Jaundice	*Turgor*
Meconium	*Umbilicus*

The practical nurse is frequently called upon to aid in the care of the newborn. During her student experience, she will be assigned to the hospital nursery. She will also care for the newborn on the children's division. After graduation, many students will marry and become parents. The older practical nurse may find a great deal of satisfaction assisting mothers with new babies in the home. This is an area in which the demand is great and the supply of nurses limited. In modern society, generations of families no longer live together. Relatives who would delight in helping with the care of a new grandchild are frequently miles away. The young mother who is new in a community is justly concerned. A practical nurse who renders such assistance to new mothers during their first weeks at home is of great value.

The stages of growth and development that are referred to throughout this text are as follows:

Fetal	conception to birth
Newborn	birth to two weeks
Infancy	two weeks to one year
Toddler	one year to three years
Preschool	three to six years
School age	six to 12 years
Adolescence	puberty to the beginning of adult life

INFANT DEATHS

Infant *mortality* is the ratio between the number of deaths of infants less than one year of age during any given year and the number of live births occurring in the same year. The rate is usually expressed as the number of deaths per thousand live births. The highest infant death rate is within the first months. The first 24 hours of life are the most dangerous. The infant mortality rate is considered one of the best means of determining the health of a country. In order to obtain accurate figures, all births and deaths must be registered. In the United States this is required by law. Each birth certificate is filed permanently with the state Bureau of Vital Statistics.

Prematurity, congenital malformations, pneumonia and influenza, birth injuries, asphyxia (suffocation) and atelectasis (incomplete expansion of the lungs at birth), are the leading causes of death in the newborn. Many measures are being taken to reduce infant mortality rates (see Chapter Two).

The practical nurse has a grave responsibility when she is entrusted with the care of the newborn. In order to do this intelligently she must known what he is like and how she can best meet his needs.

TENDER, LOVING CARE

The loving an infant receives is just as important as his physical care. Gentleness in caring for him is an expression of love, and makes physical care—his bath and feeding—a pleasure to him. He begins to develop a sense of trust. Each infant is an individual. Just as no two babies look alike, so each one is different in disposition, in activity, and in the way he responds to people and his surroundings. He soon learns that crying brings comforting help. Since mother is the usual person who answers his plea, he prefers her to others. If the infant is secure in the care which he receives from her, he will accept care from others,

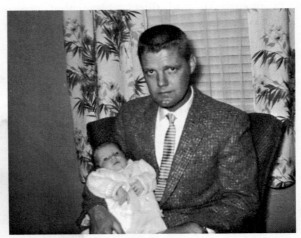

Figure 11.   The newborn is not as fragile as she looks.

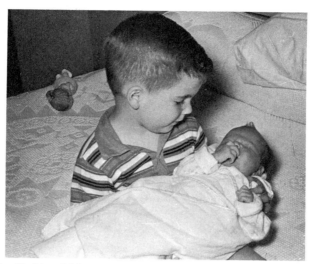

Figure 12. If older children are made to feel wanted, accepted, and cherished, their jealousy of the newborn will be kept at a minimum.

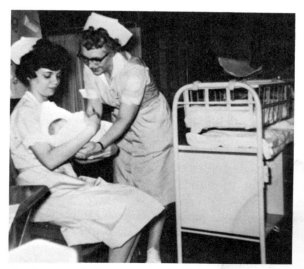

Figure 13. Student practical nurses practice how to handle the newborn in the classroom. (Courtesy of Exeter School of Practical Nursing, Exeter, N.H.)

providing it is similar. Feelings of love, affection, security, and being wanted are necessary for a healthy personality as well as for physical growth.

Brothers and sisters, or siblings, are less likely to resent their new baby as a rival if they are made to feel that the baby is theirs as well as their parents'. If the older children are made to feel wanted, accepted, and cherished, their jealousy of the newborn will be kept at a minimum.

The practical nurse should handle the newborn gently and speak to him in a soft tone of voice. She will enjoy feeding him more if she relaxes. The baby will also benefit from this relaxed manner. The nurse who keeps the baby warm, dry, and comfortably positioned will make him feel secure. After painful procedures, the nurse should hold the baby for a few minutes so that he does not associate only pain with her care.

THE FAMILY

The family is the strongest social institution in our society. Bringing up a child can be the most rewarding and satisfying experience in life; a healthy, happy baby can bring great joy to his parents. Adults mature around the lives of their children. The role of the father is honored in every Judeo-Christian society. Half of the child's heredity is transmitted through him; the newborn is a continuation of himself and his wife. A mother's love for her baby is considered to be the strongest emotional tie between two human beings.

Today's family is very different from yesteryear's family. Very often a father is away from his family for a long part of the day because of commuting to and from work or the demands of his job. This is even more pronounced when a father is in the service or travels about the country or world on business. In these cases, the mother becomes the mainstay of the family. She disciplines the children and makes the decisions. The family may be very mobile; therefore, it is common for the children to attend several schools. Many close groups form in the social life of military bases and college communities where families are all in the same situation. Both parents may work in order to meet the rising costs of living. In these cases, the father frequently helps with the housework and care of the children so that the demands of their daily schedule can be met.

It must also be said that many children are not reared by two parents. Reasons such as divorce, separation, death, or illegitimate pregnancies create many one-parent families. Children may be raised by relatives, foster parents, and, in some instances, institutions. The home into which a baby is born influences his entire life. Poverty per se is less detrimental to a child in a home where there is love and affection than in a home where there is a great deal of discord and infant rejection.

PHYSICAL CHARACTERISTICS

Head

The newborn's head is proportionately large in comparison with the rest of his body, for his brain grows rapidly before birth. The normal limits of head size range from 13.2 to 14.8 inches. The head may be out of shape from molding (the shaping of the fetal head to conform to the size and shape of the birth canal). Occasionally, a hematoma (*hemato-* blood + *-oma* tumor) protrudes from beneath the scalp. This condition usually clears up within a few weeks. Some newborns have a large amount of black hair which eventually is replaced by new hair. It is washed daily, when the baby is bathed, and brushed into place.

The *fontanels* are unossified spots on the cranium of a young infant. The anterior fontanel is diamond-shaped and located at the junction of the two parietal and two frontal bones. It usually is ossified by 12 to 18 months of age. The posterior fontanel is triangular and located between the occipital and parietal bones. It is smaller than the anterior fontanel, and is usually ossified by the end of the second month. The pulsating of the anterior fontanel may be seen by the nurse. These areas are covered by a tough membrane, and there is little chance of their being injured with ordinary care.

The features of the newborn's face are small. His mouth and lips are well developed, as they are necessary to obtain food. He can taste and smell. It is difficult to tell when he can actually see. To him, the surroundings at first are only dark or light, or a blur. When the nurse washes the face of the newborn, she uses a soft washcloth without soap. The eyes are washed from the nose outward, using a different section of the facecloth for each eye.

The newborn is deaf until his first cry. He makes some responses to

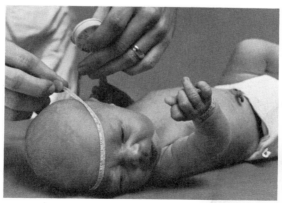

Figure 14.   The circumference of the head is measured during a routine physical examination. (From Marlow, D.: Textbook of Pediatric Nursing, 3rd Ed. 1969.)

loud noises during the first week but is not able to interpret what he hears. The ears and nose need no special attention except for cleansing during the bath with a soft cloth. Occasionally, they may be *externally* cleansed with a cotton wisp moistened slightly with water. Toothpicks or wooden applicator sticks are dangerous to use. They may cause injury to the baby if he moves suddenly.

Respiratory System

Before a baby is born, he is completely dependent on his mother for all vital functions. The fetus needs oxygen and nourishment in order to grow. These are supplied through the blood stream of the pregnant woman by way of the placenta and umbilical cord. The fetus is relieved of the waste products of metabolism through this same route. The lungs are not inflated, and are almost completely inactive. The circulatory system is adapted only to life within the uterus. Little blood flows through the pulmonary artery, due to natural openings within the heart and vessels which close at birth or shortly thereafter. When the umbilical cord is clamped and cut, the lungs take on the function of breathing in oxygen and removing carbon dioxide. The first breath taken helps to expand the collapsed lungs, although full expansion does not take place for several days. The physician assists the first respiration by holding the newborn's head down and removing mucus from the passages to the lungs. The baby's cry should be strong and healthy. The most critical period for the newborn is the first hour of life when the drastic change from life within the uterus to life outside the uterus takes place.

An identification band is placed on the newborn in the delivery room. Silver nitrate drops or antibiotic solutions are instilled in the eyes to prevent ophthalmia neonatorum, an inflammation of the conjunctiva which can lead to blindness. He is wrapped in a light blanket and carried to the nursery. The nursery nurse removes excessive blood from the baby's face and scalp with a soft, moist cloth. She weighs and measures the newborn if it has not been done previously in the delivery room. During this procedure she should observe the general condition of the newborn. She then dresses him in a diaper and shirt and places him in a bassinet on his side or abdomen. A light blanket is placed over him and the foot of the bassinet is elevated. The newborn remains in this position for the first 24 hours to promote the drainage of mucus from the respiratory passages.

The nurse refers to the patient's chart to determine whether or not there were any particular difficulties during the birth process. She also reviews the orders left by the doctor. She must observe the newborn *very closely*. Respiratory distress may be shown by the rate and character of respirations, color (watch for cyanosis), and general behavior. Mucus may be seen draining from the nose or mouth. It is wiped away with a sterile gauze square. The nurse may also use a sterile catheter attached

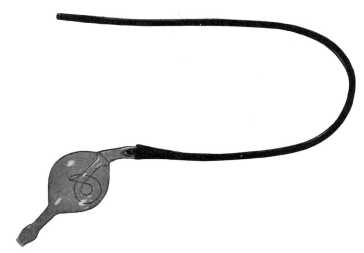

Figure 15. This type of suction catheter is used in many newborn nurseries to clear the newborn's mouth and throat of mucus. The glass mucus trap prevents the contents from being drawn into the operator's mouth. (From Davis, M. E., and Rubin, R.: DeLee's Obstetrics for Nurses. 18th Ed., 1966.)

to a glass mucus trap to suction mucus from the throat. (She places her mouth on the glass end of the apparatus and creates a gentle suction with withdraws the mucus. The trap prevents the mucus from being drawn into the nurse's mouth.) (See Fig. 15.) *Immediate* assistance is needed if this does not bring relief.

Circulatory System

The mother's blood has brought essential oxygen to each cell of the fetus during his life in the uterus, as stated previously. The obstetrician cuts off this supply when he severs the umbilical cord. From this time on the newborn has not only a systemic circulation, but also a pulmonary circulation. (There is some pulmonary circulation prior to birth, although not as great as after the lungs have expanded.)

The circulation of the fetus differs from that of the newborn in that most of the blood by-passes the lungs. Some of the blood goes from the right atrium to the left atrium of the heart through an opening (the foramen ovale) in the septum. Some of the blood goes from the pulmonary artery to the thoracic aorta by way of the *ductus arteriosus.*

In the "blue baby," part of the blood continues to by-pass the lungs and does not pick up oxygen. This lack of oxygen accounts for the cyanosis.

"Murmurs" are caused by blood leaking through openings that have not yet closed. Murmurs may be thought of as functional (innocent) or organic due to improper heart formation. Functional murmurs are due

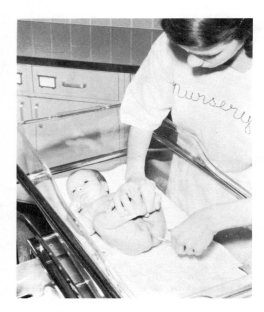

Figure 16. The baby's temperature is taken twice a day, rectally. If the baby has an elevation, the temperature should be taken every four hours. (From Davis, M. E., and Rubin, R.: DeLee's Obstetrics for Nurses. 18th Ed., 1966.)

to the sound of blood passing through normal valves. Organic murmurs are due to blood passing through abnormal openings or normal openings that have not yet closed. The majority of heart murmurs are not serious. However, they should be checked periodically to rule out other possibilities.

The newborn has an unstable heat regulating system. His temperature falls immediately after birth to about 96° F. Within a few hours it climbs slowly to a range of 98° to 99° F. His body temperature is influenced by the temperature of the room and the amount of blankets covering him. The temperature of the nursery or in the case of rooming-in, the mother's room, should be 68° to 76° F. The humidity should be 45 to 55 per cent. The air in the room needs to be fresh, but there should be no drafts. The most accurate way to determine whether a baby is warm or cool is to observe the color of his face. If it is flushed, he is too warm; if it is pale or bluish, he is too cold. The hands and feet should not be used as a guide, since the baby's extremities are cooler than the rest of his body. The newborn cannot adapt to changes in temperature. He needs to be wrapped in a blanket whenever he leaves the nursery. Since his heat perception is poor, the nurse must be very careful when applying forms of external heat such as hot water bottles or heat lamps.

The temperature of the newborn may be taken in the rectum or the axilla. If taken rectally, the nurse must be gentle to avoid injuring the rectal mucosa (see Fig. 15). When taking an axillary temperature, the thermometer is held firmly in the axilla for five minutes. During this time the baby's arm is held against his side.

The newborn's pulse and respiration are counted before his temperature is taken, since he is apt to cry when the thermometer is inserted into the rectum. The pulse rate is irregular and rapid, varying from 120 to 150 beats per minute. Blood pressure is low and may vary with the size of the cuff used. The average blood pressure at birth is 80/46. The respirations are approximately 35 to 50 per minute. Always report the following changes:

1. Temperature elevated to 100° F. or below 97° F.
2. Pulse elevated to 160 or below 120.
3. Respirations elevated to 60 or below 30.

Umbilical Cord

The umbilical cord which is attached to the placenta at birth is tied and cut by the physician. Gradually the cord stump shrinks, discolors, and finally falls off. Some doctors recommend that the umbilicus be cleansed daily with 60 to 70 per cent alcohol for its drying effect and to minimize the danger of infections. The blood vessels of the cord and their extension into the abdomen are a potential portal of entry for germs until the umbilical wound is completely healed. Redness, odor, or discharge from this area should be reported to the physician. The nurse must also observe the cord for bleeding, particularly during the first 24 hours.

If the mother has Rh negative blood, continuous sterile wet dressings are applied to the umbilical stump of the newborn until the administration of an exchange transfusion is ruled out. An exchange transfusion, which is performed through the umbilical vein, is discussed in Chapter Six under Erythroblastosis Fetalis.

Musculoskeletal System

The bones of the newborn are soft because they are made up chiefly of cartilage in which there is only a small amount of calcium. The skeleton is flexible. The joints are elastic to accommodate the birth canal. Since the bones of the child are easily molded by pressure, his position must be changed frequently. If the baby lies constantly in one place, the bones of his head can become flattened.

The movements of the newborn are random and uncoordinated. He lacks the muscular control to hold his head steady. The development of muscular control proceeds from head to foot, and from the center of the body to the periphery. The baby will therefore hold his head up before he can sit erect. In fact, his head and neck muscles will be the first ones he can control. The legs are small and short and may appear bowed. There should be no limitation of movement. Fingers clenched in a fist should be separated and observed. Most newborns appear cross-eyed because their eye muscle coordination is not fully developed. At

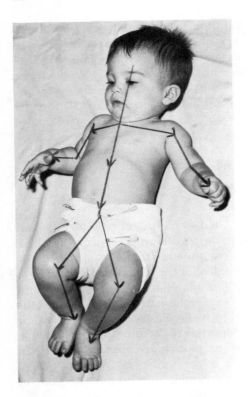

Figure 17. The development of muscular control proceeds from head to foot (cephalocaudal) and from the center of the body to the periphery. (From Marlow, D.: Textbook of Pediatric Nursing, 3rd Ed. 1969.)

first the eyes appear to be blue or gray; however, the permanent coloring becomes fixed between the third and sixth month. The baby needs freedom of movement. He stretches, sucks, and makes faces. He moves his whole body vigorously when crying. The morning bath provides him with an excellent opportunity for exercise. When handled he should not feel limp to the nurse.

Nervous System

The practical nurse will recall that the nervous system directs most of the body's activity. The newborn can move his arms and legs vigorously, but he cannot control them. The reflexes he is born with, such as winking, sneezing, gagging, sucking, and grasping, help to keep him alive. He can cry, swallow, and lift his head slightly when lying on his stomach. If his crib is jarred he will draw his legs up and fold his arms across his chest in an embrace position. This is normal, and is called the *Moro reflex.* Its absence may indicate abnormalities of the nervous system. The *rooting reflex* causes the infant to turn his head in the direction of anything that touches his cheek in anticipation of food. The practical nurse should remember this when helping a mother to breast feed her infant. If the breast touches the infant's cheek, he will turn toward it to find the nipple. The newborn requires watchful care to protect him from his environment.

The baby sleeps approximately 15 to 20 hours a day, and is awake mainly for feedings. Following feedings, he should be placed on his stomach with his head turned outward or on his right side to reduce the danger of choking from food or vomitus. Putting his head at the foot of the crib occasionally will prevent him from sleeping constantly on one side of his head. On nice days, he can sleep outdoors in his carriage.

Length and Weight

The length of the average newborn is 19 to 21½ inches. The weight varies from 6 to 8½ pounds. Girls generally weigh a little less than boys. In the first three to four days after birth about 6 to 10 ounces are lost. This may be due to withdrawal from maternal hormones, withholding of water, and the loss of feces and urine. It is expected and natural, and the mother need not be alarmed by it. Some hospitals prefer not to tell the mother the daily weight of the newborn in order to avoid upsetting her. The practical nurse should comply with this rule if it is used in the hospital where she is employed.

Procedures for measuring and weighing the infant are given on pages 24 and 25. Infants are weighed at the same time each day, when morning care is given. Breast-fed babies may also be weighed before and after feedings.

Genitourinary Tract

The kidneys function normally at birth but are not fully developed. The first urine may be voided immediately or not for several hours. The practical nurse must keep an accurate record of the frequency of each urination. Anuria, changes in color, or any unusual findings should be brought to the attention of the physician.

The genitals of the male and female are undeveloped at birth. The testes of the male descend into the scrotum before birth. Occasionally, they remain in the abdomen or inguinal canal. This condition is called *undescended testes.* The prognosis is good under proper medical or surgical treatment.

The penis is covered by a sleeve of skin called the foreskin. There is a difference of opinion in the value of retracting this daily for cleansing purposes. Some feel that the smegma or cheeselike material secreted by the head of the penis may collect and cause irritation. They advise retracting the foreskin daily, cleansing it, and returning it to its normal position. The foreskin should be retracted only to the extent that it will not cause pressure. It must be returned all the way to its normal position, because constriction may cause circulation of the penis to be impaired. Others feel that the danger of infection from smegma is slight, and no retraction is necessary. The practical nurse should be completely familiar with how to retract the foreskin if this method is to be used.

Circumcision is the surgical removal of the foreskin of the penis. It is done to prevent infection, to facilitate the discharge of urine, and to make the area easier to clean. The operation is generally performed about the fourth day of life; however, some physicians carry out the procedure in the delivery room shortly after birth when the available prothrombin (*pro* for + *thrombos* clot) of the blood is at normal levels. It is considered minor surgery; however, the nurse must watch for excessive bleeding. In some hospitals, a gauze dressing containing petroleum jelly is applied to the area to prevent irritation from diapers.

The Jewish religious rite of circumcision, comparable to baptism in the Christian faith, is performed on the eighth day after birth if the newborn's condition permits. The boy receives his name at this time.

If the baby is not circumcised during the first weeks of life, new problems may be created. Some physicians feel that it is unwise to perform this operation after the child has become aware of his body parts.

The *female* genitals may be slightly swollen. A blood-tinged mucus discharge may appear from the vagina. This is due to hormones transmitted from the mother at birth. The nurse should cleanse the vulva from the *urethra to the anus*, using a clean cotton ball or different sections of a washcloth for each stroke. This prevents fecal matter from infecting the urinary tract.

Skin

The skin of white babies is red or dark pink; the skin of Negro babies is a reddish black. It is covered with fine hair called *lanugo* which tends to disappear during the first week of life. It is more evident in the premature. *Vernix caseosa,* a cheeselike substance which covers the skin of the newborn, is made up of cells and glandular secretions, and is thought to protect the skin from infection.

Many hospitals identify newborns by footprints. The skin is so constructed with ridges and grooves that each individual has a unique pattern that never changes except to grow larger. That is why fingerprints or footprints positively identify a person.

Tissue turgor refers to the condition of the skin in regards to how well-hydrated or dehydrated the newborn is. To test tissue turgor (elasticity), the practical nurse gently grasps and releases the skin. It should spring back into place immediately. When the skin remains distorted, tissue turgor is termed poor. (See Fig. 18.)

Peeling of the skin occurs during the first weeks of life. Areas such

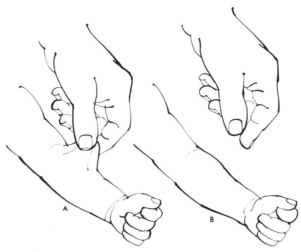

Figure 18. Testing tissue turgor. (From Leifer, G.: Principles and Techniques in Pediatric Nursing, 1966.)

as the nose, knees, elbows, and toes may break down because of friction from rubbing against the sheets. The area involved should be kept dry and the baby's position changed frequently. The buttocks need special attention. A wet diaper should be changed immediately to prevent the newborn from becoming chafed. The buttocks should be washed and dried well.

Physiologic jaundice, characterized by a yellow tinge to the skin, is caused by the rapid destruction of excess red blood cells which the baby does not need in an atmosphere that contains more oxygen than could be obtained during prenatal life. Physiologic jaundice becomes evident between the third and fifth day of life and lasts for about a week. This is a normal process and is not harmful to the baby.

Bathing the Baby. The bath is an excellent time to observe the naked newborn. Special attention must be given to areas of the skin that come in contact with each other since chafing may occur. These are found in the neck, behind the ears, in the axillae, and in the groin. They should be dried well. Powder is seldom used in the hospital since it can be irritating to the respiratory tract. The use of lotions and oil and the type of soap will vary with each institution. No bath is necessary after delivery if the excessive blood is wiped from the newborn's face and scalp, since the vernix caseosa is protective. The following method for giving a sponge bath may be used on the pediatric ward and in the home until the cord has healed. The nurse will have to adapt it to the patient's condition and the routine of her hospital.

EQUIPMENT. Linen: bath towel, washcloth, shirt, diaper, quilted pad, crib sheet, receiving blanket. Bath tray: cotton balls, mild soap, baby oil or lotion, pin holder, comb. Paper bag, wash basin, clean covergown for nurse.

METHOD

1. Bathe before midmorning feeding. Temperature of room 75° to 80° F. Temperature of water 100° to 105° F. (test with elbow or bath thermometer). Wash hands. Don clean covergown.
2. Wash baby's face with plain water and dry.
3. Clean outer nostrils p.r.n. Use a separate cotton wisp moistened with water for each side of the nose.
4. Wrap washcloth around one finger and cleanse outer ear.
5. Squeeze cheeks gently to examine mouth. Gums should be pink and clean, breath should be sweet.
6. Wash scalp by making a lather of soap on the hands. Go over the scalp thoroughly.
7. Hold head over tub, and rinse soap off with a wet washcloth. (If there is a scaly crust (cradle cap), apply oil at night and the scale will come off more readily with the next morning's shampoo.) Dry gently with a soft towel.
8. Remove diaper and cleanse diaper area with cotton dipped in water. Wash from front to back, using a separate cotton ball for each stroke.
9. Remove shirt, soap hands, and go over the entire body, front and back. Rinse with washcloth. Pay special attention to creases, folds, and genitals.
10. Pat dry and re-dress. Comb hair.
11. Apply clean crib sheet and quilted pad to crib. Cover baby with clean receiving blanket. Tidy unit. (Reline wastebasket with paper bag.)

Intestinal Tract

The intestinal tract functions as an outlet for amniotic fluid as early as the fifth month of prenatal life. The normal functions of the gastro-intestinal tract begin after birth: food is prepared for absorption into the blood, the food is absorbed, and waste products are eliminated. *Meconium,* the first stool, is a mixture of amniotic fluid and secretions of the intestinal glands. It is dark green, thick, and sticky, and is passed 8 to 24 hours following birth. The stools gradually change during the first week. They become loose, and are a greenish-yellow with mucus. These are called *transitional* stools.

The stools of a breast-fed baby are bright yellow, soft, and pasty. There may be three to six stools a day. As he grows older the number decreases. The bowel movements of a bottle-fed baby are more solid than those of the breast-fed baby. They vary from yellow to brown and are generally fewer in number. There may be one to four a day at first but gradually this decreases to one or two a day. The nursery nurse keeps an accurate record of the number and character of stools each newborn has daily.

The newborn receives nothing by mouth for 12 to 24 hours following birth. This provides sufficient time for him to become cleared of mucus, and allows both mother and child a period of rest. A baby's hunger is evidenced by crying, restlessness, sucking of fist, and the rooting reflex.

BREAST FEEDING

Most mothers can nurse their babies. If a mother feels that she would like to breast feed her newborn, she should be encouraged to try it. It is comforting to remind her that if serious difficulties result, she can always change to formula feedings. The kind encouragement and support that the nurse is capable of giving can eventually bring great satisfaction to the mother and her child.

Compared with cow's milk, breast milk contains more of the following: iron, sugar, vitamins A and C, and niacin. Breast milk has less protein and calcium than cow's milk, but the amounts present are better utilized by the baby. Breast milk is more digestible because its fat globules are smaller, and it is pure, i.e., free from bacteria. It provides the baby with greater immunity to certain childhood diseases. Breast-fed babies are less prone to intestinal upsets. In brief, the quality of mother's milk is suited to the needs of the baby.

Practical factors in favor of breast milk are: it saves time and money, it is delivered to the baby in the proper quantity, and it aids the mother physically. As the baby nurses, the mother's uterus contracts, thus hastening its return to normal size and shape. The emotional satisfaction received by mothers who nurse is also considered one of the greatest assets.

Contraindications. Conditions of the mother that contraindicate nursing are a chronic disease such as tuberculosis, heart trouble, or advanced nephritis. Conditions of the newborn that may contraindicate nursing are inability to suck due to weakness and prematurity, cleft palate, or harelip. The doctor will determine the advisability of nursing

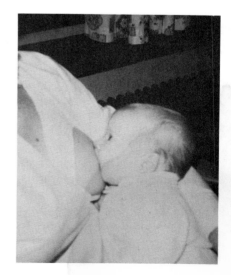

Figure 19. Breast feeding is rewarding for mother and baby.

in such cases. Breast milk can be expressed manually and given to baby by medicine dropper if necessary.

The practical nurse must keep in mind that even though breast feeding is highly recommended, she should respect the choice of the mother and never criticize her decision. The new mother tends to be especially vulnerable to rejection. She needs rest and a secure environment to prepare her for the busy duties of motherhood. Her stay in the hospital should be a pleasant one, unmarred by thoughtless conversation or personality conflicts.

Technique

Breast milk, slightly bluish and thin, appears on the third or fourth day after birth. It is preceded by *colostrum* which is watery and yellowish. The newborn is generally put to breast immediately or from four to 12 hours following delivery. The suckling of the newborn stimulates the production of milk; therefore, many doctors suggest that the mother nurse from both breasts at each feeding, if there is no contraindication to this remedy. The *let-down* reflex by which the milk is squeezed into the large ducts and nipples is stimulated by the infant's sucking or, sometimes, crying. The mother feels a vague tingling sensation in her breasts when this occurs. If she is tense or tired this feeling can be inhibited. A good fluid intake, an ample diet with extra milk, an adequate vitamin intake, and moderate rest and exercise will eliminate most difficulties. Factors to be emphasized are:

1. The mother should wash her hands thoroughly with soap and water before nursing. She should also cleanse her nipples.
2. She should be in a comfortable sitting or lying position. When lying down she should be on her side with her arm supported comfortably.
3. Allow the breast to gently touch the infant's cheek so that he will turn in that direction to suck (rooting reflex). The baby should grasp the whole nipple and areola with his mouth, and should remain awake. (The nipple should be on top of his tongue.)
4. The baby gradually increases his nursing from three to seven minutes the first three days, and from 10 to 20 minutes thereafter. The mother retracts the breast tissues from his nostrils so that he may breathe easily.
5. Burp the baby at least twice during the feeding (see p. 49).
6. To remove the baby from the breast, gently press his cheeks together or have the mother insert her finger into the baby's mouth to break the suction. The room should be quiet and the mother should not be disturbed while breast feeding her baby.

Weaning is usually begun about the sixth month or when the infant can use a cup. It is done gradually. Extra attention is given to the baby before and after the use of the cup so that pleasure is associated with it. This helps to compensate for the loss of satisfaction from sucking. Weaning should not be attempted when the baby is ill. Complementary or relief bottles may be used throughout the period of nursing, or occasionally; the mother should consult her doctor for specific instructions. If the mother becomes pregnant, she should discontinue breast feeding, since this would place added strain on her.

BOTTLE FEEDING

Newborns who are not breast-fed are placed on formula. Modern scientific information has made such feedings safe and nutritionally adequate. The doctor prescribes a preparation of cow's milk, sugar, and water in proportions appropriate for the individual baby. He will instruct the mother as to changes in the original formula and how much to offer. Cow's milk may be pasteurized, homogenized, evaporated, condensed, or powdered.

Recent studies have indicated that babies tolerate cold milk equally as well as milk that has been heated slightly. If cold milk is used, there is no chance of burning a baby from overheated milk, the milk does not sour as rapidly, and time and energy are conserved. The practical nurse should follow the routine advised by the pediatrician on the division in which she is employed.

The mother or nurse needs to be relaxed and comfortable when feeding the newborn. His head and back are supported in the left arm. He should be warm and dry. Propping the bottle on a pad deprives the baby of the pleasure of being held and loved, and is dangerous because the baby may choke if the flow of milk is too rapid.

Preparation of the Formula

Formulas must be sterile and accurate, otherwise they can be a source of infection to the newborn, whose gastrointestinal tract is unstable and sensitive. In the formula room, personnel wear gowns, caps, and masks. In the home, the mother wears a clean dress or coverall apron. The hands must be washed thoroughly. There are two basic ways of preparing formula: the aseptic and the terminal heat methods.

In the *aseptic method* all articles, bottles, and nipples are sterilized beforehand, and the sterile formula ingredients are mixed and poured into sterile bottles.

The *terminal heat method* is used in many hospitals and homes for formulas that can stand the degree of heat necessary for this form of sterilization. The formula is prepared in *clean* utensils and poured into *clean* bottles. Nipples and caps are applied. Formula, bottles, and nipples are then sterilized. This eliminates the danger of contamination of the formula during its preparation. In the hospital, the bottles are placed in racks and sterilized in the autoclave. In the home, a sterilizer may be obtained to serve essentially the same purpose. Specific instructions for its use are included by the manufacturer.

Currently many hospitals are using commercially prepared formulas. This eliminates the need to prepare formulas in the formula room. The mother can also purchase these in disposable containers at her local drugstore.

The practical nurse learns how to make each of these formulas during her experience in the formula room. Regardless of the method used, all bottles, nipples, caps, and other utensils must be thoroughly cleansed. Bottles and nipples are scrubbed with a bottle brush in hot, soapy water and rinsed well in hot, clear water. Water is squeezed through nipple holes during washing and rinsing. Bottles are placed upside down on a rack to drain. Nipples and caps are put in a clean jar or an area especially designated for them. It is helpful to rinse bottles and nipples immediately following each feeding to prevent the milk from forming a film.

Most nipples come with one or three holes or a cross cut, and should be firm. The size of the hole required is determined by the condition of the newborn. To enlarge a nipple hole, insert the blunt end of a darning needle into a cork. Hold the point of the needle in a flame until it is red hot. Puncture the nipple, then place it in cold water to harden the rubber. Test the flow. Most hospitals keep a small supply of nipples in a sterile container in the nursery. The practical nurse uses sterile forceps to remove one from the container. She must remember to hold the forceps' tongs down when removing sterile equipment of any type from a container.

Nipple covers, made of assorted materials, including paper, are used for the purpose of keeping nipples sterile. If screw cap bottles are used, the disc is used to push the shoulder of the nipple through the cap. The disc is then removed and the cap put on the bottle.

Feeding Method

The following points should be observed when feeding the baby by bottle:

1. Wear a covergown.
2. The baby wears a bib. Change diaper p.r.n. Wash hands following.
3. Hold the baby unless contraindicated. If a baby cannot be removed from his crib, sit by him and elevate his head and shoulders.
4. Check the patient's indentification band with the name on the formula cap. Observe the amount of formula in the bottle.
5. Let a few drops of formula fall on the inner aspect of your wrist to test:
   Temperature: Should be warm but not hot.
   Size of nipple hole: Formula should drop but not flow in a steady stream. If the holes are too small, the weak newborn will tire and fail to finish the feeding. If they are too large, he may choke or miss the satisfaction he receives from sucking.
6. Do not contaminate the nipple.
7. Hold the bottle so that the nipple is full of formula. This prevents the baby from swallowing air.

8. Burp the baby halfway through the feeding and at the end by one of the following methods:
   a. Place a diaper or small towel over your shoulder to protect your gown. Place the baby firmly against your shoulder and pat his back.
   b. Place the baby in a sitting position. Put a towel beneath his chin. Support his chest and head with one hand. Gently rub his back with the other.
9. The feeding should take 15 to 20 minutes. Do not hurry the baby or force him to eat too much.
10. Leave the baby clean and dry. Place him on his abdomen or right side to promote digestion and prevent aspiration of regurgitated milk or vomitus.
11. Chart the amount of formula offered, the amount taken and retained, regurgitation or vomiting,* how the formula was taken, and whether or not the baby appeared satisfied following the feeding.

In the hospital, newborns are placed on individualized scheduled feedings. The majority are fed every three or four hours. In the home, the baby who is fed when he is hungry ("demand feedings") will soon adopt a schedule similar to the scheduled feedings just mentioned, with a few reasonable alterations. Prompt fulfillment of the baby's needs assures him that the world is a good place in which to live.

Vitamins

Babies need extra vitamins D and C. Breast milk contains sufficient vitamin C if the mother's diet is rich in citrus fruits and certain vegetables. Vitamin D may be added to milk and is labeled "vitamin D milk." Commercial concentrated preparations that contain vitamins D, C, and A may also be prescribed by the doctor. The fluid is drawn up in the dropper to the prescribed amount (0.3 or 0.6 cc.) and placed directly into the baby's mouth. This is given each morning at a regular time.

CARE OF THE PATIENT'S UNIT

Babies in the newborn nursery are usually placed in small, transparent bassinets that are equipped with a bath tray which can be pulled out. On the children's ward the baby may be placed in the same type of bassinet or in a crib. When making a crib, the nurse places the baby at the foot of it and tucks the clean sheet in at the top of the mattress. She then reverses the procedure. The nurse must guard the infant when the cribside is down. If the crib is large, it may be easier to place the baby on the far side of it and apply the clean sheet lengthwise. The nurse tucks in the side closest to her, raises the cribside, and remakes the other side of the crib.

Each unit is restocked daily with the necessary articles of linen which include diapers, shirts, crib sheets, receiving blankets, and quilted or

---

*Regurgitation is an overflow of milk which occurs shortly after feeding. Vomiting means bringing up a more substantial amount.

flannel pads. Some hospitals keep small trays in the bedside stands of each baby. Included on them are such items as safety pins, comb or brush, cottonballs, soap, thermometer in holder, and water. This tray is cleaned daily and whenever necessary. Cribs and stands in the rooms of discharged babies are terminally disinfected according to hospital procedure.

ROOMING-IN

Rooming-in is the term given to the hospital unit available in a limited number of hospitals whereby the mother keeps her newborn by her bedside and takes as much care of him as her condition permits and she desires. Its advantages are that the newborn receives individual attention from his mother and father and becomes better acquainted with his parents, and the mother need not worry that her baby is being neglected in the busy nursery. It also provides an excellent opportunity for the medical staff to teach parents many aspects of infant care.

BAPTISM

If the condition of a newborn is poor, most Christian parents will want to have him baptized. The minister or priest should be notified. In an emergency, the nurse may perform the baptism by pouring water on the baby's forehead while saying "I baptize thee in the name of the Father, and of the Son, and of the Holy Spirit." Should there be any doubt as to whether the baby is alive, the baptism is given conditionally: "If you are capable of receiving baptism, I baptize you in the name of the Father, and of the Son, and of the Holy Spirit."

Occasionally parents will pin small medals to the baby's blankets or clothing. The nurse must be extremely careful not to lose these since they are of great sentimental value to the parents, particularly if the baby dies.

CLOTHING

The newborn in the hospital needs to wear merely a shirt and a diaper and to be covered with a light blanket. A shirt that ties or snaps on in a double-breasted fashion is easy to put on and gives added warmth to the chest. The diaper may be folded in a triangle or rectangle and pinned at the hips. The female baby needs the thickness of the diaper low under her buttocks when lying on her back and in front when lying on her stomach. The male needs padding over the penis. The nurse should slip two fingers of one hand between the baby's body and the pin to prevent injuring him.

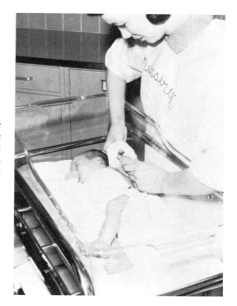

Figure 20. The simplest way to dress the newborn is to put your hand through the sleeve, grasp the baby's hand and pull it through gently. (From Davis, M. E., and Rubin, R.: DeLee's Obstetrics for Nurses. 18th Ed., 1966).

DIAPER PAIL

Each newborn should have a diaper pail for diapers soiled with feces. The doctor will want to observe the type and character of the newborn's stool, particularly if there is a disorder of the gastrointestinal tract. If the nurse places a small amount of water in the rim around the top of the pail, she will create a suction which will prevent the escape of odors. Pails with foot pedals and closely fitted tops are also available. This pail is emptied each day following the physician's visit. The diapers are emptied into the hopper, rinsed in cold water, and sent to the laundry.

PREVENTING INFECTION

Infections that are relatively harmless to an adult may be fatal to the newborn. The practical nurse caring for the newborn should review the ways in which germs enter and leave a person's body. Briefly, the portals of entry are the respiratory tract, the gastrointestinal tract, the genitourinary tract, and breaks in the skin. The portals of exit are the same as those just mentioned, and the germs are in the excretions from the various systems: sneezes, sputum, vomitus, feces, saliva, urine, and discharges from the skin and mucous membrane.

Very often patients in pediatric units are placed on *protective precautions.* The meaning is implied by the name—the physician wishes to protect the particular child from undue exposure to germs. Prematures, newborns, and infants are frequently on this type of precaution. Because they are highly susceptible to infection, children with burns or with diseases in which the white blood cells of the body are reduced are also protected in this manner. Protective precautions differ from isolation technique in that the child is being protected from the nurse. No one with a cold or similar malady should come in contact with the patient. A mother does this in the home by keeping outsiders away from the baby.

HANDWASHING

One of the most effective procedures employed in the prevention of infections is proper handwashing. The nurse must conscientiously wash and rinse her hands and forearms before she handles each baby and before and after handling equipment. Although most germs are transmitted by direct contact, some are capable of remaining alive for a time outside of the body, and may be transferred indirectly through articles. No rings should be worn since bacteria may collect on them. Personnel entering the newborn nursery scrub their hands with an antiseptic such as pHisoHex. In other areas of the hospital the hands are washed with soap under running water. Parents and relatives should be taught the importance of this simple but highly effective procedure.

EQUIPMENT.   Running water, soap, paper towels.
METHOD
1. Keep the hands lowered over the basin throughout the entire procedure.
2. Wet the hands.
3. Soap hands well, working up a lather.
4. Rinse the bar of soap, leaving it clean for the next use.
5. Use friction. Rub well between the fingers and around the nails. Wash the entire hands, wrists, and forearms; rinse well.
6. Repeat steps 2, 3, 4, and 5 three times.
7. Dry the hands well following.

CLOTHING OF PERSONNEL

When the practical nurse cares for newborns, infants, and other patients prone to infection, she wears a covergown over her uniform i.e., for protective precautions. This gown is generally hung in the patient's cubicle, and is replaced daily and whenever necessary. Gowns are hung by the neckband, inside out, so that the area which comes in contact with the baby is kept clean. Do not wear gowns in the corridor. Some institutions require that personnel also wear masks. They are considered of limited value.

In the nursery, special scrub dresses are worn by personnel. The use of caps and masks varies with each institution. If the nurse leaves the nursery, she wears a covergown over her scrub dress. Physicians, technicians, and non-nursery personnel should wear a gown, cap, and mask when on duty in the nursery.

HEALTH EXAMINATIONS OF PERSONNEL

Health examinations of personnel before employment and annually minimize the spread of infection from unhealthy persons. Many hospitals require throat cultures and stool examinations for personnel assigned to specific areas, e.g., the nursery. The practical nurse who has signs of a cold, earache, skin infection, or intestinal upset should not work in the nursery or care for the ill child.

SYMPTOMS OF INFECTION IN THE NEWBORN

The following signs and symptoms of infection in newborns and infants should be reported:

1. Temperature elevated to 100° F.
2. Refusal to take formula.
3. Rashes or skin lesions.
4. Loose, watery stools.
5. Discharge from eyes, nose, umbilicus.
6. Vomiting.

The newborn is removed from the nursery and placed in an isolated room or special isolation nursery. Persons who care for an infected baby must not enter the regular newborn nursery.

HOSPITAL DISCHARGE

The mother is given a 24 hour supply of formula upon discharge. She should also receive an instruction booklet on formula preparation to supplement the information she has received in the hospital. An appointment is made for an examination of both her and the baby in approximately six weeks. The pediatrician and the obstetrician will see her to answer any specific questions she may have.

All infants should remain under medical care by a family physician, pediatrician, or those in charge of child health conferences. The location of the nearest conference may be obtained by calling the health department or visiting nurse association. Its main purpose is to provide health supervision for infants and children who would not otherwise receive this service. Here under the supervision of competent physicians and public health nurses, healthy infants are weighed, examined, and given immunizations. Mothers are given guidance in regard to the physical and emotional health of their child. The practical nurse should become acquainted with the health and welfare facilities in her town or city. The classified section of her telephone book is a good place to begin investigations, should she be in a new community. Many agencies are listed under social service.

HOME CARE

The new baby should have a room of his own if possible. Simple, durable, easy-to-clean furnishings are necessary. A crib with a firm mattress is a suitable place for the infant to sleep for several years. Mattress covers of thin rubber large enough to tuck in at the sides may be used. *Plastic bags are never used for this purpose.* Contour sheets are convenient. Blankets of lightweight cotton or wool are warm and easy to launder. The newborn does not require a pillow.

Attach pictures securely to the wall with wall tapes. Thumbtacks may be swallowed by the growing child. A chest of drawers for clothing, an adult chair—preferably a rocker—and some type of flat-topped table for baby's changes are necessary. A bathinette will serve this purpose as well as that of the bath. The baby needs his own bathtub, which may be merely a plastic basin. Scales are nice to have but are not essential. A tray containing articles frequently used will save time and energy. This might include safety pins, hairbrush and comb, cotton balls, orange wood stick, baby oil or lotion, and powder if desired. A diaper pail is also necessary.

Clothing must be soft, washable, and of the proper size. It should be easy to put on and take off. Nightgowns with draw-string necks are to be avoided because they may be dangerous. Buttons need to be sewed on tightly. Grip-fasteners are safer. If the mother does not have a clothes dryer, she will need a clothes rack to dry the infant's garments when the weather is inclement.

Diapers are made of gauze, knitted cotton, bird's-eye, or cotton flannel. Contour and prefolded types are available, and are convenient if a diaper service is used. However, they take longer to dry when laundering at home and are more costly. Disposable diapers are handy. The newer ones are more absorbent and have an outer waterproof sheet which eliminates the need for rubber pants. Diaper liners are specially treated tissues which are placed within the diaper. When diapers are soiled, the stool is rinsed into the toilet. The diapers are soaked in cold water, washed with a mild soap, rinsed thoroughly, and dried outdoors in the sun. Diapers that have been improperly washed and rinsed may aggravate rashes. Waterproof pants should be loose and so cut that air can circulate through them. They are not used when the skin is irritated.

If a rash is present, leave the buttocks exposed to the air as much as possible. External heat may also be used. An electric light bulb (40 to 60 watts) placed in a gooseneck lamp and directed to the involved area is sufficient treatment in most cases. Place the bulb 12 to 16 inches away from the buttocks to avoid burning the baby. Do not apply ointment to the area when the light is being used. The light is applied for 10 to 15 minutes three or four times a day until the rash disappears.

The quantity of items that the mother will need is determined by her washing facilities and the climate where she lives. It is wise to obtain sufficient amounts of the few articles that have to be changed often, e.g., three or four dozen diapers, six shirts and blankets, six nightgowns, and two or three sweater sets.

STUDY QUESTIONS

1. What is meant by the term infant mortality?
2. Define the following: meconium, vernix caseosa, fontanels, Moro reflex, rooting reflex.
3. It is feeding time and you have just brought Mrs. Webster and Mrs. Jones their babies. Mrs. Webster is nursing her baby; Mrs. Jones' baby is bottle-fed. They are discussing feedings and ask your opinion. What would your reply be in this situation?
4. List the advantages of breast feeding.
5. What care is given to the umbilicus of the newborn? Why is this care important?
6. Define circumcision. When is it usually performed?
7. What measures must the practical nurse take to prevent infection of the newborn in the newborn nursery? On the children's ward? In the home?
8. How can the nurse on the busy pediatric unit satisfy the needs of the baby for tender, loving care?
9. Baby Rand is crying loudly in her bassinet. List several discomforts that might be the cause of her unhappiness. What can the nurse do to alleviate them?
10. Define skin turgor. How does the nurse test for good skin turgor?

BIBLIOGRAPHY

American Red Cross: Home Nursing Textbook. New York, Doubleday & Co., Inc., 1963.
Anthony, C.: Structure and Functions of the Body. 3rd Ed. St. Louis, The C. V. Mosby Co., 1968.
Blake, F.: The Child, His Parents and the Nurse. Philadelphia, J. B. Lippincott Co., 1954.
Blake, F., and Wright, F.: Essentials of Pediatric Nursing. 7th Ed. Philadelphia, J. B. Lippincott Co., 1963.
Bleier, I.: Maternity Nursing. 2nd Ed. Philadelphia, W. B. Saunders Co., 1966.
Culver, V. M.: Modern Bedside Nursing. 7th Ed. Philadelphia, W. B. Saunders Co., 1969.
John Hancock Mutual Life Insurance Company: You and Your Baby, 1961.
Marlow, D.: Textbook of Pediatric Nursing. 3rd Ed. Philadelphia, W. B. Saunders Co., 1969.
Spock, B.: Baby and Child Care. 9th Ed. New York, Duell, Sloan and Pearce, Inc., 1968.
United States Department of Health, Education, and Welfare: Infant Care. Children's Bureau Publication No. 8, 1967.

Chapter 5

THE PREMATURE

VOCABULARY

Antibody	*Lanugo*
Aspiration	*Oxygen analyzer*
Fetus	*Placenta*
Gestation	*Resuscitation*
Immaturity	*Twitch*
Incubator	

Prematurity is the leading cause of death in the newborn period. The nursing care of the premature requires experience and skilled training. The practical nurse who is interested in this type of nursing will need specialized instruction in a premature nursery. No amount of textbook learning can take the place of actual supervised practice. The material presented in this chapter serves only to acquaint the student with the premature so that she may appreciate his struggle for survival and the intense responsibility of those who specialize in his care.

A newborn is considered "premature" if he weighs five and one half pounds (2500 gm.) or less at birth, regardless of the period of gestation. The lower the birth weight, the greater the chances that death may occur. Twelve to 20 per cent of premature babies do not live.

CAUSES OF PREMATURITY

The predisposing causes of prematurity are numerous, and in many cases, the cause is unknown. Prematurity may be caused by multiple births such as twins or triplets, illness of the mother (e.g., malnutrition, heart disease, diabetes mellitus, and infectious conditions), and the hazards of pregnancy itself (e.g., toxemias, placental abnormalities which may result in premature rupture of the membranes, placenta previa [the placenta lies over the cervix instead of higher in the uterus], and premature separation of the placenta). Recent studies also indicate that there may be a relationship between smoking and prematurity. Adequate prenatal care to prevent these births is recognized as extremely important. Each day the fetus remains in the uterus his chances for survival become better.

PHYSICAL CHARACTERISTICS

Premature birth deprives the newborn of the complete benefits of intra-uterine life. The baby the practical nurse views in the incubator will

56

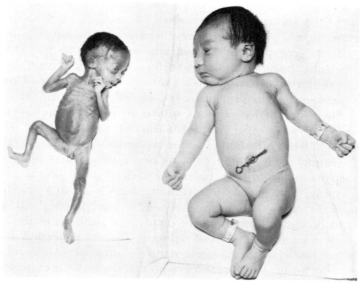

Figure 21. The premature baby, on the left, was 28 days old when this picture was taken. He lived and is normal. The baby on the right is a full-term newborn. (From Davis, M. E., and Rubin, R.: DeLee's Obstetrics for Nurses. 18th Ed., 1966.)

resemble pictures of a fetus of seven or eight months' gestation (see Fig. 18). The organs are immature and the body systems are not functioning to capacity. Respiration is handicapped by an incomplete development of the alveoli of the lungs and by weakness of the thoracic cage and muscles of respiration. Red blood cells are easily destroyed, and even a slight loss of blood is of great significance.

The premature has poor control of body temperature due to a lack of insulating subcutaneous fat and excessive heat loss by radiation from a surface area that is large in proportion to body weight. The heat regulation center of the brain is immature. Fine hair called *lanugo* covers the forehead, shoulders, and arms. The small capacity of the stomach and weakness or absence of sucking and swallowing reflexes makes eating a problem. The kidneys are not functioning to capacity.

The premature is more susceptible to infections than the full-term newborn, for protective antibodies from the mother may not have been transferred. His skin and mucous membranes are not functioning as effectively as they would at full term. Antenatal storage of minerals and vitamins is low or absent. The management of the premature is based upon his physical immaturity.

At Birth

The doctor appraises the physical status of the premature at delivery. Resuscitation is performed if indicated. The baby is given cord and eye care and properly identified. Weighing is sometimes omitted until later if the condition of the baby is poor. He is placed in an incubator naked and taken to the nursery. A report is given to the nurse in charge concerning the general condition of the premature, and she is notified of the type of delivery and any complications that may have occurred. Many hospitals today transfer their prematures to special premature centers which are geared to the care of this type of patient.

The Incubator. The premature is placed in an incubator in order to maintain environmental conditions similar to those of the uterus. It is designed to provide proper heat, humidity, oxygen, and mist; isolation; and protection from infection. The top of the incubator is transparent to enable personnel to view the premature clearly at all times. Some models include alarms to indicate overheating or lack of circulating air, facilities for positioning, and a scale to weigh the baby without removing him from his warm environment (see Fig. 22). The practical nurse must understand how to use the types of incubators available in the nursery where she is assigned. She should request assistance if needed.

Heat is essential for the premature's survival. An incubator is prepared and preheated whenever a premature birth is expected. The

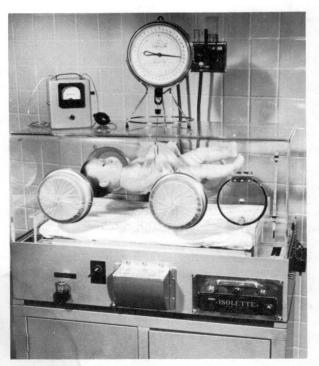

Figure 22. When oxygen is being administered, the oxygen content must be checked at regular intervals with an oxygen analyzer shown here at the left on the Isolette. In the center of the Isolette is a specially designed scale that allows weighing of the baby without removing him. (From Bleier, I. J.: Maternity Nursing, 1966.)

temperature is generally kept at 85° to 95° F. The nurse records the temperature of the incubator every four hours. The doctor may ask the nurse to regulate it from time to time in an effort to *stabilize* the body temperature of the premature. A relative humidity of 60 per cent or higher is desirable. The doctor will leave specific orders for the exact temperature and humidity levels he desires for the individual premature.

If oxygen is used, its concentration should not exceed 40 per cent. An oxygen analyzer is used to determine actual oxygen concentration (see Fig. 22). *Retrolental fibroplasia* may result from oxygen poisoning in the premature (see Fig. 26). It affects the blood vessels of the eye and is a cause of blindness in the newborn. To prevent this condition, oxygen therapy is given only when the premature is in immediate need of it, and then only in low concentrations and for short periods of time rather than continuously. Newer models of the Isolette have an oxygen concentration control that limits the amount of oxygen within the Isolette to 40 per cent. (See Fig. 23.) Another way to insure that the premature will

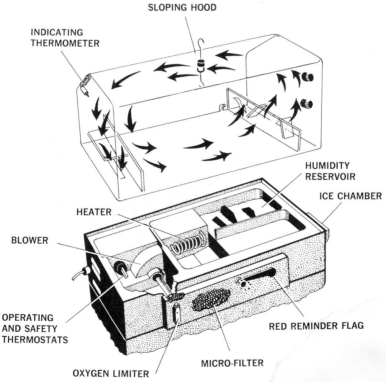

Figure 23. The oustanding features of the Isolette. Microfiltered nursery air is drawn into the incubator and circulated by the blower, with or without oxygen. The air is forced around the heating element and over the humidity reservoir. Incoming oxygen is filtered and concentrations limited automatically to 40 per cent. Unique red flag assembly delivers higher concentrations if prescribed for periods of respiratory emergency and serves as a constant reminder to attending personnel. (Courtesy of Air Shields, Inc. Hatboro, Pa.)

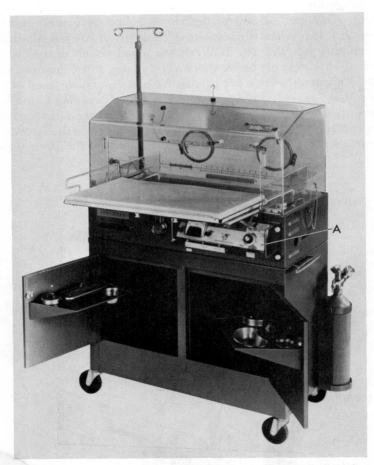

Figure 24. Isolette infant incubator—intensive care model. The Isolette shown above has an optional servo-control unit (*A*). (Courtesy of Air Shields, Inc. Hatboro, Pa.)

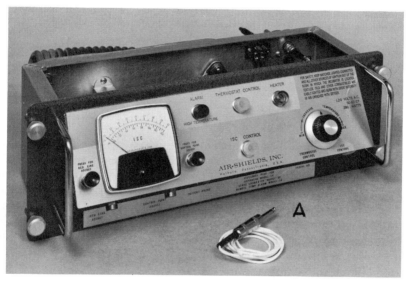

Figure 25. Isolette Servo-Control (ISC) power unit. A special temperature sensing thermistor termed a "patient probe" (*A*) is taped to the baby's abdomen and connected to the unit. This detects changes in skin temperature and regulates the heat of the Isolette in accordance. Thus the infant acts as a thermostat to the unit. (Courtesy of Air Shields, Inc. Hatboro, Pa.)

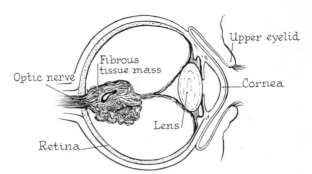

Figure 26. *Retrolental fibroplasia.* In small prematures who have been exposed to too much oxygen for too long, an overgrowth of retinal blood vessels may result. This vascular mass may convert to scar tissue, block the passage of light from the lens to the retina, and produce blindness. (From Geddes, A. K.: Premature Babies, 1960.)

receive only the proper amount of oxygen is to use a combination of 40 per cent oxygen and 60 per cent nitrogen.

Close Observation

The doctor examines the premature when the patient's condition permits. He writes specific orders concerning treatment and nursing care. When he leaves the nursery, he relies on the nurses to keep him informed of any significant changes in the baby's condition. The experienced nurse in the premature nursery observes and charts care and treatment with great accuracy. For example, a chapter could be spent on her observations of the premature's behavior during feedings. The following is a list of *general* observations to serve as a guide in his care. Sudden changes are reported immediately.

Color	pale, cyanosis, jaundice.
Respirations	regularity, apnea, sternal retractions, labored.
Pulse	rate and regularity.
Abdomen	distention.
Stools	frequency, color, consistency.
Skin	rashes, irritations, pustules, edema.
Cord	discharge.
Eyes	discharge.
Feeding	sucking ability, vomiting, regurgitation, degree of satisfaction.

Mucous membranes	dry lips and mouth, signs of thrush.
Voiding	particularly the first.
General activity.	increase, decrease, lethargy, twitching, frequency and quality of cry, hyperactivity.

PREVENTING INFECTION

Merely placing the premature in an incubator will not assure freedom from infection. The nurse must wash her hands meticulously before and after handling the newborn or equipment used in his care. Each baby should have his own supplies. The premature is handled very gently and as little as possible to prevent infection and to conserve his energy. Germs may be transferred to the premature by contaminated nipples, formula, bottles, and other feeding utensils; improperly sterilized linen; improper cleansing of the baby's anal area; and exposure to personnel who harbor infections.

NUTRITION

The premature is given nothing by mouth for 24 to 72 hours, or until his air passages are cleared of mucus. The first few feedings may consist of merely clear fluids. As he progresses, he will be placed on a formula, which is generally high in protein and low in fat. The doctor will calculate the exact proportions and amounts to be given each premature. The way in which he is fed depends on his size and strength. Prematures are not removed from their incubators for feedings until the doctor has given permission. They are fed by gavage, medicine dropper with rubber tip, and special premature bottles and nipples. The bottles hold one and one half ounces of formula.* The nipples are small and soft. Gavage or tube feedings are not administered by student practical nurses because of the dangers that can result from improper placement of the tube.

It is very difficult for the small premature to handle any type of feeding. He needs to be fed small amounts slowly. Overfeeding is dangerous. The hazards of aspiration are increased in the premature because his gag and cough reflexes are weak and it is difficult for him to clear his airway. The baby needs to be burped frequently. His head may be elevated for 45 minutes following feedings to decrease the changes of regurgitation. The doctor will order additional vitamin C to prevent scurvy and vitamin D to prevent rickets. Supplementary iron is also

*Bleier, p. 145.

given after the second month of life, since prematures are particularly prone to iron deficiency anemias.

POSITION

If the premature has a great deal of mucus, he is placed in the head-down position, otherwise he is turned from side to side at least every two hours. He should not be left in one position for long periods of time, as it is uncomfortable and may be harmful to the lungs.

HOSPITAL DISCHARGE

The parents need guidance throughout the hospitalization period to help prepare them for this new experience. They may be disheartened by the unattractive appearance of the premature. It is difficult for a mother to leave the hospital without her baby. She needs to be encouraged to visit him whenever possible. She is very concerned with her ability to care for such a small, helpless creature, and to see her baby graduate from the incubator to a bassinet is very gratifying. She should be taught aspects of his daily care such as feeding and bathing. Emphasis is also placed on the protective care of the infant at home, as well as on good hygiene and safety.

The doctor will carefully evaluate the premature before he is discharged. In general, the parents can take him home when his weight is five to five and one half pounds. Continued medical supervision is important. The services of the public health nurse are indicated in many cases. She visits the home before the baby arrives and helps to aid the mother with necessary preparations. The handicaps of prematurity become less limiting as the child grows older.

STUDY QUESTIONS

1. List the characteristics of a premature baby.
2. What is an incubator?
3. How does the nursing care of the premature differ from that of the full-term newborn?
4. Define the following: premature, retrolental fibroplasia, sternal retractions, oxygen analyzer, servo-control.
5. What is the cause of retrolental fibroplasia?.
6. Close observation is extremely important in the care of the premature. List several significant changes that should be reported to the nurse in charge.
7. What problems confront the parents of the premature? In what ways might the practical nurse help to allay their fears?

BIBLIOGRAPHY

Bleier, I.: Maternity Nursing—A Textbook for Practical Nurses. 2nd Ed. Philadelphia, W. B. Saunders Co., 1966.

Broadribb, V.: Foundations of Nursing. Philadelphia, J. B. Lippincott Co., 1967.

Davis, M., and Rubin, R.: DeLee's Obstetrics for Nurses. 18th Ed. Philadelphia, W. B. Saunders Co., 1966.

Geddes, A.: Premature Babies. Their Nursing Care and Management. Philadelphia, W. B. Saunders Co., 1960.

Hasselmeyer, E. G.: Behavior Patterns of Premature Infants. United States Department of Health, Education and Welfare. Public Health Serive Publication No. 840, U. S. Government Printing Office, 1961.

Marlow, D.: Textbook of Pediatric Nursing. 3rd Ed. Philadelphia, W. B. Saunders Co., 1969.

Ross Laboratories: The Premature Infant. Nursing Education Service, 1959.

Chapter 6

DISORDERS OF THE NEWBORN

VOCABULARY

Congenital	*Irritable*
Dehydration	*Prognosis*
Epidemic	*Pustule*
Hypostatic	*Restraint*
Incontinent	*Swelling*
Inherited	*Transfusion*

Many disorders of the newborn that formerly led to death or a lifetime of invalidism can now be cured, or corrected so that the patient may lead a reasonably normal life. These conditions are generally divided into several large groups. Included are:

Congenital Anomalies. These are malformations present at birth, some of which are inherited. They are the result of defects in the development of the fetus, and may be slight or so severe that they are not compatible with life. An example of a congenital anomaly is a cleft lip and palate.

Birth Injuries. This term includes both avoidable and unavoidable trauma at birth. An example of a birth injury is a fractured clavicle.

Respiratory Complications. These may develop before, during and after the birth process. Atelectasis, or incomplete expansion of the lungs, is an example of this condition.

Infections. Infection of the newborn may be acquired before birth, during passage through the birth canal, and through contact with contaminated personnel or supplies. Syphilis is an example of an infection acquired before birth. Thrush, a disease that infects the mouth of the newborn, is acquired as the baby passes through the birth canal.

Congenital Anomalies

NERVOUS SYSTEM

Hydrocephalus

Description. Hydrocephalus (*hydro-* water + *cephalo-* head) is a congenital anomaly characterized by an increase of cerebrospinal fluid in the ventricles of the brain, which results in an increase in the size of the head and pressure changes in the brain. It is most commonly caused by an obstruction such as a tumor or improper formation of the ventricles.

The practical nurse will recall that the brain and spinal cord are surrounded by fluid, membranes, and bone. The three membranes, called *meninges*, are the dura mater, arachnoid, and pia mater. The arachnoid or middle membrane resembles a cobweb, with its spaces filled with fluid. Cerebrospinal fluid is also found in spaces of the brain called *ventricles*. This fluid is continually forming and being reabsorbed into the blood.

Symptoms. The most obvious symptom is an increase in head size. This is accompanied by strabismus, or crossed eyes, and the sclera of the eye may be seen above the iris. The scalp is shiny and the veins dilated. The infant is helpless and lethargic. The patient's body becomes thin, and the muscle tone of his extremities is often poor. His cry is shrill and high pitched. Irritability, vomiting, and anorexia are present, and convulsions may occur.

Treatment. Ventriculography may be done as a diagnostic aid prior to surgery. This is an x-ray examination of the ventricles of the brain, after air or some other suitable substance has been injected. After careful evaluation of this and other preoperative tests, the doctor decides whether or not to operate. The surgeon attempts to by-pass or *shunt* the point of obstruction. The cerebrospinal fluid may thus be

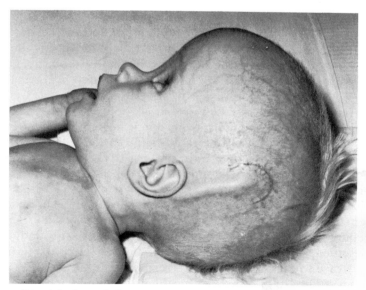

Figure 27. A hydrocephalic infant on whom a ventriculoperitoneal shunt was performed. Note the presence of the tube as it emerges from the skull and passes under the skin of the scalp and the chest. (From Marlow, D.: Textbook of Pediatric Nursing, 1969.)

carried to another area of the body, where it will be absorbed and finally excreted. This is accomplished by inserting special tubing which is replaced at intervals as the child grows (see Fig. 27). The prognosis of this condition has improved with modern drugs and surgical techniques. If the brain is not seriously damaged before the operation, mentality may be preserved. Motor development is sometimes slower, if the child cannot lift his head like a normal infant. Death may occur, however, from extreme malnutrition or infections during early childhood.

Nursing Care. The practical nurse may be called upon to give preoperative care in the hospital for the infant or child with hydrocephalus or to give supportive care in long-term inoperable conditions. The surgery required for this condition is highly intricate; therefore, the majority of the postoperative care will be given by the professional nurse. The practical nurse may assist the professional nurse during the convalescent period following surgery if the child is progressing well.

The general nursing care of an infant with hydrocephalus who has not undergone surgery presents several problems. The child may be barely able to raise his head. His mental development is delayed. Lack of appetite, a tendency to vomit easily, and poor resistance to infections present challenging problems.

The position of the patient must be changed frequently to prevent hypostatic pneumonia and pressure sores. Hypostatic pneumonia occurs when the circulation of the blood in the lungs is poor and the patient remains in one position too long. It is particularly prevalent in patients who are poorly nourished or weak, or who have a debilitating disease. When the practical nurse turns the patient with hydrocephalus, she must always support his head. To turn the patient in bed, the weight of the head should be borne in the palm of one hand, and the head and body rotated together to prevent a strain on the neck. When lifting the patient from his crib, the head may be supported by the nurse's arm and chest.

Pressure sores may occur if the patient's position is not changed at least every two hours. The tissues of the head and ears, as well as the bony prominences, have a tendency to break down. A pad of lamb's wool or sponge rubber placed under the head may help to avoid these lesions. If the skin becomes broken, it should be given immediate attention to prevent infection. The patient must be kept dry, especially around the creases of the neck where perspiration may collect.

In most cases the nurse may hold the infant to feed him. She should sit with her arm supported, since the head is heavy. A calm, unhurried manner is necessary. The room should be as quiet as possible. Following the feeding the infant is placed on his side. Do not disturb him after he is once settled, since he vomits easily. The practical nurse must organize her daily care so that it does not interfere with his meals.

Observations to be charted include: type and amounts of food taken, vomiting, condition of skin, motor abilities, restlessness, irritability, and changes in vital signs. Symptoms of increased pressure within the head are evidenced by an increase in blood pressure and a decrease in pulse and respiration. Signs of a cold or other infection are reported to the nurse in charge immediately and recorded.

Spina Bifida

Description. Spina bifida is a congenital defect in which there is an imperfect closure of the spinal canal. Portions of the spine may be completely or partially lacking. It is most common in the lumbosacral portion of the vertebrae. As a result of this condition the membranes may protrude through the opening. This is called a meningocele (*meningo-* membrane + *-cele* tumor). It contains portions of the membranes and cerebrospinal fluid. The size varies from that of a walnut to that of the head of a newborn.

More serious is a protrusion of the *membranes* and *cord* through this opening, or a *meningomyelocele.* Although it resembles a meningocele, there may be associated paralysis of the legs and poor control of bowel and bladder functions. Hydrocephalus may also be present.

Treatment. The prognosis of these conditions depends on the extent of the structures involved. If the defect involves only the vertebrae, i.e., spina bifida, there is no need for treatment unless neurological symptoms appear. In a meningocele, with no weakness of the legs or

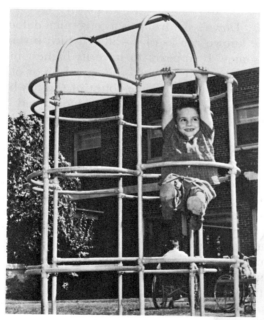

Figure 28. Dave, a victim of spina bifida, proves that handicapped persons are not necessarily bedridden. (Courtesy of Crotched Mountain Foundation, Greenfield, N.H.)

sphincter involvement, surgical correction is performed with excellent results. Surgery is also indicated in a meningomyelocele for cosmetic value and to help prevent infection. In some cases it may improve neurological symptoms. Currently surgery is being performed as early as possible, preferably in the first 24 hours of life. By doing this, some patients retain a degree of movement which is found in the legs at birth but which is lost thereafter. Rehabilitation following surgery is necessary since the legs remain paralyzed and the patient is incontinent of urine and feces. The aim of rehabilitation is to minimize the child's disability and put to constructive use the normal parts of his body. Every effort is made to help the child to develop a healthy personality so that he may have a happy and useful life. Eventually, the child can be taught to use a wheel chair and possibly to walk with braces and crutches.

Nursing Care. The practical nurse will need demonstrations and careful explanations when assisting with the care of these infants in the hospital. The main objectives of the extensive nursing care required include: prevention of infection or injury to the sac; correct position to prevent pressure on the sac and to prevent deformities; good skin care, particularly if the baby is incontinent of urine and feces; adequate nutrition; tender, loving care; accurate observations and charting; education of the parents; continued medical supervision; and rehabilitation.

Down's Syndrome (Mongolism)

Description. Down's syndrome is a congenital defect of the embryo. There are three known causes of it—all of which involve abnormalities of the chromosomes. It appears to have its highest incidence in newborns of mothers who have reached the age of 35 or older. In the most common type the total chromosome count of the newborn is 47 rather than the normal count of 46. Sometimes a mongoloid baby is the first-born of a young mother. In such cases, subsequent children are usually normal.

Symptoms. The signs of this condition, which are apparent at birth, are: an oriental appearance (see Fig. 29), close-set and upward-slanting eyes, small head, round face, flat nose, protruding tongue which interferes with sucking, and mouth breathing. Also, the hands of the baby are short and thick, and the little finger is curved. There is a wide space between the first and second toes. His undeveloped muscles and loose joints enable him to assume unusual positions. Physical growth and development may be slower than normal. He is mentally retarded; the maximum mental level will be about that of a seven year old. Congenital heart deformities may be associated with this condition.

This happy-go-lucky child is very lovable. He is restless and somewhat more difficult to train than the normal youngster. His resistance

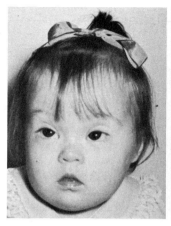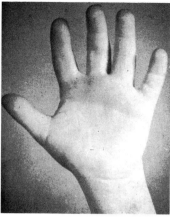

Figure 29. *A,* typical facial appearance of young child with Down's syndrome. *B,* typical broad, spadelike hand of Down's syndrome in a 12 year old boy. Note the shortness of all fingers. (From Nelson, W. E. (Editor): Textbook of Pediatrics, 1969.)

to infection is poor; many die before puberty. The lifespan of this patient has been increased with the widespread use of antibiotics. The child is trained to live as normal a life as possible within his capacity.

Attitude of the Practical Nurse. The practical nurse needs to be aware of her own feelings before she can give effective support to the handicapped child and his parents. She must have patience and understanding. The child is encouraged to help himself within his ability, even though it may take more time. This is especially true when he is ill and hospitalized.

The decision as to whether to keep the newborn or place him in an institution is an agonizing one. Sometimes parents cannot accept the fact that their baby will be retarded, and are ashamed to tell anyone of the baby's condition. The nurse must not be alarmed by the mother's need to cry. It takes exceptional strength to accept this diagnosis. Empathy on the part of the nurse is of particular importance. For further discussion of the mentally retarded child, see page 252.

CARDIOVASCULAR SYSTEM

Congenital Heart Disease

General Description. A baby born with congenital heart disease has a defect in the structure of his heart or in one or more of the large blood vessels which lead to and from the heart or in both. The heart or vessels have failed to develop properly. You will recall that the heart of the

Table 6-1.   *Diagnostic Tests Useful in Congenital Heart Defects*

Test	Definition	Value
Angiocardiography* (selective)	Serial x-rays of the heart and great vessels following the injection of an opaque substance. A radiopaque catheter is moved into the heart chambers and the medium injected in specific areas.	Abnormal communications in the heart can be observed. The course of the blood through the heart and great vessels can be traced.
Aortography	X-rays of the aorta after the injection of an opaque material.	Useful in revealing patent ductus arteriosus.
Barium swallow	Barium given by mouth.	Shows indentation of the esophagus by the aorta or other vessels.
Cardiac catheterization	A radiopaque catheter is passed through a cutdown site directly into the heart and large vessels.	Reveals blood pressure within the heart. Doctor can examine the heart closely with the tip of the catheter to detect abnormalities. Blood samples can be obtained to determine oxygen content.
Chest x-ray	————	Provides a permanent record. Shows abnormalities in shape and position of heart.
Cineangio-cardiography*	Motion pictures of images recorded by fluoroscopy.	Useful record and monitoring device.
Electrocardiogram	Tracing of heart action by electrocardiography.	Detects variations in heart action and shows the condition of the heart muscle. May also be used as a monitoring device during cardiac catheterization.
Fluoroscopy	Method of x-ray in which the image is focused on a radio-sensitive screen.	Shadows may be directly studied by radiologist. Physician can determine size, shape, and position of beating heart.

*These procedures are now considered by many to be a part of cardiac catheterization.

fetus is completely developed during the first eight weeks of pregnancy. A mother who contracts German measles early in her pregnancy or who is poorly nourished may bear a child with a faulty heart. Heredity and unknown factors are also responsible for the defect. Heart defects are the principal cause of death among the congenital anomalies during the first year of life. It is important, therefore, that the practical nurse stress the need for good prenatal care and impress upon the parents the value of well baby clinics. Many organic heart murmurs have been detected

Table 6-2. *General Signs and Symptoms of Congenital Heart Abnormalities**

Infants

1. Dyspnea
2. Difficulty with feeding
3. Stridor or choking spells
4. Pulse rate over 200
5. Recurrent respiratory infections
6. Failure to gain weight
7. Heart murmurs
8. Cyanosis
9. Cerebral vascular accidents
10. Anoxic attacks

Children

1. Dyspnea
2. Poor physical development
3. Decreased exercise tolerance
4. Recurrent respiratory infections
5. Heart murmur and thrill
6. Cyanosis
7. Squatting
8. Clubbing of fingers and toes
9. Elevated blood pressure

*Ross Laboratories: A Study Guide to Congenital Heart Abnormalities, 1961.

early in infancy at the baby's periodic checkup. The symptoms, as indicated in Table 6-2, depend upon the location and type of heart defect. Some patients have mild cases and can lead a fairly normal life under medical management. Others are taken care of medically until the optimum time for surgery.

Surgical Progress. Many exciting advances are taking place in the field of cardiac surgery. Better techniques and finer monitoring devices are being perfected. The *thoracotomy* is widely performed with fewer complications; thus, the risk of entering the chest cavity is decreased. The *cardiopulmonary bypass machine* takes over the function of the heart and lungs. While keeping other vital tissues of the body alive this machine gives the surgeon more time and a clearer field in which to operate. Another technique used in heart surgery is *hypothermia* (*hypo-* under + *therme-* heat). This procedure reduces the temperature of the body tissues which in turn decreases their need for oxygen. It may be done through the use of cooling agents in the heart-lung machine. Complete heart transplants, although in their infancy, may offer another avenue of hope for the child with a congenital heart defect which is incompatible with life.

Classification. For purposes of clarification, heart defects are divided into two broad groups: *cyanotic* or those conditions in which the patient has cyanosis, and *acyanotic* or those conditions in which the patient does not have cyanosis. Frequently, more than one abnormality is present, or complications develop which could alter the degree of cyanosis. The following conditions are followed by the nursing considerations which are relative to the care of the child with a congenital heart defect.

Acyanotic Defects

1. Patent Ductus Arteriosus. As previously mentioned on pages 37 and 38, the circulation of the fetus differs from that of the newborn in

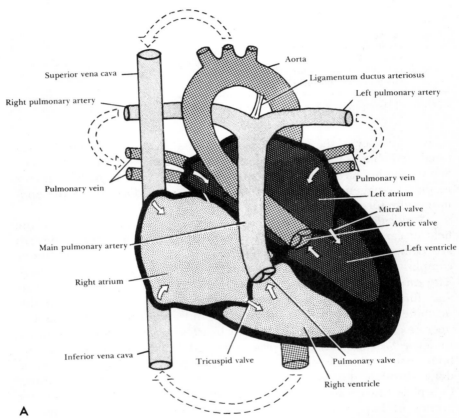

A

Figure 30. *A*, the normal heart. *B*, interatrial septal defect. *C*, interventricular septal defect. *D*, tetralogy of Fallot. *E*, patent ductus arteriosus. *F*, coarctation of the aorta. (*A* from clinical education aid No. 7, Ross Laboratories, Columbus, Ohio. *B* and *C* from Ingalls, A.: Maternal and Child Health Nursing. C. V. Mosby Co., 1967. *D* from Ross Laboratories, Columbus, Ohio. *E* and *F* from Diagnosis of Congenital Cardiac Defects in General Practice. Used with the permission of the American Heart Association.)

(*Figure continues on opposite page.*)

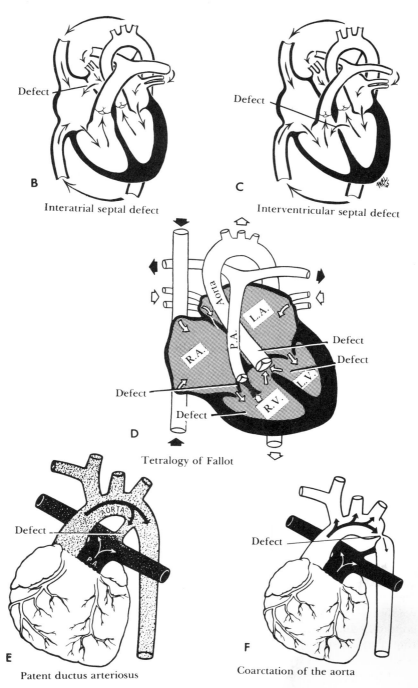

B
Interatrial septal defect

C
Interventricular septal defect

D
Tetralogy of Fallot

E
Patent ductus arteriosus

F
Coarctation of the aorta

Figure 30. *Continued.*

that most of the blood bypasses the lungs. The *ductus arteriosus* is the passageway by which the blood crosses from the pulmonary artery to the aorta and avoids the deflated lungs. This vessel closes shortly after birth; however, when it does not close, blood continues to pass from the aorta, where the pressure is higher, into the pulmonary artery. This causes oxygenated blood to recircle through the lungs, overburdening the pulmonary circulation. This makes the heart pump harder.

Patent ductus arteriosus is one of the most common cardiac anomalies. The word patent means "open." It occurs twice as frequently in females as in males. Closed heart surgery is performed in all diagnosed cases if there are no other complications. If this condition is left uncorrected, the patient could eventually develop congestive heart failure or endocarditis. The opening is closed by ligation or by division of the ductus. This is done between the second and fifth years, if there is a choice. The prognosis is excellent (see Fig. 30).

2. Coarctation of the Aorta. The word coarctation means a "tightening." In this condition, there is a constriction or narrowing of the aortic arch or of the descending aorta. The patient may not develop symptoms until later childhood. Since the graft will not grow but the aorta will, the best time for surgery is between the ages of eight and fifteen. The surgeon resects the narrowed portion of the aorta and joins its ends. The joining is called an *anastomosis*. If the section removed is large, an end-to-end graft using tubes of dacron or similar material may be necessary. As in patent ductus arteriosus, closed heart surgery is performed because the structures are outside of the heart. The prognosis is favorable, if there are no other defects.

3. Interatrial Septal Defect. This is one of the more common congenital heart anomalies. The incidence is higher in females than in males. There is an abnormal opening between the right and the left atria. Blood which contains oxygen is forced from the left atrium to the right atrium. This type of arterial venous shunt does not produce cyanosis, unless the flow is reversed by heart failure. Less serious types of this defect can be corrected by open heart surgery. With the use of the heart-lung bypass machine, the condition can be corrected in a dry or bloodless field. The hole is then sutured or patched. The prognosis depends upon the location of the atrial defect in the septum.

4. Interventricular Septal Defect. As the name suggests there is an opening between the right and left ventricles of the heart. Blood passes directly from the left to the right ventricle. A loud harsh murmur combined with a systolic tremor is characteristic of this defect. The condition may be mild or severe. Surgical risk is high during infancy; therefore, postponement is advised until early childhood. The correction is similar to that of interatrial septal defects. A *staged* procedure by way of closed heart surgery is sometimes done on babies to provide relief from symptoms until the optimum time for definitive surgery.

Cyanotic Defects

1. Tetralogy of Fallot. "Tetra" means four. In this condition, there are four defects: (a) stenosis or narrowing of the pulmonary artery which decreases the bloodflow to the lungs, (b) hypertrophy of the right ventricle; the right ventricle becomes enlarged since it has to work harder in order to pump blood through the narrow pulmonary artery, (c) dextraposition (*Dextra-* right + position) of the aorta; the aorta is displaced to the right and blood from both ventricles enters it, and (d) ventricular septal defect.

When venous blood enters the aorta, severe heart trouble is evident in the infant. Cyanosis increases with age, and clubbing of the fingers and toes is seen. The child rests in a "squatting" position so that he can breathe more easily. Feeding problems, growth retardation, frequent respiratory infections, and severe dyspnea upon exercise are prevalent. The red blood cells of the body increase polycythemia (*poly-* many + *cyth-* cells + *hema-* blood) in an effort to compensate for the lack of oxygen. Iron deficiency anemias, due to poor appetite, are common. Blackouts and convulsions may occur. In some cases, mental retardation develops because there is a lack of oxygen reaching the brain. The child is treated medically until he can endure surgery. Staged surgery may be done to increase the flow of blood to the lungs. For correction of the problem, open heart surgery is being perfected.

CONGESTIVE HEART FAILURE

An infant with a severe heart defect may develop congestive heart failure. The practical nurse must constantly be on the alert for signs and symptoms of this condition. Some of these are cyanosis, pallor, rapid respirations, rapid pulse, feeding difficulties, fatigue, failure to gain weight, edema, and frequent respiratory infections.

Cyanosis. When observing the baby's color, the nurse notes whether the cyanosis is general or localized. If it is localized, she records the exact location in her notes, i.e., hands, feet, lips, or around the mouth. Is the cyanosis deep or light? Is it constant or transient? Sometimes a baby's color improves when he cries, sometimes it gets worse; this is significant. If overt cyanosis is not apparent in the Negro infant, observe the palms of the hands and bottoms of the feet. Clubbing of the fingers and toes as a result of pooling of the blood in the capillaries of the extremities may be evident. The infant may be very pale or have a mottled appearance.

Rapid Respirations. Over 60 respirations per minute in a newborn at rest indicate distress. The amount of dyspnea does vary; in more acute cases, it is accompanied by flaring of the nostrils, mouth breathing, and sternal retractions. The baby has more trouble breathing when he is flat in bed than when he is being held upright. Air hunger is indicated, if the patient is irritable and restless. His cry is weak and hoarse.

Rapid Pulse. This is termed *tachycardia.* A pulse rate of over 150 beats per minute is significant. The heart is pumping harder in an effort to get sufficient oxygen to all parts of the body.

Feeding Difficulties. When the nurse tries to feed the infant, he tires easily. He may refuse to suck after a few ounces. When placed in his crib, he cries and appears hungry. He may choke and gag during feedings; the pleasure of sucking is spoiled by his inability to breathe.

Poor Weight Gain. The patient fails to gain weight. A sudden increase in weight may indicate the beginning of heart failure.

Edema. Watch for puffiness about the eyes and, occassionally, in the legs, feet, and abdomen.

Frequent Respiratory Infections. The baby's resistance is very low. Slight infections can be very dangerous, since the heart and lungs are in distress already.

Nursing Goals

The nursing goals significant to the care of the afflicted newborn can be adapted to all children with heart defects. These are: (1) to reduce the work of the heart, (2) to improve respiration, (3) to maintain proper nutrition, (4) to prevent infection, (5) to reduce the anxiety of the patient, and (6) to support and instruct the parents.

The nurse must organize her work so that the baby is not unnecessarily disturbed. The patient needs a great deal of energy. A complete bath and linen change are luxuries that an infant with a serious heart defect cannot afford. He should be fed early if crying and late if asleep. The doctor will order the position in which the infant should be placed. In some cases, the knee chest position facilitates breathing; in other cases, a slanting position with the head elevated may be helpful. Older babies may be placed in infant seats.

A low salt formula such as Lonalac may be prescribed. This will help prevent retention of fluids in the tissues. Cereal, as well as new foods which are added to the child's diet, is selected in terms of salt content. In some cases, nasogastric tube feedings are advantageous since they are less tiring for the patient. Oxygen is administered to relieve dyspnea. As breathing becomes easier, the baby begins to relax. A soft voice with gentle care will soothe the patient. Whenever possible, the infant is held and loved during feedings. Preventing infection is paramount; this is discussed on pages 51 to 53.

Digitoxin and digoxin are common oral digital preparations used for infants. Their action is to slow and strengthen the heart beat. The nurse counts the patient's pulse before administering them. A resting apical pulse is most accurate (see page 19). If the pulse of a newborn is below 100, the medication is withheld and the doctor is notified.

Tachycardia and irregularities in the rhythm of the pulse are significant and should be reported. Symptoms of toxicity include nausea, vomiting, anorexia, irregularity in rate and rhythm of the pulse, or a sudden change in pulse. If the baby is discharged while on this medication, the parents are taught how to take the pulse and what significant factors they should be aware of when administering it. Diuretics such as mercaptomerin (Thiomerin) or Diuril are useful in reducing edema. Proper recording of the number of voidings each day and the weight of the baby will help the doctor to determine the effectiveness of the diuresis. Morphine is given for relaxation.

Complications other than *cardiac decompensation* (heart failure) may arise before or following surgery. Due to the increased numbers of red blood cells circulating within the body, i.e., polycythemia, the blood becomes sluggish and prone to clots. When this is accompanied by dehydration, the threat of cerebral thrombosis may become a reality. An accurate record of intake and output is essential. Signs of dehydration, such as thirst, fever, poor skin turgor, apathy, sunken eyes or fontanel, dry skin, dry tongue, dry mucous membranes, and a decrease in urination, should be brought to the immediate attention of the nurse in charge. Pneumonia can occur rapidly. Fever, irritability, and an increase in respiratory distress may indicate this condition. The nurse insures that the patient's position is changed regularly to help prevent this setback.

The parents of the child need support and understanding over a long period of time. A mother's fears and dependencies come to the surface when she gives birth to a defective baby. Since the heart is the body's vital organ, this type of diagnosis causes a great deal of apprehension. The physician has to reassure the parents without minimizing the danger involved. If the infant's condition permits, he is sent home under medical supervision until the preferred age for surgery. Every effort must be made by the family to provide him with a normal environment that is within his limits. It is easy for parents to become overpermissive since they do not wish the child to become excited unnecessarily. The child senses this and soon gains control of the home. This is difficult for everyone but is especially exhausting and confining for the mother. A program of discipline and guidance with some modifications is desirable.

The patterns formed during infancy will set the framework of a healthy personality for the patient. The child with a heart condition who is well-integrated into family life has a decided advantage over the child who is made to think he is an invalid. Routine naps and early bedtime will provide adequate rest for most patients. As the child grows, he usually sets his own limits on the amount of activity he can handle. Substitutions can be made for strenuous activities, such as bicycle riding, and for rigorous competitive games. The child receives the usual childhood immunizations. Prompt treatment of infections is important. A suitable diet with adequate fluids is necessary. It is not essential for all patients to be on salt-free diets. Dental care should be regular. All-day attendance in school may be too tiring for the child; therefore, special provisions in this area may be necessary. The child will need careful evaluation before any type of minor surgery, such as a tonsillectomy, is performed.

Some children will need hospitalization occasionally for various tests or problems. Simple explanations must be given to the patient regarding his condition. He should be allowed to handle and to see hospital equipment prior to its use whenever feasible. Cardiac surgery is generally performed at a regional medical center where the necessary costly equipment is available. The American Heart Association has established standards and recommendations for centers which care for children with congenital heart defects. The immediate pre- and post-operative care of this type of patient is not within the realm of the student practical nurse. She may, however, be called upon to assist the registered nurse and doctor as needed. Whenever possible, a continuum of nursing care by an experienced registered nurse who follows the patient throughout his hospitalization is desirable for both the physical and psychological welfare of the patient. The physician may refer the baby to a local crippled children's service for evaluation and follow-up. The financial burden to the parents throughout the years for medical and surgical necessities is phenomenal. All avenues for financial aid should be explored by qualified personnel.

THE BLOOD

Erythroblastosis Fetalis

Description.   Erythroblastosis fetalis (*erythro-* red + *blast-* a formative cell + *-osis* diseased condition) is a condition that becomes apparent late in fetal life or soon after birth. It is one of many congenital hemolytic diseases which is found in the newborn. There is an excessive destruction of the red blood cells of the baby, which is due to an incompatibility between the red blood cells of the mother and those of the fetus.

One of the substances that causes this condition is the Rh factor. For a long time, doctors had suspected that the cause of many transfusion reactions was due to specific differences in the blood, other than the four main blood groups (A, B, AB, O). About 1940, investigators discovered a factor in the blood of Rhesus monkeys that influenced the outcome of transfusions. They called this the Rh factor, after the Rhesus monkey.

Eighty-five per cent of the white population of the United States have the Rh factor in their blood. They are said to be Rh positive. Fifteen per cent of the population do not possess this factor and are called Rh negative. It is relatively rare in Negro and Asian women. Rh incompatibility occurs when the father is Rh positive and the mother is

Rh negative. It could also occur if the mother was repeatedly administered blood transfusions of Rh positive blood.

If the fetus inherits the dominant Rh positive factor from his father, his body produces Rh positive blood cells. These cells may pass from him through the placenta to the mother's blood. Since this is a foreign substance to the mother, her blood starts to manufacture antibodies. (Antibodies are the body's source of defense, since they act against invaders.) These antibodies are brought through the placenta to the fetus by way of the umbilical cord. Here they begin to destroy the red blood cells of the fetus. If it is the first or second pregnancy of the mother, destruction of this type may not occur, since the number of antibodies manufactured by her may not be sufficient enough to cause harm. However, the mother accumulates antibodies with each pregnancy; therefore the chances that complications may occur increase with each pregnancy. If large number of antibodies are present, the baby may be severely anemic or dead at birth.

The prevention of erythroblastosis fetalis begins in the prenatal period. In anticipating the problem, the doctor can make the necessary advance preparations. All pregnant women should have their blood typed. Women who are Rh negative can then have further blood tests to determine the presence of Rh antibodies. Not every Rh negative woman is threatened with erythroblastotic babies. Some never become sensitized, even though they bear several Rh positive children.

Symptoms. The symptoms of erythroblastosis fetalis vary with the intensity of the disease. Anemia and jaundice are present. The jaundice, termed *pathological,* differs from *physiologic* jaundice in that it becomes evident within 24 hours following delivery. Its presence should be reported immediately to the doctor. Other congenital diseases may cause jaundice of this type; however, erythroblastosis fetalis is generally responsible.

Enlargement of the liver and spleen and extensive edema may develop. The circulating blood usually contains an excessive number of immature nucleated red blood cells. Severe jaundice may cause serious damage to the brain called *kernicterus,* which is fatal in nine out of ten cases, or leaves the newborn mentally retarded or spastic.

Treatment and Nursing Care. The pediatrician examines the baby immediately following birth. Blood specimens are sent to the laboratory. After careful evaluation of the condition of the newborn and the results of the blood work, the course of therapy is determined. An exchange transfusion may be indicated. A plastic catheter is inserted into the umbilical vein of the cord, and small amounts (10 to 20 ml.) of blood are withdrawn, and equal amounts of Rh negative blood injected, until approximately 500 ml. of blood has been replaced. In this way, healthy cells are added and antibodies are removed. Repeated small transfusions may be necessary later. Antibiotics may be given to prevent infection.

Many fascinating advances are being made in the prevention and treatment of this problem. Today a physician may perform an *amniocentesis* on the pregnant mother to determine the condition of the fetus. A needle is placed into the uterus and a specimen of amniotic fluid is obtained for analysis. With this knowledge, the doctor may induce labor early to save the newborn or he may perform an intrauterine exchange transfusion. In this relatively new procedure, the doctor inserts a needle into the abdomen of the fetus. The position of the needle is verified by x-rays, and a transfusion is given. Repeated transfusions may be required. A material called Rhogam is now available which when given intramuscularly to a mother, provided she has not been previously sensitized, within three days after delivery of an Rh positive baby will prevent her from developing the harmful antibodies.

The registered nurse assists the physician in setting up and administering the exchange transfusion. She keeps an accurate record of the amounts of blood withdrawn and injected. She observes the baby's condition closely during and after treatment. An exchange transfusion may last for one to two hours. An incubator and oxygen are made ready to receive the newborn following the transfusion. He is observed for lethargy, increased jaundice, cyanosis, edema, convulsions, color changes of the urine, and changes in vital signs. The prognosis of this condition is excellent when treatment has been prompt.

The practical nurse is usually responsible for the following: observing the newborn's color and reporting any evidence of jaundice during the first and second day; applying wet, sterile compresses to the umbilicus as ordered until an exchange transfusion is ruled out; stressing to mothers the importance of good prenatal care; helping to interpret the treatment to mothers by giving reassurance as needed; and assisting the registered nurse and doctor when necessary.

GASTROINTESTINAL SYSTEM

Cleft Lip (Harelip)

Description. A cleft lip is characterized by a fissure or opening in the upper lip, and is a result of the failure of the embryonic structures of the face to unite. This disorder appears more frequently in boys than in girls and may occur on one or both sides of the lip. The extent of the defect may vary from slight to severe. Sometimes it is accompanied by a *cleft palate*, a fissure in the midline of the roof of the mouth. Cleft lip and palate are common congenital anomalies.

Treatment and Nursing Care. The initial treatment is surgical repair. The cleft lip is repaired first because it interferes with the infant's ability to eat. The baby cannot create a vacuum in his mouth and is unable to suck. Surgery not only improves the infant's sucking, but also greatly improves his appearance. Indirectly, this affects the amount of

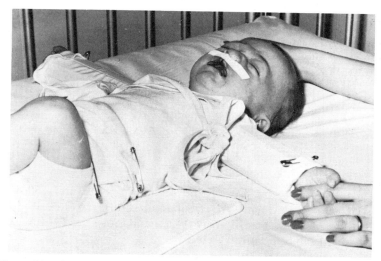

Figure 31. Appearance of a two month old infant after repair of a cleft lip. A Band-aid is used to hold the suture line together. Elbow restraints prevent the infant from rubbing his face. The mother remained with this child throughout his hospitalization. (From Marlow, D.: Textbook of Pediatric Nursing, 1969.)

affection he will receive, since most people refrain from cuddling a baby who is obviously disfigured. Currently the operation is performed any time after birth, if the infant's general health is good and he is free from infection (see Fig. 31). Most surgeons operate between 10 days and 2 months; however, it can be scheduled for the first day of life.

The infant who is to have plastic surgery for the repair of a cleft lip is admitted several days in advance. He is given a complete physical examination and blood tests are made. Photographs may also be taken. Any signs of infection such as a cold should be reported to the head nurse. The doctor may order restraints to prevent the patient from scratching his lip, and to accustom him to them, since they will be necessary postoperatively. An Asepto syringe with a rubber tip is used to feed the baby before and after surgery since motions must be avoided to decrease tensions on the suture line.

FEEDING METHOD. The following feeding method may be used for babies with both a cleft lip and palate. The nurse will need to allow herself more time than the usual 20 minutes required for bottle feedings.

Equipment. Sterile medicine dropper with rubber tip or Asepto syringe with rubber tip, warmed formula, covergown for nurse, bib.

Procedure
1. Check to see that the baby is dry and warm. Change the diaper p.r.n. Wash your hands following. Leave restraints on during feeding.
2. Hold in sitting position. Draw the formula into an Asepto syringe or medicine dropper.

3. Place the rubber tip of the feeder just inside the lips, and on the opposite side of the mouth from the cleft or repaired area.
4. Exert gentle pressure on the bulb of the feeder, allowing a small amount of fluid to drop into the mouth.
5. Allow the baby to swallow before giving more. Prevent sucking motions as much as possible.
6. Bubble frequently. Sit the baby up and gently pat his back with one hand while supporting his chest with the other. NOTE: The doctor may wish to have the formula followed by a small amount of sterile water to cleanse the mouth.
7. Following the feeding, return the baby to his crib. He is placed on his right side. Support his back with a rolled blanket or small pillow.
8. Chart: time of feeding, method, amount offered, amount taken and retained, untoward results, e.g., vomiting.

Aftercare of Equipment. Wash the feeder in cold water followed by warm, soapy water, and rinse. Use a small brush if necessary. Boil for 10 minutes, then place in a sterile tray. Wash and rinse the formula bottle. Place the soiled bib in a laundry chute.

The practical nurse student is not usually asked to care for the infant in the immediate postoperative period. In following his progress, however, she will note that the nursing emphasis is placed on (1) preventing the baby from sucking and crying, which could cause tension on the suture line, (2) careful positioning (never on the abdomen) to avoid injury to the operative site, (3) cleansing of the suture line to prevent crusts from forming which could cause scarring, (4) applying restraints to prevent injury to the operative site, and (5) cuddling and other forms of affection to provide for the infant's emotional needs, which is of particular importance because he is unable to obtain the usual satisfactions from sucking.

The infant remains on feedings by dropper until the wound is completely healed, which is from one to two weeks. The mother who has fed her baby preoperatively and been allowed to assist with his feedings during hospitalization will not find it too difficult to continue after discharge. The infant receives his usual daily vitamins. The immediate improvement as a result of this surgery is very encouraging to the parents, particularly if the child must have further surgery for cleft palate repair.

Cleft Palate

Description. A cleft palate is more serious than a cleft lip. It forms a passageway between the nasopharynx and the nose, which not only complicates feeding, but leads easily to infections of the respiratory tract and middle ear and is generally responsible for speech difficulties which occur in later life. Unlike cleft lip, it is more common in females than in males.

Treatment. Surgery to correct this condition is now done anytime after 10 months. Many surgeons operate before 18 months if at all possible, so that speech patterns will not be affected. To facilitate communication, a dental speech appliance may be used if surgery has been deferred or if it has been contraindicated because of extensive malformation. This appliance must be changed periodically as the child grows.

The management of the child with a cleft palate requires expert teamwork over a long period of time. The emotional problems that sometimes occur with this condition require more extensive attention than the repair itself. In large cities, special cleft palate clinics are available where several specialists can work together under convenient consultation. The parents should be instructed as to the resources available in the state in which they live. Financial assistance is usually indicated because of the length of treatment required.

Postoperative Management

NUTRITION.   The patient is fed with an Asepto syringe with a rubber tip (gravity feeder). If he is old enough he may be taught to use this himself. His diet is progressive. At first it consists of clear fluids and then full fluids. By the second postoperative week a soft diet can generally be taken, and subsequently a regular diet is allowed. Hot foods and liquids should be avoided to prevent injury to the operative site. The patient must not suck on a straw. When feeding with a spoon, place only its side into the mouth. Do not allow the spoon to come in contact with the roof of the mouth.

ORAL HYGIENE.   The mouth is kept clean at all times. Feedings should be followed by a little water. The doctor may prescribe a mild antiseptic mouthwash.

RESTRAINTS.   Elbow restraints are generally sufficient. They should be removed one at a time periodically to prevent constriction of circulation and to allow normal movement. In the home they may be made out of rolled cardboard tied with a string. Prevent the child from placing his fingers or objects in his mouth. Teach him to keep his tongue away from the sore part of his mouth.

SPEECH.   Speak slowly and distinctly to the child and encourage him to pronounce his words correctly. Children who have had extensive repairs, or who have associated deafness, need the help of a speech therapist. Others require a minimum of help from their parents.

DIVERSION.   Crying is to be avoided as much as possible. Play should be quiet, particularly in the immediate postoperative period. Read to the child or help him to color.

COMPLICATIONS.   Earaches and dental decay may accompany this condition. The mother must be instructed to take the child to his physician at the first signs of earache. Visits to the dentist should be regular.

MUSCULOSKELETAL SYSTEM

Clubfoot

Description.   Clubfoot, one of the most common deformities of the skeletal system, is a congenital anomaly characterized by a foot that has

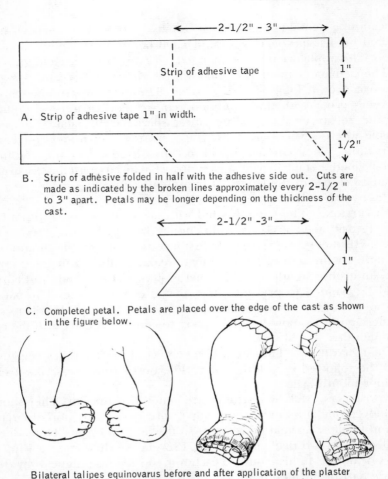

A. Strip of adhesive tape 1" in width.

B. Strip of adhesive folded in half with the adhesive side out. Cuts are made as indicated by the broken lines approximately every 2-1/2 " to 3" apart. Petals may be longer depending on the thickness of the cast.

C. Completed petal. Petals are placed over the edge of the cast as shown in the figure below.

Bilateral talipes equinovarus before and after application of the plaster casts. Adhesive petals have been placed around the ends of the casts.

Figure 32.   Method of applying adhesive petals around the edges of a cast to prevent plaster from irritating the skin. (From Marlow, D.: Textbook of Pediatric Nursing, 1969.)

been twisted inward or outward. Many mild forms are due to improper position in the uterus and clear up with little or no treatment when the extremity is allowed unrestricted activity. In contrast, true clubfoot does not respond to simple exercise. Although the cause is subject to controversy, many feel that it is due to an abnormal degree of compression and molding of the infant's feet in the uterus.* Several types are recognized. Talipes (*talus*- heel + *pes*- foot) equinovarus (*equinus*- extension + *varus*- bent inward) is seen in 95 per cent of cases (see Fig. 32). The feet

*Farrow, R. and Forest, D.: The Surgery of Childhood for Nurses. Baltimore, The Williams and Wilkins Co., 1968.

are turned inward and the child walks on his toes and the outer borders of the foot. It generally affects both feet.

Treatment.   The treatment of clubfoot should be started as early as possible, otherwise the bones and muscles will continue to develop abnormally. During infancy, conservative treatment consisting of manipulation and casting to hold the foot in the right position is carried out. A *Denis Browne splint* may also be used, usually for children under one year of age. This is made up of two foot plates attached to a cross bar. When it is fitted to the shoes, the feet may be put in various positions of angulation by sets of screws. When the infant kicks, his feet are automatically forced into the correct position. If these methods are not effective, surgery is indicated.

The infant with a clubfoot is under medical care for a long period of time and is hospitalized frequently. The psychological effects on this baby may sometimes be more hazardous than the physical disability.

Cast Care.   A cast is made of plaster of Paris bandage. This consists of crinoline which has powdered plastic in its meshwork. It is placed in warm water before being applied over wadding or stockinet. The wet plaster of Paris hardens as it dries.

If the patient returns to the ward before the cast is dried, it must be left uncovered and protected from pressures that could cause a dent in it. If the doctor orders the leg and foot elevated on pillows to prevent swelling, the nurse who assists must use the palms of her hands, not her fingers, to hold the cast. Indentations made in a wet cast by fingers can press on the underlying skin and cause damage. The cast dries in about 24 hours.

The toes are left exposed for observation. The nurse checks them for signs of poor circulation, which are pallor, cyanosis, swelling, coldness, numbness, pain, or burning sensations. She should also report irritations of the skin around the edges of the cast, and lack of movement of the toes. Adhesive petals may be placed around the edges of the cast to prevent skin irritation (see Fig. 32).

It is difficult to keep a child's cast free from food particles which cause skin irritation. He needs careful supervision during mealtime to prevent him from placing bits of food under the edges of the cast. Powder and oil are not used following the bath as they may cause irritation.

When surgery has been performed, the nurse must also observe the cast for evidence of bleeding. If a discolored area appears on the cast, it is circled and the time recorded. Further bleeding will enlarge the circle, and the approximate amount of bleeding can be estimated. If bleeding is noted, the patient's vital signs are also checked and compared with his preoperative readings. The cast is changed following surgery about every three weeks to bring the foot gradually into position. When it is removed for the final time, exercise and special shoes may be indicated.

Emotional Support.   The practical nurse is an important figure in

the care of the long-term patient because of her close daily contact with
the patient and his parents. She should review the normal growth and
development of children in her patient's age range, to anticipate some of
his problems.

In general, children from birth to four years of age suffer the most
from being separated from their parents. They cry loudly when visiting
hours end and need the nurse to console them. They may be slow in
developing certain motor abilities, and in many cases regress to their
baby ways. This is particularly true of bowel and bladder control. The
nurse should not shame a child if an "accident" occurs.

The mother can give much beneficial information about her child.
Be a good listener. Mothers should be encouraged to participate in the
care of their hospitalized children, for it will bring them emotional relief
and will reassure the child.

Financial burden of hospitalization, surgery, special shoes, and continued medical supervision poses a real problem. If the practical nurse
suspects that the parents need financial help, she should report it to the
nurse in charge.

Congenital Dislocation of the Hip

Description.   Congenital dislocation of the hip is a common orthopedic deformity. The head of the femur is partly or completely displaced from a shallow hip socket or *acetabulum.* The exact cause of this
condition is unknown, but it is believed to be inherited. It is seven times
more common in females than in males. Newborn infants seldom have a
complete dislocation. When the baby begins to walk, the pressure exerted on the hip causes a complete dislocation. Accordingly, the practical
nurse can understand why early detection and treatment is of particular
importance in this condition.

Symptoms.   A dislocated hip is frequently discovered at the periodic
health examination of the baby during its first or second month of life.
One of the most reliable signs is a limitation of abduction of the leg on
the affected side. When the infant is placed on his back with his knees
and hips flexed, the doctor can press the femur of the normal hip back
until it almost touches the examining table. This can only partially be
accomplished on the affected side. The knee on the side of the dislocation is lower and the skin folds of the thigh are deeper. When the infant
is prone, one hip is higher than the other (see Fig. 33). The child who is
walking and who has had no treatment displays a characteristic limp.
Bilateral (*bi*- two + *latus*- side) dislocation may occur; however, unilateral
(*uni* one + *latus* side) dislocation is more common. X-rays will confirm the
diagnosis.

Treatment.   The treatment is begun immediately upon detection of
the dislocation. The physician attempts to form a normal joint by
keeping the head of the femur within the hip socket. This constant
pressure enlarges and deepens the acetabulum; thus, it corrects the

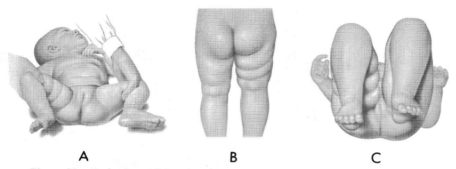

Figure 33.   Early signs (dislocation of right hip). *A,* limitation of abduction. *B,* asymmetry of skin folds. *C,* shortening of femur. (From Clinical Education Aid No. 15, Ross Laboratories, Columbus, Ohio.)

dislocation. The nurse will recall that the bones of small children are fairly pliable because they contain more cartilage than bones of adults.

There is some discrepancy over the exact course of treatment; however, some device to maintain abduction of the hips is used (see Fig. 34). If the dislocation is severe or has not been detected until the child has begun to walk, it may be necessary to put the child in traction. This pulls the head of the femur down to the correct position opposite the acetabulum. Casting in a frog-like position is then achieved. This type of cast is shown in Figure 35. The length of time that the patient remains in a cast varies according to his progress, growth, and the condition of the cast; however, it is usually from five to nine months. During this time, the cast may be changed about every six weeks. Sometimes surgery is required. In this case, open reduction of the dislocation or repair of the shelf of the hip bone is done. A cast is applied following surgery to keep the femur in the correct position.

Nursing Care.   A nursery nurse carefully observes each infant during the morning bath to detect signs of a dislocated hip. When the baby is prone, the nurse observes the buttocks for variation in size. The legs of the infant should be equal in length. The infant should be kicking both legs, not just kicking one leg. There should be no difference in the depth of the skin folds of the baby's upper thighs. In the well baby clinic, the nurse notices the posture and gait of older children. She records her findings.

Infants who progress well with the Curtis or Fredjka splint or similar brace remain at home. The mother and baby visit the physician regularly. The parents need assurance that they may hold the baby and sit him in a chair. They should be encouraged to ask questions of the clinic nurse and doctor.

The child who is admitted to the hospital with a diagnosis of a congenital dislocated hip should be given as much personal attention as

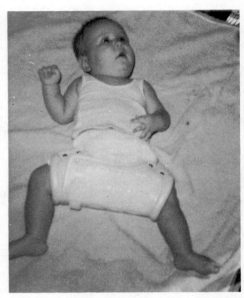

Figure 34. Jeanine and Curtis Splint. This three and one-half month old baby was born with a complete dislocation of the right hip. A splint was used to maintain abduction of the hips. She is now 16 months and walking without problems. Hospitalization was not required.

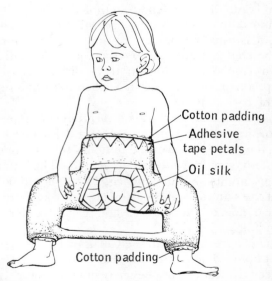

Figure 35. A body (Spica) cast. This body cast maintains the legs in a frog-like position and is used to treat congenital dislocation of the hip. Note that the child is able to move her toes freely. Yellow oil-silk protects the cast from moisture in the diaper area. All edges are padded with cotton and protected by adhesive "petals." (From Leifer "Principles and Techniques in Pediatric Nursing." W. B. Saunders Co., 1965.)

possible. The first admission will set the pattern for future hospitalization; therefore, it is important that the child make a satisfactory adjustment. The nurse should familiarize herself with the child's Habit and Care Sheet (pages 20 and 21). Every effort should be made to provide patients who are hospitalized for many weeks with a home-like environment.

The type of cast which is used is called a *body spica*. It encircles the waist and extends to the ankles or toes. General cast care is discussed on pages 87 and 88 and should be reviewed at this point. Other aspects pertinent to this particular type of cast are discussed in the following paragraphs.

The nurse prepares the bed for the patient's arrival by placing bedboards beneath the mattress. If this is not done, the extra weight of the cast will cause the mattress to sag. Firm plastic-covered pillows are required. These are placed beneath the curvatures of the cast for support. Older children may benefit from an overhead bar and trapeze. The room should be adequately ventilated. A fracture pan should be available in the bedside table.

A newly applied cast is left uncovered to facilitate drying. This takes place in about 24 hours. After the cast is fully dried, some physicians apply shellac, varnish, or a clear plastic spray in an effort to protect the cast from becoming soiled and to prolong its usefulness.

The head of the patient's bed is slightly elevated so that urine or feces will drain away from the body of the cast. Do not elevate the head or shoulders of a child in a body cast by means of pillows, as this thrusts the patient's chest against the cast and will cause discomfort or respiratory difficulty. The child who is not toilet trained may be placed on a Bradford frame to facilitate nursing care (page 180). Frequent change of position is important; bed patients need to be turned often. Infants may be held in the nurse's lap after the cast has dried. A ride on a stretcher to the playroom or around the hospital provides a change of position as well as a change of scenery.

Turning a Child in a Body Cast*

Two people, one on each side of the bed, are needed to turn a child in a body cast.

1. Move the child to the edge of the bed as far as possible, so that the nurse who will receive the child is farthest away from him.
2. The nurse nearest to the child places one hand under his head and back and one hand under the leg part of the cast and turns the child to the midway point on his side.
3. The nurse farthest away then accepts the support of the child and cast as he is turned completely onto his abdomen.

*Leifer, G.: Principles and Techniques in Pediatric Nursing. Philadelphia, W. B. Saunders Co., 1965, p. 143.

The supporting bar between the legs should not be used as a lever when turning the child. All body curvatures should be supported with pillows or sheet rolls. Whenever possible, the older child should be on his abdomen during mealtime to facilitate swallowing and self-feeding. When placing a child in a body cast on a bedpan, support the upper back and legs with pillows so that body alignment is maintained.

Itching is a particular problem with patients in a body cast. If at all possible, prior to applying the cast, a strip of gauze is placed beneath the cast to be used as a scratcher. The gauze extends from the top of the cast to the opened area required for toilet needs. It is gently moved back and forth beneath the cast to provide relief from itching. When the strip becomes soiled, a clean one is tied to one end of the soiled gauze and pulled through the cast; the soiled portion is removed. Other methods which might cause injury to the skin beneath the cast are discouraged, since any break in the skin under a cast is very difficult to heal.

The child with a long-term disability such as this needs help in meeting the everyday needs of life. Dressing and clothing is a problem. The child cannot fit into regular furniture nor much of the play equipment enjoyed by other children. Transportation is difficult. The national and local chapters of Crippled Children and Adults, Inc. can be of particular service to the parents. Their services, plus the aid of a social worker, public health nurse, and medical team, either on an in- or out-patient basis are a must for the child and his family.

GENITOURINARY SYSTEM

Wilms' Tumor

Description. Wilms' tumor or nephroblastoma (*nephro-* kidney + blastoma) is one of the most frequent malignancies of early life. It is an embryonal adenosarcoma (*adeno-* glandular + *sarcoma-* cancer of connective tissue). During the early stages of growth, as with some other malignancies, there are few or no symptoms. About two-thirds of these growths occur before the child is three years old. A mass in the abdomen is discovered generally by the mother or by the physician during a routine checkup. X-rays of the kidneys indicate a growth and verify the fact that the remaining kidney is normal. It seldom affects both kidneys.

Treatment and Nursing Care. The treatment is surgical. The kidney and tumor are removed as soon as possible after the diagnosis has been confirmed. Actinomycin D, an antibiotic which seems to be effective in such cases, is given pre- and postoperatively. Irradiation therapy is given before and after surgery. The prognosis of a hopeless situation has improved somewhat with prompt diagnosis and treatment.

General nursing measures for the comfort of the patient are accomplished. One factor pertinent to this condition is that all unnecessary handling of the abdomen is to be avoided as it can cause the disease to spread. The doctor explains this to the mother and in the hospital a sign is placed on the crib or child—"Do not palpate abdomen." The practical nurse must consider this extremely important and refrain from bathing the affected side. The lungs are the most common site of metastasis for this disease. Observations of bloody urine and elevated blood pressure are reported immediately. The emotional support to parents and child by the nurse in conditions which may be fatal is discussed on page 242.

Birth Injuries

NERVOUS SYSTEM

Intracranial Hemorrhage

Description. Intracranial hemorrhage, the most common type of birth injury, may result from trauma or anoxia. It occurs more frequently in the premature, because his blood vessels are so fragile. Blood vessels within the skull are broken and bleeding occurs into the brain. When the diagnosis is made, the specific location of the hemorrhage may be noted, i.e., subdural, subarachnoid, and so forth. This injury may also occur during precipitated delivery or prolonged labor, and when the newborn's head is large in comparison to the mother's pelvis.

Symptoms. The symptoms of intracranial hemorrhage may occur suddenly or gradually. Some or all are present, depending on the severity. They include: inability to move normally, lethargy, poor sucking reflex, irregular respiration, cyanosis, twitching, forceful vomiting, a high-pitched, shrill cry, and convulsions. The fontanel may be tense and under pressure, rather than soft and compressible. One pupil of the eye is apt to be small and the other large. If the symptoms are mild, complete recovery may occur. Death results if there is a massive hemorrhage. The infant who survives an extensive hemorrhage may suffer residual defects such as mental retardation or cerebral palsy. The diagnosis is established by the history of the delivery, evidence of an increase in pressure of the cerebrospinal fluid, and the symptoms and course of the disease.

Treatment and Nursing Care. The newborn is placed in an incubator which allows proper temperature control, ease in administering oxygen, and continuous observation. He is handled gently and as little as possible. The head is elevated. The doctor may prescribe vitamin K to control bleeding and phenobarbital if twitchings or convulsions are apparent. Prophylactic antibiotics may also be used, as well as daily vitamins. The baby is fed carefully since his sucking reflex may be affected. He vomits easily. The nurse observes the baby for signs of increased intracranial pressure (see page 68) and convulsions.

If a convulsion occurs, observation of its character by the nurse will aid the doctor in diagnosing the exact location of the bleeding. The following are of particular importance: Were the arms, legs, or face involved? Was the right or left side of the body involved? Was it mild or severe? How long did it last? What was the condition of the infant before and after the seizure? The nurse records her observations in the nurses' notes.

Respiratory Complications

Atelectasis

Description.   The lungs are collapsed during fetal life and their failure to expand after birth is known as atelectasis. With the first breath some expansion must take place, although full development does not occur until days later. *Primary* atelectasis in which the *alveoli* fail to expand is common in prematures and infants with damaged brains. *Secondary* atelectasis occurs when the lungs collapse after they have once inflated. This collapse may be caused by pressure from misplaced organs or from pulmonary disease. Since this condition is highest among prematures, babies born by cesarean section, and those born by difficult labor and delivery, the prevention depends somewhat on proper prenatal care and delivery.

Symptoms.   The infant exhibits irregular, rapid respirations. These may be accompanied by a respiratory grunt and flaring of the nostrils. The skin is cyanotic and mottled. Inter-rib and sternal retractions may be noticeable. X-rays confirm the diagnosis. The prognosis depends on the general condition of the baby and the cause; however, death is frequent.

Treatment and Nursing Care.   The patient is placed in an incubator where increased humidity and oxygen can be easily administered. This maintains the correct body temperature, which is important. The doctor may administer carbon dioxide in an effort to stimulate respirations. Caffeine and sodium benzoate may be given by injection. Antibiotics are given to prevent secondary infection. The nurse observes and records the patient's vital signs, skin color, and the amount of respiratory distress. An open airway must be maintained; aspiration of mucus from the nose may be indicated. Upper respiratory infection must be avoided, since it could result in the death of the patient. The patient's position is changed frequently to help expand the collapsed areas; short periods of crying will aid this. The head of the infant may be slightly elevated. The baby is fed slowly and burped frequently to avoid abdominal distention, which would further inhibit breathing. Crying periods should not be encouraged following feedings, as vomiting with aspiration could occur. Gavage feedings may be in order. Organized nursing care will afford the infant sufficient rest.

Infections

GASTROINTESTINAL TRACT

Thrush

Description.   Thrush is an infection of the mucous membranes of the mouth caused by the fungus *Candida*. This organism is normally present in the mother's vagina and is nonpathogenic. However, the altered conditions in the vagina produced by pregnancy may lead to the development of *monilial vaginitis*. The mucous membranes of the baby's mouth may become infected by direct contact with this infection during delivery, or by contact with the mother's or nurse's contaminated hands. Cross-infection of other newborns may then result.

Symptoms.   White patches that resemble milk curds are visible on the tongue, inner lips, gums, and oral mucosa. These are painless but will not wipe away. Anorexia may be present. The systemic symptoms are mild if the infection remains in the mouth; however, it can pass along the mucous membranes into the gastrointestinal tract causing inflammation of the esophagus and stomach.

Treatment and Nursing Care.   This infection responds well to local application of antibiotic suspensions. Nystatin, for example, may be applied by swab. A 1 per cent aqueous solution of gentian violet is also used. It causes the mouth to become quite purple, but this is temporary. This has been explained to the mother previously so that she is not alarmed. The nurse places a bib on the baby to save on clothing. The mouth is swabbed three or four times a day between feedings with a sterile applicator moistened with the prescribed solution. Under proper care, the condition disappears within a few days following its onset.

Newborns suspected of having thrush should be isolated. Individual feeding equipment is essential, and is washed, rinsed and sterilized before it is returned to the formula room. Nipples require scrupulous cleansing, because they come in direct contact with the lesions. Practical nurses who care for the newborn with infectious conditions should not give daily care to other healthy babies.

The prevention of this infection begins in the prenatal period. Mothers suspected of having this infection can then be properly treated.

Effective handwashing to prevent reinfection from the mother is necessary. This is particularly true if she is breast feeding her infant. Nurses and other personnel must maintain a high quality of nursing care to prevent cross-infection.

Diarrhea

Description.   Despite improved care of the newborn, infectious diarrhea continues to be a serious problem in many areas of the world. It is highly contagious and may be fatal. Diarrhea may be caused by a variety of organisms, and often the offender cannot be identified. Its course may last from a few days to several weeks. *Functional* diarrhea differs from infectious diarrhea in that it is due to an organic disease rather than an infection.

Symptoms.   The symptoms of diarrhea may be mild or extremely severe. The stools are watery and are expelled with force. They may be yellowish-green in color. The baby becomes listless, refuses to eat, and loses weight. The temperature may be elevated, and the infant may vomit. Dehydration is evidenced by sunken eyes and fontanel, and dry skin, tongue, and mucous membranes. The frequency of urination may decrease. In severe cases, acidosis results.

Treatment and Nursing Care.   Newborns suspected of having diarrhea are isolated immediately. A warm stool specimen is sent to the laboratory for culture. If the causative organism is identified, specific chemotherapy is begun with sulfonamide drugs or various antibiotics. Supportive treatment designed to combat the loss of water and salts is initiated. The baby is given nothing by mouth until the vomiting ceases. Intravenous fluids may be required. As the baby's condition improves, he is given sips of fluid often, to replace the fluids lost through vomiting and diarrhea. When the sulfonamide drugs are used, the nurse must observe the infant's urine carefully. Red or chocolate-brown urine is reported immediately to the head nurse. The sulfonamides tend to be irritating to the kidneys and adequate amounts of fluid must be ingested to offset this toxic effect.

The gastrointestinal tract of the newborn is especially vulnerable to infection. The nurse must constantly seek to protect him against exposure to pathogenic organisms and must adhere strictly to nursery routines. The preparation of formula requires undivided attention to prevent germs from being carried to the newborn through this medium. Careful feeding techniques are necessary. If a nipple becomes contaminated, a new one must be applied. Proper handwashing is essential. If clothing or blankets touch the floor they must be relaundered before being used.

Constant observation of each newborn in the nursery is of utmost importance. If diarrhea is suspected, it is reported immediately and the baby isolated. The skin of the buttocks must receive special care to prevent excoriation. Removing the diaper and exposing the area to the air may be helpful. It may be necessary to soak the diapers in a disinfectant before sending them to the laundry. They should be placed in a special container and properly marked before being sent from the division.

The nurse must describe the stools accurately in the nurses' notes as to consistency, frequency, presence or absence of blood, mucus, or pus, and the color, odor, and forcefulness with which the stool is expelled.

New babies must not be admitted to the nursery when acute cases of diarrhea are present. Separate personnel are needed to care for uninfected newborns. When the epidemic has ceased, the nursery must be thoroughly scrubbed, and all equipment cleaned and sterilized according to hospital procedure.

THE SKIN

Impetigo

Description. Impetigo is an infectious disease of the skin caused by staphylococci or streptococci. The newborn is susceptible to this infection because his resistance to skin bacteria is low. Impetigo tends to spread from one area of skin to another and is contagious.

Symptoms. The first symptoms of this lesion are red papules (pimples). These eventually become small vesicles or pustules surrounded by a reddened area. When the blister breaks, the surface beneath is raw and weeping. The lesions occur in moist areas of the body, such as the creases of the neck, axilla, and groin. In older children a crust may form.

Treatment and Nursing Care. Antibiotic preparations are applied to the skin, and antibiotics may also be given parenterally. The prognosis under proper treatment is good. The nursing care consists primarily of preventing this disease by proper aseptic methods. Once the diagnosis is made, the baby is isolated to prevent other newborns from becoming infected.

Staphylococcus Aureus

Description. The genus of bacteria called *Staphylococcus* comprises very common bacteria which are found in dust and on the skin. Under normal conditions they do not present a problem to the healthy body defenses. If the number of organisms increases markedly or increases in premature and newborns whose general resistance is low, skin infections may occur. An abscess may form, and in some cases infection may enter the blood stream. This condition is called *septicemia.* Pneumonia, osteomyelitis, or meningitis may result. Primary infection of the newborn may develop in the umbilicus or circumcision wound. It generally occurs while the newborn is in the hospital, but may appear after discharge. This infection spreads readily from one infant to another. Small pustules on the newborn must be reported immediately.

Treatment and Nursing Care.   Antibiotics effective against the particular strain are administered. Some doctors recommend that other babies in the nursery be treated similarly as a prophylactic measure. Daily pHisoHex baths are given. Ointments may be applied locally.

In recent years, the staphylococci that invade the body have developed resistance to the antibiotics in current use. In some hospitals, serious epidemics have occurred in the newborn nursery and among surgical patients. It is difficult to control the spread of this infection since personnel act as carriers. The chief reservoir is the nose.

In order to prevent staphylococcal infections, no one with a skin infection should be allowed to visit mothers or enter the nursery. Mothers or newborns who have acquired this infection must be isolated. Strict standards must be upheld in the nursery: adequate space must be provided for each bassinet to avoid overcrowding, and each baby should have individual equipment. The number and quality of personnel and their health status is also an important factor. The hands of all personnel must be scrubbed thoroughly with pHisoHex or other bactericide before entering the nursery. Handwashing between patients and before and after handling equipment is *essential.* Medical supervision of all discharged babies must be continued to detect latent cases.

THE EYES

Ophthalmia Neonatorum

Description.   Ophthalmia neonatorum is an acute conjunctivitis of the newborn caused by the gonococci of gonorrhea, a venereal disease. Although no longer common in the United States, this condition is a leading cause of blindness in the world today. It is acquired during the birth process by direct contact with the infected vagina.

Prevention.   State laws require that all babies receive preventive treatment for this condition at birth. This is accomplished by instilling a 1 per cent silver nitrate solution into the newborn's eyes at birth. Recently, penicillin and other antibiotics have been also used for this purpose. Good prenatal care to discover the presence of this disease in the mother is essential. She can then be given penicillin or other antibiotics to rid her of the infection, and thus prevent her newborn from contracting this condition.

STUDY QUESTIONS

1. Define congenital anomaly, birth injury, atelectasis.
2. What is the most obvious symptom of hydrocephalus?

3. What complications may arise from neglecting to turn the patient with hydrocephalus?
4. List the symptoms of increased intracranial pressure.
5. Define rehabilitation. What is the practical nurse's role in rehabilitative nursing?
6. What factors must be charted when a convulsion has been witnessed?
7. Baby Jones has just been admitted to the newborn nursery. His mother has Rh negative blood. Why are moist, sterile dressings applied to the umbilical stump? The nurse must observe the baby for what symptoms?
8. What is the most effective procedure carried out by the practical nurse in preventing the spread of infection?
9. What care is given to the buttocks of the infant with diarrhea? List five characteristics of the baby's stool which the nurse must record.
10. Describe the method for feeding the patient with a cleft lip and palate.
11. What resources are available in your community for speech training of the child with a cleft palate?
12. Define clubfoot. Why is it necessary to begin treatment early?
13. Billy, who has congenital clubfoot, had his cast changed in the early morning. List several signs of impaired circulation that might occur.
14. Define the following: patent, anastomosis, acyanotic heart defect, polycythemia, cardiac decompensation.
15. What modern methods are being used for the repair of congenital heart defects?
16. Baby Rico has been admitted with the diagnosis of congenital dislocated hip. List the signs and symptoms of this orthopedic disorder.
17. How are staphylococcal infections spread?

BIBLIOGRAPHY

Avery, M. E.: The Lung and Its Disorders in the Newborn Infant. Vol. 1. Philadelphia, W. B. Saunders Co., 1964.
Benz, G. S.: Pediatric Nursing. St. Louis, C. V. Mosby Co., 1967.
Blake, F., and Wright, F. H.: Essentials of Pediatric Nursing. 7th Ed. Philadelphia, J. B. Lippincott Co., 1963.
Bleier, I.: Maternity Nursing. Philadelphia, W. B. Saunders Co., 1966.
Broadribb, V.: Foundations of Pediatric Nursing. Philadelphia, J. B. Lippincott Co., 1967.
Davis, M. E., and Rubin, R.: DeLee's Obstetrics for Nurses. 18th Ed. Philadelphia, W. B. Saunders Co., 1966.
Farrow, R., and Forrest, D.: The Surgery of Childhood for Nurses. 3rd Ed. Baltimore, The Williams and Wilkins Co., 1968.
Ingalls, A.: Maternal and Child Health Nursing. St. Louis, C. V. Mosby Co., 1967.
Kalafatich, A.: Pediatric Nursing. New York, G. P. Putnam's Sons, 1966.
Latham, H., and Heckel, R.: Pediatric Nursing. St. Louis, C. V. Mosby Co., 1967.
Leifer, G.: Principles and Techniques in Pediatric Nursing. Philadelphia, W. B. Saunders Co., 1965.

Marlow, D.: Textbook of Pediatric Nursing. 3rd Ed. Philadelphia, W. B. Saunders Co., 1969.

Mason, M.: Basic Medical-Surgical Nursing. New York, The Macmillan Co., 1967.

Nelson, W. (Editor): Textbook of Pediatrics. 9th Ed. Philadelphia, W. B. Saunders Co., 1969.

Physician's Desk Reference. New Jersey, Medical Economics, Inc., 1969.

Pidgeon, V. The Infant with Congenital Heart Disease. Amer. J. Nurs. 67:290-293.

Ross Laboratories: A Study Guide to Congenital Heart Abnormalities, 1961.

Chapter 7

THE INFANT

VOCABULARY

Canines	Incisors
Deciduous	Insecure
Development	Intelligence
Environment	Mature
Fear	Molars
Growth	Origin

GENERAL CHARACTERISTICS

Children, unlike adult patients, are in the process of growing while they are hospitalized. In order to give total patient care, the practical nurse must be able to recognize her patient's needs at various stages of growth and development. She must try to meet these effectively, as well as to administer the specialized nursing care required for the particular patient.

Each baby develops at his own rate. Although growth is continuous, there are slow and rapid periods. The first year of life is a period of rapid growth and development. The infant is completely dependent on adults during the first months of life, and gives little in return. His behavior is not consistent. Sucking brings him comfort and relief from tensions. This phase of personality development, the *oral stage,* is important for the infant's physical and psychological development. Gradually, the baby begins to put his fingers into his mouth. When he can use his hands more skillfully, he will not suck his fingers as much, but will be able to derive pleasure from other sources. When the infant's teeth appear, he learns to bite and enjoys objects that he can chew. The practical nurse, knowing the importance of sucking to the baby, holds him during feedings, and allows him sufficient time to suck. When he is warm and comfortable he will associate food with love. The baby who is fed intravenous fluids should be given added attention since he is denied the satisfaction received from sucking.

Love and security are vital needs of the infant. He requires the continuous affection given by his mother. She need not be afraid of spoiling him during his first year, when she attends promptly to his wants. Loving adults assure the infant that the world is a good place in which to live. Each day, he becomes impressed by our actions and learns to imitate and trust persons about him. We should not expect too much or too little from him. The baby will accomplish various activities easily, if they are not forced upon him before he is mature enough. In the same respect, we should not hold him back when he shows a readiness to learn a particular task.

The constant care of an infant is a strain on the most exemplary parents. The mother, in particular, needs and deserves the understanding of her husband and the kind support from her relatives at home and from the nurse in the hospital situation. A short break from pressures will give her renewed energy in which to enjoy her baby. A short trip to the store, a stroll with the baby in the carriage, or coffee with the neighbors affords stimulation and a change of environment for the baby as well as for the mother. The infant who is left constantly in his crib and who is not introduced to a variety of learning experiences may become shy and withdrawn.

If a mother is unable to room-in with her hospitalized infant, personnel should try to imitate her care by prompt fulfillment of the infant's physical and emotional needs. In the nursery the baby who appears hungry is fed first, rather than adhering to a specific routine. Change wet diapers as soon as possible. Soothe the child who is crying. The exactness of bathing or feeding the infant is not as important as the way in which it is done. Warmth and affection or the lack of it are easily recognized.

TEETH

Deciduous Teeth. The development of the 20 deciduous or baby teeth begins about the fifth month of intra-uterine life. The health and diet of the expectant mother affects their soundness. They appear during the first two and one-half years of life. It is a normal process and is generally accompanied by little or no discomfort. Wide individual differences occur in tooth eruption in normal, healthy infants. A delay in teething is significant if other forms of immaturity or illness are present. The physician evaluates the process of teething during the baby's regular health checkups. The first tooth generally appears about the seventh month. The one year old has about six teeth, four above and two below. The order in which the teeth appear is almost always the same (see Fig. 36). They are shed in about the same way in which they appear, i.e., lower central incisors first and so forth.

Parents and nurses must not neglect baby teeth, thinking that they will be lost eventually. A two year old who wants to brush his teeth when Mommy does should be encouraged to do so. The deciduous teeth serve not only in the digestive process, but in the development of the jaw. When the deciduous teeth are lost early because of neglect, the perma-

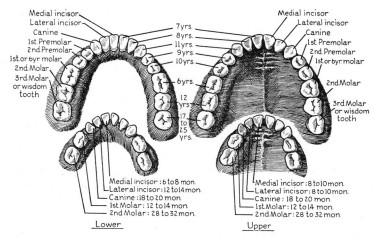

Figure 36. Permanent and deciduous teeth. (From Baillif, R. H., and Kimmel, D. L. Structure and Function of the Human Body. J. B. Lippincott Co., 1945.)

nent teeth become poorly aligned. The nurse should check that all patients three years of age and older have toothbrushes. Children sometimes need to be reminded of oral hygiene at bedtime.

Permanent Teeth. The 32 permanent teeth develop just before birth and during the first year of life. They do not erupt through the gums, however, until the sixth year of life. Nutrition and general health during the first year of life affect the formation of permanent teeth, a process that is not completed until the wisdom teeth appear about the age of 18 to 23. The first permanent teeth, which do not replace any of the deciduous teeth, but come in behind the deciduous molars, are important teeth, since the whole denture develops around them. Cavities in them are frequently neglected, because they are mistaken for baby teeth.

Oral Hygiene. Good dental care begins with proper diet to supply adequate nutrients while the teeth are developing in the jaws, especially during the prenatal period and the first year of life. Many essential elements found in milk include calcium, phosphorus, vitamins A and B complex, and protein. Vitamin D, the sunshine vitamin, and vitamin C, found in citrus fruits, are also valuable. Between-meal eating of sweets should be discouraged. Instead, substitute fresh fruits or raw vegetables.

Of most importance in the prevention of caries is the administration of fluoride by mouth. Ideally, flourides may be present naturally in the water supply or may be added to it. Many doctors advise giving fluorides to infants and children until at least eight years of age. Many fluoride preparations are available, often incorporated with vitamins. These tablets are obtained by prescription and should not be interchanged among children of various ages, as too much fluoride may cause the teeth to "mottle." Fluoride may also be applied directly to the teeth by the dentist.

FACTORS THAT INFLUENCE GROWTH AND DEVELOPMENT

Growth and development are influenced by many factors such as heredity, nationality, race, sex, and environment.

Hereditary Traits.   Characteristics derived from our ancestors are determined at the time of conception by countless *genes* within each chromosome. Each gene is made up of a chemical substance called *DNA*, which plays an important part in determining inherited characteristics. Examples of these inherited traits are the color of eyes and hair, and physical resemblances within families. Currently, many exciting advances are taking place in the field of *genetics;* it may prove to be an effective weapon of preventative medicine in the future.

Nationality and Race.   Many physical differences between nations and races formerly distinguished with ease have become less apparent in our age of common environment and customs. For instance, one thinks of a person of Japanese origin as being short of stature. However, Japanese children living in America compare favorably in height with children of the United States.

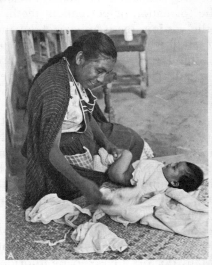
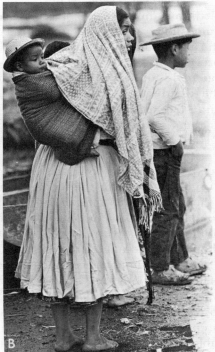

Figure 37.   Customs of child care differ with nationality and race. (From "South of the Border," Baby Talk Magazine, March 1969. p. 29. Courtesy of Peggo Cromer.)

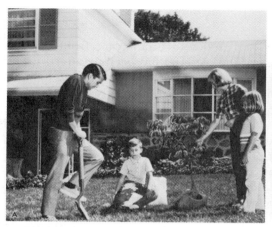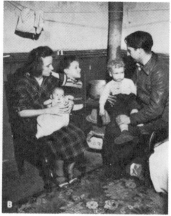

Figure 38. Children are influenced physically and mentally by their home life. They come from vastly different financial backgrounds. This must be considered by the practical nurse who attends to the needs of the hospitalized child and his family. (Courtesy of H. Armstrong Roberts.)

Sex. The male infant weighs more and is longer than the female. He grows and develops at a different rate.

Environment. The physical condition of the newborn is influenced by his prenatal environment. The health of the mother at the time of conception, and the amount and quality of her diet during pregnancy, is important for proper fetal development. Infections or diseases may lead to malformations of the fetus. A healthy and strong newborn can adapt easily to his surroundings.

The home greatly influences the infant's physical and emotional growth and development. If a family is financially strained by an added member, and the parents are unable to provide nourishing foods and suitable housing, the infant is directly affected. An uneducated mother may not know the proper methods of cooking foods to preserve their nutritional value. Immunizations and other medical attention may be neglected. The baby senses tension within the family and is affected by it.

In contrast, when the surroundings are secure and stable, the infant feels wanted and loved, and his energies are not wasted by fright and insecurity. Intelligence plays an important role in social and mental development. Potential intellect is believed to be inherited, but is greatly affected by environment.

These and other factors are closely related and dependent on one another in their effect on growth and development. They make each person unique. If a child is ill, physically or emotionally, his developmental process may be slowed down.

INFANT CARE

On the following pages are guides to infant care from the first month of life to the first year. The material has been arranged under headings and in chronological order so that it may be referred to easily by the student. Though this is convenient, it is merely a summary of data. Some of the aspects of care are important throughout the entire year, e.g., daily vitamins and safety measures. The practical nurse should not get the impression that physical patterns can be separated from social patterns or that abrupt changes will take place with each new month. The development of humans cannot be separated into specific areas any more than the body's structure can be separated from its function. No two infants are just alike at a certain age. However, individual variations range about central norms that serve as guides in the evaluation of an infant's or child's progress. The addition of the various solid foods to the diet and the time of immunizations vary slightly depending on the baby's health and his doctor. The types, nevertheless, remain the same.

Guides to Infant Care

ONE MONTH

Physical Development

Weighs approximately eight pounds. Has regained weight lost after birth. Gains about one inch in height per month for the first six months.

Lifts head slightly when placed on stomach. Pushes with toes. Turns head to side when prone. Head wobbles. Clenches fists. Stares at surroundings.

Social Behavior

Makes small, throaty noises. Cries when hungry or uncomfortable. Sleeps 20 out of 24 hours. Awake for 2 A.M. feeding.

Care and Guidance

Sleep. On stomach with head turned to side, following feedings. If prefers side-lying position, support back with blanket roll. Use a firm mattress. No pillow.

Diet. Breast milk or sterilized formula every four hours as baby indicates need. Vitamins A, D, and C every day. When giving vitamin C

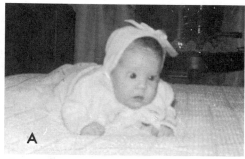

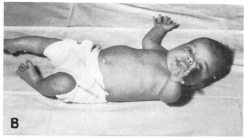

Figure 39. *A*, one month old Sandy stares at her surroundings. Her eyes appear crossed at times. Her head wobbles. *B*, the infant weighs about eight pounds. (*B* from Marlow, D., Textbook of Pediatric Nursing, 1969.)

in the form of orange juice, give at room temperature. Do not boil or add hot water, since vitamin C is destroyed by heat. Plain, boiled water may be given between feedings. Bubble baby well.

Exercise. Allow freedom from the restraints of clothing before bath. Provide fresh air and sunshine whenever possible.

Support head and shoulders when holding infant. Attend promptly to physical needs. Observe baby frequently.

TWO MONTHS

Physical Development

Posterior fontanel closes. Tears appear. Can hold head erect in midposition. Follows moving light with eyes. Holds a rattle briefly. Legs are active. *likes music*

Social Behavior

Smiles in response to mother's voice. Knows crying will bring attention. Awakes for 2 A.M. feeding.

Care and Guidance

Sleep. Develops own pattern, may sleep from feeding to feeding.
Diet. First solid foods. Fine cereals or strained fruits are usually

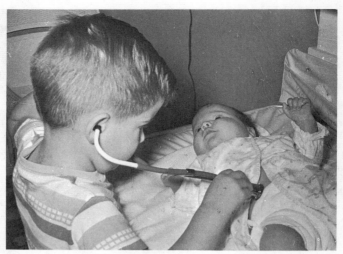

Figure 40. Two month old Karen receives her medical check up.

a flexiable routine

given. Offer only small amounts at first (1 tsp.). Place food on the back of his tongue. Be sure baby wears a bib. Cereal is diluted with formula; fruits should be given at room temperature. The consistency and amounts are gradually increased as the infant becomes more familiar with solid foods. <u>Give one new food at a time, when the infant is hungriest</u>.

Exercise. <u>Provide a safe, flat place for him to kick and be active.</u>

Physical examination by the family doctor, well baby clinic, or pediatrician.

Immunization. <u>First DPT</u>, an inoculation against diphtheria, whooping cough, and tetanus. <u>Oral polio vaccine</u> (Trivalent OPV) may also be started.

Still completely dependent on adults for physical care. Needs a flexible routine throughout infancy and childhood.

THREE MONTHS

Physical Development

Weighs 12 to 13 pounds. Stares at hands. Reaches for objects, but misses them. Carries hand to mouth.

Can follow an object from right to left and up and down when it is placed in front of his face. <u>Supports head steady</u>.

Social Behavior

Cries less. Can wait a few minutes for attention. <u>Enjoys having people talk to him. Takes impromptu naps</u>.

Begins to coo + smile

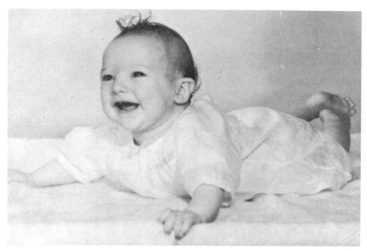

Figure 41. Three month old Mary Ellen supports her head well and smiles obligingly for her photographer.

Care and Guidance

Sleep. Yawns, stretches, naps in mother's arms.

Diet. Add bland green and yellow vegetables, strained meat. Gradually takes larger amounts.

Exercise. May have short play period. Enjoys playing with his hands.

Immunization. Second DPT.

FOUR MONTHS

Physical Development

Weighs about 13 to 14 pounds.

Drooling indicates appearance of saliva.

Lifts head and shoulders when on abdomen, and looks around. Turns from back to side. Sits with support. Begins to reach for objects he sees. Coordination between eyes and body movements.

Moves head, arms, and shoulders when excited. Extends his legs, and partly sustains his weight when held upright.

Social Behavior

Coos, chuckles, gurgles. Laughs aloud. Responds to others. Likes an audience. Sleeps through the night. May show preference for certain foods.

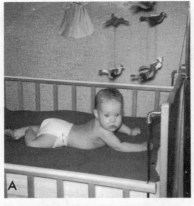
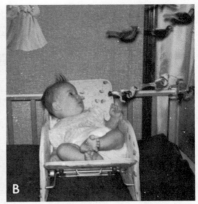
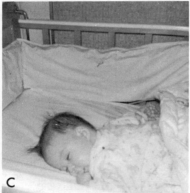

Figure 42. *A*, Sandy at four months can lift her head and shoulders and look around when on her abdomen. *B*, Sandy sits with support. She sees the birds and tries to reach them. *C*, she sleeps through the night.

Care and Guidance

Sleep. Stirs about in crib. Will sleep through ordinary household noises—avoid tiptoeing around.

father + other children

Diet. Add boiled egg yolk. Egg white is not given until later. Soup may also be tried. Avoid showing own dislikes for certain foods. If the baby refuses a certain food, omit it temporarily. Keep mealtime pleasant. Do not introduce new foods when baby is ill. The amount of food consumed is determined by the individual baby. Consult your doctor as to advisability of continued sterilization of formula. Always boil raw milk.

Exercise. Plays with rattles and dangling toys. Start acquainting him with a playpen where he can roll with safety.

Immunization. Third DPT and polio (see p. 259 for booster inoculations).

Elimination. One or two bowel movements per day. May skip a day.

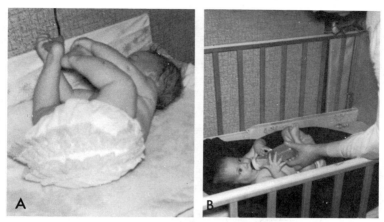

Figure 43. *A*, at five months Sandy grasps her toes in play. Natural exercise is important for proper growth and development. *B*, she tries to hold her bottle.

FIVE MONTHS *Changes very rapidly.*

Physical Development

<u>Doubles birth weight</u>. <u>Sits with support</u>. <u>Holds head well</u>. Grasps objects handed to him. <u>Puts everything into his mouth</u>.

Social Behavior

<u>Talks to himself</u>. Seems to know whether persons are familiar or unfamiliar.

May sleep through 10 P.M. feeding. Tries to hold bottle of orange juice at feeding time.

Care and Guidance

Sleep. Takes two or three naps daily in crib.
Diet. Custard and simple puddings may be given for variety.
Exercise. Provide space to pivot around. Makes jumping motions when held upright in lap.
Safety. Check toys for loose buttons and rough edges before placing them in playpen.

SIX MONTHS

Physical Development

Gains about 3 to 5 ounces per week during next six months. Grows about one-half inch per month.

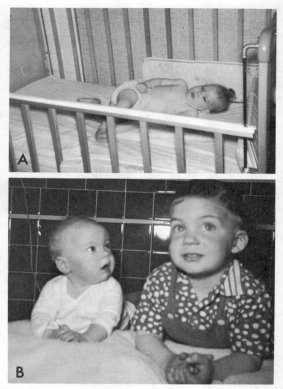

Figure 44. *A,* at six months Sandy turns completely over in her crib. *B,* Debbie shows her interest in the world about her.

Sits alone momentarily. Springs up and down when sitting. Turns completely over. Hitches (moves backward when sitting). Bangs table with rattle. <u>Pulls himself to a sitting position.</u>

Social Behavior

Cries loudly when interrupted from play. Increased interest in world around him. Babbles and squeals. Sucks food from spoon. Awakes happy.

Care and Guidance

Sleep. Needs his own room. Should be moved from parent's room if not previously done. Otherwise, as he becomes older he may become unwilling to sleep away from them.

Diet. Includes cereal, egg yolk, and a variety of fruits, meat, and vegetables. A low feeding table for meals is safe and convenient. May begin weaning from breast to cup gradually. Allow to hold plastic cup with a small amount of milk.

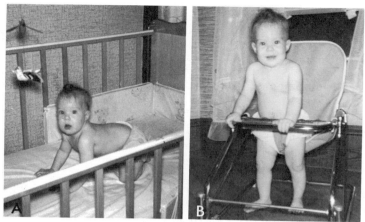

Figure 45. *A*, at seven months Sandy begins to crawl. *B*, she also shows interest in standing, and bounces actively in her chair.

Exercise. Enjoys splashing about in tub.

Immunization. Oral polio vaccine.

Provide a chewable object such as a teething ring or piece of cloth for his enjoyment.

SEVEN MONTHS

Physical Development

Two lower teeth appear. These are the first of the deciduous teeth, the central incisors.

Begins to crawl. Can grasp objects more easily. Appears interested in standing. Holds an adult's hands and bounces actively while standing. Struggles when being dressed.

Begins to preferr is mother.

Social Behavior

Shifts moods easily—crying one minute, laughing the next. Shows fear of strangers.

Anticipates spoon feeding. Sleeps 11 to 13 hours at night.

Care and Guidance

Sleep. Fretfulness due to teething may appear. This is generally evidenced by lack of appetite, and wakefulness during the night. In most cases, merely soothing and offering a cup of water are sufficient.

Diet. Add finger foods, such as toast or zwieback.

Exercise.   Enjoys lying on back; kicks, pulls off booties.

EIGHT MONTHS

Physical Development

<u>Sits steadily</u> alone. Uses index finger and thumb like pincers. Pokes at objects, enjoys dropping articles into a cup and emptying it.

Social Behavior

Plays pat-a-cake. Enjoys family life. Amuses himself longer. Reserved with strangers.

Indicates need for sleep by fussing and sucking thumb. Impatient, especially when food is being prepared.

Plays pik-a-boo

Care and Guidance

Sleep.   Takes two naps a day.

Diet.   Continue to add new foods slowly. Baked potato, macaroni, gelatin, and cottage cheese may be offered.

Let him eat by his himself

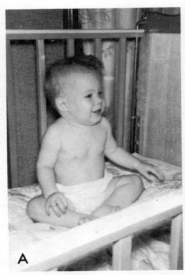 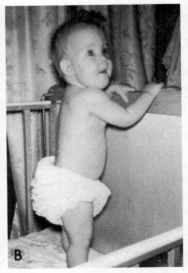

Figure 46.   *A,* Sandy sits alone steadily at eight months. *B,* she shows an increased interest in standing.

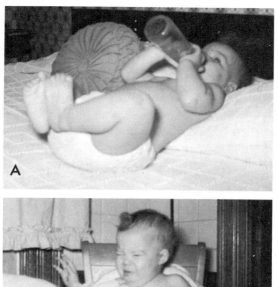

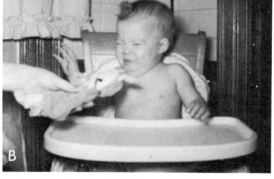

Figure 47. *A*, at nine months Sandy holds her own bottle. *B*, she cries when scolded.

Exercise. Enjoys jump chair. Rides in stroller. Stuffed toys or those that squeak or rattle are appropriate.

Safety. Remain with baby at all times during bath in tub. Protect him from chewing paint from window sills or old furniture. Paint containing lead can be poisonous.

NINE MONTHS

Physical Development

Shows preference for the use of one hand. Can raise himself to a sitting position. Holds his bottle.

Social Behavior

Tries to imitate sounds, e.g., says "Ba Ba" for bye-bye. Cries if scolded.

Drops food from high chair at mealtime. Falls asleep after 6 P.M. feeding.

Care and Guidance

Sleep. Has generally begun to sleep later in the morning.

Diet. Introduce chopped and mashed foods. Place newspaper beneath feeding table. Use unbreakable dishes. Allow him to pick up pieces of food by hand and put them into his mouth.

Exercise. Is busy most of the day exploring his surroundings. Provide sufficient room and materials for safe play.

Help him to learn. See that he doesn't get into trouble. In this way punishment is limited—avoid excessive spankings and "No's".

TEN MONTHS

Physical Development

Pulls himself to a standing position in the playpen. Throws toys to floor for mother to pick up. Cries when they are not returned. Walks around furniture while holding on to it.

Social Behavior

Knows his name. Plays simple games such as "peek-a-boo." Feeds himself a cookie. May cry out in sleep without waking.

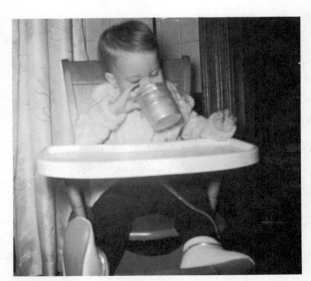

Figure 48. Sandy takes orange juice and water from a cup at 10 months. She spills it frequently.

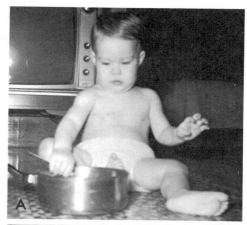

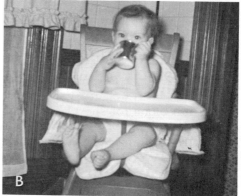

Figure 49. *A*, at 11 months Sandy enjoys playing with an empty pan and spoon. *B*, she blows bubbles in her milk and still spills the contents.

Care and Guidance

Sleep. Avoid strenuous play before bedtime. A night light is convenient for mother, and makes his surroundings more familiar. Pajamas with feet are warm, for he becomes uncovered easily.

Diet. Takes orange juice and water from cup. Solid foods in general are taken well.

Exercise. Tours around room holding adult's hands. Daytime clothing should be loose, so as not to interfere with movement.

ELEVEN MONTHS

Physical Development

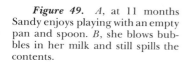

Stands upright holding on to adult's hand.

Social Behavior

Understands simple directions. Impatient when held. Enjoys playing with empty dish and spoon following meals.

Care and Guidance

Sleep.   Greets mother in A.M. with excited jargon.
Diet.   Still spills from cup. Enjoys blowing bubbles.
Exercise.   Plays with toys in tub. Enjoys gross motor activity. Creeps, kicks, pulls himself up.
Safety.   Cover electrical outlets with tape. Put household cleaners and medicines out of reach if not previously done. Needs to be sat down in playpen at times, since he tends to stand until he becomes exhausted.

TWELVE MONTHS

Physical Development

Pulse 100-140. Respirations 20-40 per minute.
Triples birth weight. Height is 29 inches.
Stands alone for short periods. May walk. Puts his arm through his sleeve, as an aid to being dressed.
Six teeth (four above and two below). Drinks from a cup, eats with a spoon with supervision.

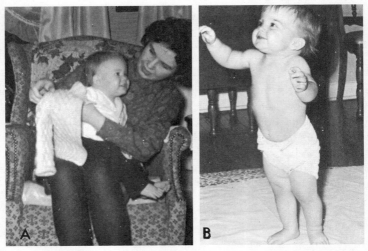

Figure 50.   *A,* at twelve months Sandy puts her arm through her sleeve as an aid to being dressed. *B,* she can stand alone for a few minutes or longer. (*B* from Marlow, D.: Textbook of Pediatric Nursing, 1969.)

Social Behavior

Friendly. Will repeat acts that bring about a response. Good or bad. Recognizes "No. No." Verbalization slows, owing to his concentration on getting about. Enjoys rhythmic music.

Shows emotions such as fear, anger, jealousy. Will react to these emotions by adults.

Plays with food, removes it from his mouth.

Care and Guidance

Sleep. May take one long nap daily.

Diet. Gradually add egg white and fish (baked, steamed, or boiled). Drain oil from tuna or salmon. Interest in eating dwindles.

Exercise. Plays in playpen in back yard for an hour in A.M. Enjoys putting clothespins in a basket and then removing them. Places objects on his head.

Distraction is an effective way to deal with his determination to do what he wants regardless of the outcome.

Immunization. Live measles vaccine, tuberculin test.*

STUDY QUESTIONS

1. Why must the pediatric nurse be able to recognize the various stages of growth and development in the infant?
2. Of what value is "sucking" to the baby?
3. Mrs. Jones tells you that she always props baby Sue's bottle, since it saves her so much time. What would you reply?
4. What is the value of attending to the needs of an infant promptly and cheerfully during his first year?
5. Define: chromosome, gene, heredity, DNA.
6. How does the infant's environment affect his physical growth and development? Mental hygiene?
7. Define immunity.
8. List the immunizations given during the first year of life. What diseases do they prevent?
9. Tommy is six months old. Prepare a day's menu for him.
10. What are deciduous teeth?
11. Prepare diagrams showing the eruption of the deciduous and permanent teeth. Label the teeth and include the approximate month or year that they appear.
12. Jay is eight months old. You are giving him cottage cheese for the

---

*Smallpox vaccination is given between 15 and 18 months of age. Keep site uncovered except for clothing.

first time. How would you introduce this to him? List four factors to keep in mind in regard to adding solid foods to baby's diet.

13. Discuss the needs of the newborn. How do these needs change during the first year?

14. Observe a three month old infant on the children's ward. How does his physical growth and development compare with that of the healthy three month infant?

15. Jean, seven months old, shows a fear of strangers. Discuss various ways in which to handle this problem in the home. In the hospital.

BIBLIOGRAPHY

Blake, F.: The Child, His Parents and the Nurse. Philadelphia, J. B. Lippincott Co., 1954.

Blake, F., and Wright, F. H.: Essentials of Pediatric Nursing. 7th Ed. Philadelphia, J. B. Lippincott Co., 1963.

Gesell, A.: How a Baby Grows, A Story In Pictures. New York, Harper & Brothers, 1945.

Gesell, A., and Ilg, F.: Infant and Child in the Culture of Today. New York, Harper & Brothers, 1943.

Marlow, D.: Textbook of Pediatric Nursing. 3rd Ed. Philadelphia, W. B. Saunders Co., 1969.

Nelson, W. (Editor): Textbook of Pediatrics. 9th Ed. Philadelphia, W. B. Saunders Co., 1969.

New Hampshire State Department of Health: Child Development Chart. Maternal and child health.

Ross Laboratories: The Phenomena of Early Development, 1962.

Spock, B.: Baby and Child Care. Rev. Ed. New York, Duell, Sloan and Pearce, Inc., 1968.

United States Department of Health, Education, and Welfare: Infant Care. Children's Bureau Publication No. 8, 1963.

Chapter 8

DISORDERS OF THE INFANT

VOCABULARY

Allergic	*Hypertrophy*
Aqueous	*Instilled*
Aspirate	*Ointment*
Congestion	*Purulent*
Diarrhea	*Suppository*
Hemoglobin	*Virus*

During infancy, rapid physical and emotional development takes place. Hospitalization during this period is a frustrating experience for the baby. He is used to getting what he wants when he wants it, and shows his displeasure quickly when illness restricts his desires. The baby who is breast fed at home may be unable to continue his regime if it creates undue hardship for the mother. He misses the continuous affection of his parents. His daily schedule is upset. The infant who drinks well from a cup at home may refuse it entirely when hospitalized.

Nursing personnel must try to meet the needs of these little patients by protecting them from excess frustration. It is not wise to expect them to develop new habits when they need their energies to cope with their illness and strange environment. Forcing them to eat or sleep leads only to further difficulties. Gentleness, patience, and ingenuity are not merely qualities attributed to a nurse but a dire necessity in caring for children.

During convalescence, the infant's needs change. One must try to recognize his need for play and social interaction. A warm, continuous relationship with the nurse is important. The parents need reassurance that their services are still needed. Occasionally, a situation occurs in which the nurse actually competes with the parents for the child's affection. This occurs most often with the long-term patient. It is natural for the nurse to become attached to a baby, but never to the extent that she makes the parents feel rejected or inadequate. Sometimes she may do this unintentionally, especially if the child's care is such that the parents cannot assist directly. The thoughtful nurse, during her conversation with the parents, remembers to mention how happy the infant looks when he sees them, or something equally as comforting.

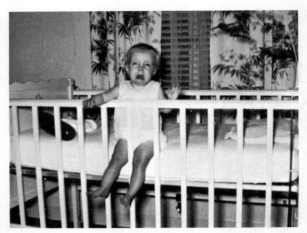

Figure 51. Charla cries when she is tired, hungry, frightened, or desires attention. Her plea should not be ignored, particularly in the hospital situation.

The Ear

OTITIS MEDIA

Description. Otitis media (*ot-* ear + *-itis* inflammation of + *media* middle) is an inflammation of the middle ear. The middle ear is a tiny cavity in the temporal bone. Its entrance is guarded by the sensitive tympanic membrane, or "eardrum," which transmits sound waves through the oval window to the inner ear, which contains the organs of hearing and balance. The middle ear opens into air spaces, or *sinuses,* in the mastoid process of the temporal bone. It is also connected to the throat by a channel called the eustachian tube. These structures—the mastoid sinuses, the middle ear, and the eustachian tube—are lined by mucous membranes. As a result, an infection of the throat can easily spread to the middle ear and mastoid.

Otitis media may be secondary to an upper respiratory infection, and sometimes accompanies scarlet fever and measles. It is caused by a variety of organisms. The bacteria involved are usually those that cause a sore throat or tonsillitis (hemolytic streptococci or pneumococci). Infants are more prone to this infection, for their eustachian tube is shorter, wider and straighter than that of older children and adults (see Fig. 52). Since babies lie flat for long periods, germs have easy access from the eustachian tube to the middle ear. This is thought by some to be a contributing factor. In the older child, infected adenoids may be responsible.

Symptoms. The symptoms of otitis media are pain in the ear, often very severe, irritability, and interference with hearing. Fever (which may

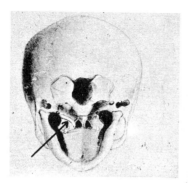

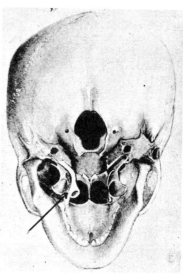

Figure 52. Diagram showing the position and direction of the eustachian tube in the infant and adult. The infant's eustachian tube is shorter, wider, and straighter. (From Wright, F. H., and Blake, F. G.: Essentials of Pediatrics. 7th Ed. J. B. Lippincott Co., 1963.)

run as high as 104°) headache, and vomiting may also accompany it, as well as diarrhea, and febrile convulsions. The nurse may suspect an earache in the infant who rubs his ear frequently or pulls at it. He may also roll his head from side to side and cry piercingly. The older child can point to the place that is tender.

If an abscess forms, a rupture of the eardrum may result and pus drains from the ear. When this happens, the pressure is relieved and the patient is more comfortable. The doctor can also incise the tympanic membrane to prevent a tear by spontaneous rupture. This is called a myringotomy (*myringo-* eardrum + *-tomy* incision of). It is not done as frequently today as in past years.

Complications of an ear infection include: deafness, mastoiditis, chronic otitis media, and meningitis. These are rare under modern treatment. Prevention lies in prompt treatment of respiratory infections or infected tonsils and adenoids.

Treatment and Nursing Care. The patient is isolated, and treatment is directed toward finding the causative organism and relieving the symptoms. A throat culture may be taken. Antibiotics are given initially until the specific germ is determined. These and the sulfonamides have proved very effective. They should be given until the infection has completely subsided. Aspirin is given to relieve pain. Codeine may also be necessary.

Nose drops. The doctor may prescribe Neo-Synephrine 0.25 per cent nose drops every four hours to relieve congestion of the nasal passages and to open the blocked eustachian tube. (Oily nose drops are to be avoided since there is danger of aspiration which could result in a

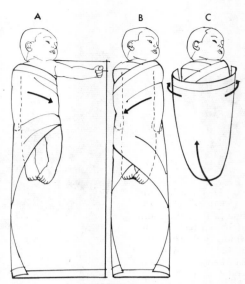

Figure 53. The mummy restraint. (From Leifer, G.: Principles and Techniques in Pediatric Nursing. Philadelphia. W. B. Saunders Co., 1965.)

type of pneumonia.) To be effective, nose drops must reach the inner and upper nasal passages. The liberal use of nose drops in the home is to be discouraged, since delicate membranes may become irritated, and the procedure is upsetting to the small child. The older child can tilt his head back to enable the nurse to instill the drops. The infant or toddler generally has to be restrained. The following method is appropriate; however, it may not be necessary in all cases. The nurse's approach should be gentle, to prevent frightening the child.

Equipment: sheet for restraint, nose drops, tissues.
Method

1. Immobilize the infant with mummy restraint (see Fig. 53).
2. Wipe excess mucus from nose with a tissue.
3. Place infant on his back with his head over the side of the mattress or his head extended over a rolled blanket.
4. Encircle infant's cheeks and chin with left arm and hand.
5. Instill drops with right hand.
6. Keep infant in this position for one-half to one minute to allow the drops to reach the proper area.
7. Remove restraints. Make infant comfortable.
8. Chart: time, name of nose drops, strength, number of drops instilled, how the patient tolerated the procedure, untoward reactions.

LOCAL HEAT. An electric heating pad or covered hot water bottle may be applied locally (temperature of hot water bottle 115°). Because a heating pad may become overheated, close observation is necessary.

EAR DROPS. The doctor may prescribe a drug or oil to be instilled into the ear to relieve pain. It is warmed to body temperature unless ordered otherwise. The infected ear is drawn down and back and the correct number of drops instilled. The patient remains lying down for a few minutes to permit the fluid to be absorbed. After this procedure, the patient is turned to his affected side to promote drainage. The nurse charts the following: time, name of drug or oil, number of drops administered, the area, i.e., right or left ear, untoward reactions, and whether or not the patient obtained relief.

The skin around the ear needs to be protected from drainage to prevent it from breaking down. Cold cream or other suitable lubricants are sufficient. If *sterile* cotton is to be placed in the ear, it must be inserted loosely to prevent infected material from being forced into the mastoid area. Some doctors do not advise its use, for they feel that it interferes with free drainage.

Respiratory System

THE COMMON COLD

Description. A cold, the most common infection of the respiratory tract, is caused by one or a number of viruses, which are spread from one child to another by sneezing, coughing, and direct contact. Droplets remain suspended in the air and on dust particles for short periods of time. The infection is transferred mainly during the initial stage. Bacteria such as pneumococci and staphylococci are the cause of the second phase of a cold, during which the nasal drainage becomes thicker and purulent. Factors that contribute to the individual's susceptibility include age, state of nutrition, general health, fatigue, and emotional upsets. Chilling of the body reduces the temperature of the nasal mucous membrane, thereby lowering its defense mechanism.

As the child becomes exposed to more children, the number of colds he contracts increases. Parents may notice this particularly during the child's first few years of school, since he has had little opportunity to build up resistance. The older the child, the better he is able to resist infection.

Symptoms. The symptoms of a cold in infants and small children are different from those in an adult. Children's air passages are smaller and more easily obstructed. Fever as high as 104° F. is not uncommon under three years of age. Nasal discharge, irritability, sore throat, cough, and general discomfort are present, and there may be vomiting and diarrhea. The diagnosis is complicated by the fact that many infectious diseases resemble the common cold during their onset, for example measles and poliomyelitis. Complications of a cold include bronchitis, pneumonitis, and ear infections.

Prevention. To prevent the child from catching a cold, avoid exposing him to children with this virus as much as possible. Infants under six months of age can acquire this infection so they too must be protected from infected persons. Be sure to provide nourishing foods and see that the child gets sufficient rest.

Treatment and Nursing Care. There is no cure for the common cold. When a cold is suspected, treatment should be started early. The treatment is designed to relieve the symptoms. Rest, fluids, and proper diet are important. If anorexia is present, food should not be forced upon the child. His appetite will gradually improve with his condition. When high fever accompanies a cold, the doctor must be consulted. Aspirin will reduce the temperature, but the correct dosage should be prescribed, particularly when the infant is under one year of age. From one to five years of age, one tablet of baby aspirin (1¼ grains) every four hours during the day is sufficient. This is given only during the first or second days of a cold, since overuse of aspirin can be toxic. Aqueous nose drops will relieve nasal congestion. The older child can help squeeze the bulb of the dropper when they are instilled. The infant needs nose drops mainly before feedings and at bedtime. When drops are instilled 10 to 15 minutes before nursing, the nasal passages are cleared and he can suck easily. Each child needs his own bottle of nosedrops to prevent cross infection.

Moist air soothes the inflamed nose and throat. An electric vaporizer is safe and convenient. If one is not available, a shallow pan containing water may be placed on a radiator in the child's room. Its effects are limited, however. If a lot of moisture is indicated, as for croup, the infant may be taken to a small room, such as the bathroom, and all of the hot water faucets turned on to create sufficient steam.

The older child is taught the proper way to remove nasal secretions from his nose. The mouth is opened slightly and secretions are blown gently through both nostrils at the same time. This method prevents infection from being forced into the eustachian tubes. When there is a large amount of nasal discharge, the nurse protects the upper lip by the application of cold cream or petroleum jelly.

In the hospital, the child is isolated. During the initial stage of the fever he is kept in bed. Frequent change of position is necessary. In the home it is difficult to keep a child with a cold away from other members of the family. He must be taught to cover his mouth and nose when sneezing, and to wash his hands following. Tissues must be properly discarded and burned. A mother need not be embarrassed at turning the neighborhood children away from the door when Johnny has a cold. Not only is she doing her community a favor, but she is also protecting him from further infection.

Avoid fatigue immediately after a cold, and allow a day or two for convalescence.

Gastrointestinal Tract

INGUINAL HERNIA

Description.   An inguinal hernia is a protrusion of part of the abdominal contents through the inguinal canal in the groin. It is more common in boys than in girls. The hernia may be present at birth (congenital) or acquired, and varies in size. A hernia is termed *reducible* if it can be put back into place by gentle pressure; if this cannot be done, it is called an *irreducible* hernia.

Symptoms.   The infant with a hernia may be relatively free from symptoms. Irritability, fretfulness, and constipation are sometimes evident. The diagnosis is made when physical examination shows a mass in the inguinal area, which reappears from time to time, particularly when the child cries or strains. A *strangulated* hernia occurs when the intestine becomes caught in the passage and the blood supply is diminished. This happens more frequently during the first six months of life. Vomiting and severe abdominal pain are present. Emergency surgery is necessary if a strangulated hernia occurs, and in some cases a bowel resection is performed.

Treatment and Nursing Care.   Today most inguinal hernias are repaired successfully by the surgical operation called *herniorrhaphy* which is relatively simple and tolerated well by the child. The postoperative care is directed toward keeping the wound clean until it has completely healed. Waterproof collodion dressings may be used for this purpose. Diapers are left open to prevent the wound from becoming contaminated. The practical nurse checks and records frequently the temperature, pulse, respiration, blood pressure (optional, depending on the age of the patient), and bandage during the first 24 hours following surgery. She measures and records the patient's intake and output. Infants may be held for feedings. After the operation has been performed, the first voiding is of particular importance. If a patient has not voided from 8 to 12 hours following surgery, catheterization may be necessary. The patient's gown and linen are changed when necessary. His position is turned frequently to avoid respiratory complications.

UMBILICAL HERNIA

Description.   An umbilical hernia is a protrusion of a portion of intestine through the umbilical ring (an opening in the muscular area of

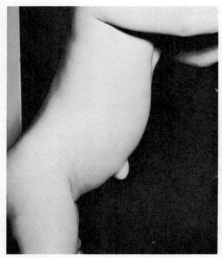 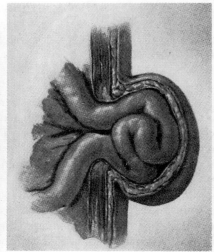

Figure 54.   *A,* Side view of infant with an umbilical hernia. *B,* Diagrammatic representation of an umbilical hernia. (Copyright, The Ciba Collection of Medical Illustrations, by Frank H. Netter, M.D.)

the abdomen where the umbilical vessels passed through). This type of hernia is common in the Negro race, and appears as a soft swelling covered by skin which protrudes when the infant cries or strains. Most of the small umbilical hernias disappear spontaneously during the first year of life. This type of hernia is not known to become strangulated or cause other complications.

Treatment.   The treatment of this condition is controversial. In general, surgery is not advised unless the hernia causes symptoms, becomes strangulated or enlarged, or persists until the child is three to five years of age.

HYDROCELE

Description.   A hydrocele (*hydro-* water + *-cele* tumor), an excessive amount of fluid in the sac that surrounds the testicle, causes the scrotum to swell. Its appearance in the newborn is not uncommon, and in many cases the condition corrects itself as the baby grows.

Treatment.   If a chronic hydrocele persists in the older child it is corrected by surgery.

VOMITING

Description.   Vomiting, a common symptom during infancy and childhood, is the result of sudden contractions of the diaphragm and the muscles of the stomach. It must be evaluated in relation to the child's total health status. Occasional vomiting is to be expected. Persistent vomiting requires investigation, since it results in dehydration and electrolyte imbalance. The continuous loss of hydrochloric acid and sodium chloride from the stomach can cause *alkalosis*. In this condition the acid-base balance of the body becomes disturbed and there is a dangerous excess of alkali (base) in the body's system, which will result in death if not treated.

The well child vomits from various causes. Some of them stem from improper feeding techniques. The practical nurse should ask herself the following questions when the infant vomits: Was he fed too fast? Too much? Was he bubbled frequently? Was he properly positioned following the feeding? Has there been a recent formula increase? Did he vomit any previous feedings? Sometimes the difficulty lies with the formula. If the fat content is too high it can slow down the emptying process of the stomach. The introduction of foods of a different consistency may also precipitate this symptom. The infant sometimes instigates vomiting by gagging himself with his fingers or objects of play.

Other factors that cause vomiting are ear, nose, and throat infections. Vomiting is seen in the primary stages of many communicable diseases. Specific disorders such as increased intracranial pressure, strangulated hernia, and various bowel obstructions are also responsible. In these conditions, the vomiting is not necessarily associated with feedings. When the cause of the illness is discovered and properly treated, the symptom disappears. Aspiration and aspiration pneumonia are serious complications of vomiting. Vomitus becomes drawn into the air passages upon inspiration, and causes immediate death in extreme cases.

Treatment and Nursing Care. To prevent vomiting, the nurse must carefully feed and bubble the baby, especially if he is ill. The nurse must be relaxed and the surroundings should be peaceful. Treatments are avoided immediately following feedings. The baby should be handled as little as possible at this time. To prevent aspiration of vomitus, the nurse places the infant on his stomach or right side following feedings. When a child begins to vomit, his head is turned to one side, and an emesis basin and tissues are provided. The nurse can relieve some of the strain involved if she supports the patient's head firmly. When the vomiting has ceased, the basin is removed from sight. The nurse rinses the patient's mouth with cold water or a mild antiseptic solution. His hands and face are bathed with warm water. Particular attention is given to the creases of the neck and behind the ears. When the practical nurse changes the patient's position, she turns him slowly and gently, because motion tends to increase nausea. A clean gown is applied, and the bed linen is changed if necessary. The window to the room is opened slightly to provide ventilation and minimize the odor.

The nurse may estimate the amount of material vomited by filling a similar basin with water to about the same level as the vomitus and measuring the water. Factors to be charted include: time, amount, color (bloody, bile stained), consistency, force, frequency, and whether or not it was preceded by nausea. The diet following vomiting is prescribed by the doctor. In the hospital, intravenous fluids may be given. Oral fluids are withheld for a short time to allow the stomach to rest. Gradually sips of water are given according to the infant's tolerance and condition. The patient's intake and output is carefully recorded so that the doctor is able to compare the kidney output with the total fluid intake.

When vomiting is persistent, drugs such as Thorazine or Phenergan may be prescribed. They are available in rectal suppository form. The nurse lubricates the suppository and inserts it well into the rectum where it dissolves. Slight pressure is exerted over the anus for a short time to ensure that the suppository is not expelled. Charting includes the time, name of suppository, and whether or not relief from vomiting was obtained.

PYLORIC STENOSIS

Description.   Pyloric stenosis (narrowing) is a disorder of the digestive tract. The pylorus, the lower end of the stomach, becomes partially blocked, so that food does not empty properly into the duodenum. This is due to an overgrowth of the circular muscles of the pylorus. The stomach muscles above the obstructed area also enlarge in their attempt to force material through the narrowed passage. An abnormal increase in the size of an organ or part, such as this, is called *hypertrophy.* This condition is commonly classified as a congenital anomaly; however, its symptoms do not appear until the baby is two or three weeks old. Its incidence is higher in males than in females, with a tendency for it to be inherited. It is the most common surgical condition of the digestive tract in infancy.

Symptoms.   Vomiting is the outstanding symptom of this disorder. The force progresses until most of the food is ejected for a considerable distance. This, termed *projectile* vomiting, occurs before and after feedings, and the vomitus contains mucus and may be blood-streaked. The baby is constantly hungry, and will eat again immediately after vomiting has occurred. Dehydration, as evidenced by sunken fontanelle, inelastic skin, and decreased urination, and malnutrition are present. In severe cases, the fat pads of the cheeks disappear, giving the patient a withered "old man" look. An olive-shaped mass may be felt by the physician in the right upper quadrant of the abdomen. X-rays confirm an enlarged stomach. It is difficult for the barium to pass into the duodenum. In severe cases, the outline of the distended stomach and peristaltic waves are visible during feedings. (See Fig. 55). The urine and blood are alkaline, since the fluid being lost from the body is mostly hydrochloric acid from the stomach juices. Bowel movements gradually decrease, since little or no food passes into the intestine.

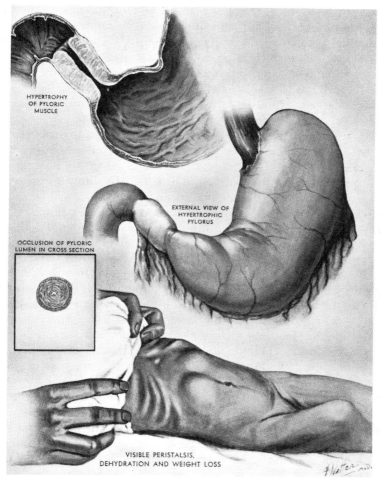

HYPERTROPHY
OF PYLORIC
MUSCLE

EXTERNAL VIEW OF
HYPERTROPHIC
PYLORUS

OCCLUSION OF PYLORIC
LUMEN IN CROSS SECTION

VISIBLE PERISTALSIS,
DEHYDRATION AND WEIGHT LOSS

Figure 55. Pyloric stenosis. (Copyright, The Ciba Collection of Medical Illustrations, by Frank H. Netter, M.D.)

Treatment. There are two methods used to treat pyloric stenosis, one medical and the other surgical. Medical treatment is not generally carried out in this country, since the results from surgery are excellent. Also, if medical treatment is not successful, the patient's condition becomes worse, and his changes for surviving surgery are poorer. Medical treatment consists of thickening the formula with cereal to make it less easy to vomit, refeeding after vomiting, gastric lavage (emptying of the stomach to prevent further distention) and the administration of atropine or its derivatives to lessen the spasms of the pyloric muscle. The nurse watches the patient for toxic symptoms of this drug, which are an increase in pulse, fever, flushing of the face, and dilation of the pupils. Phenobarbital is also given for its quieting effects on the overactive baby. The operation performed for pyloric stenosis is called a *pyloromyotomy* (*pyloro-* + *myo-* muscle + *-tomy* incision of). The surgeon incises the pyloric muscle in such a way that the opening is enlarged and food may again pass easily through it.

Nursing Care. The dehydrated infant is given intravenous fluids preoperatively to restore fluid and electrolyte balance. If this is not done, shock may occur during surgery. A blood transfusion may be indicated in order to correct anemia. Parenteral administration of thiamine and ascorbic acid may be given to assist in the healing of the wound. Vitamin K is administered. Thickened feedings are given until the time of operation in hopes that some nourishment will be retained. The doctor prescribes the degree of thickness of the formula, which is given by teaspoon or through a nipple with a large hole. The infant is bubbled *before* feedings as well as during to get rid of any accumulated gas in the stomach. He is fed slowly and handled gently and as little as possible. He is placed on his stomach or right side following feedings. The pylorus is on the right side of the abdomen; thus drainage into the intestine is facilitated. The head of the bed may be raised slightly. If vomiting occurs, the nurse may be instructed to refeed the infant. Charting of the feeding includes: time, type and amount offered, amount taken and retained, and type and amount of vomiting. The nurse also notes whether the baby appeared hungry following the feeding.

The nurse weighs the patient at about the same time each morning and records it. Other factors to be charted include the type and number of stools and the color and frequency of voiding. The infant's position is changed frequently, since he is weak and vulnerable to pneumonia. All procedures designed to protect him from infection must be strictly carried out.

The care of the patient following surgery includes such procedures as careful observation of vital signs and administration of intravenous fluids. The wound site is inspected frequently for bleeding. Signs of shock are an increase in pulse and respiration; pale, cool skin; and restlessness. In addition, the baby is observed for vomiting. He is placed on his stomach or right side to prevent the aspiration of vomitus. His position is changed gently. When indicated, the doctor prescribes oral feedings of small amounts of sugar and water that gradually increase in amount until a regular formula can be taken and retained. As soon as intravenous feedings are discontinued and oral fluids tolerated, the baby is held and fed from a bottle. The nurse must avoid overfeeding the patient. Vomiting is seen following surgery; however, it is not as severe and gradually diminishes. The diaper is placed low over the abdomen to prevent infection of the wound.

CYSTIC FIBROSIS

Description

Cystic fibrosis is a generalized disorder of the outward secreting or exocrine glands, in particular the mucous and sweat glands. This disease affects many parts of the body but particularly the lungs and pancreas. It occurs in about 1:1000 to 1:2000 live births. It is an inherited congenital disorder, the exact cause of which is unknown. The condition is believed to be inherited as a *mendelian recessive trait* from both parents. The parents, *carriers* of this disease, do not show any symptoms. When two *genes* for the disease combine in their child at the time of conception, cystic fibrosis results. It affects both sexes equally but is rare in the Negro race. Adolescents and young adults who previously would have died in childhood are now being treated.

Symptoms

LUNG INVOLVEMENT. Cystic fibrosis is considered the most serious lung problem in the United States. The air passages of the lungs become clogged with mucus. There is a widespread obstruction of the bronchioles. It is hard for the patient to breathe; expiration is especially difficult. Increased air becomes trapped in the lungs (obstructive emphysema) and small areas of collapse (atelectasis) may occur. Eventually, the chest assumes a barrel-shape appearance with increased diameter across the front and back. The right ventricle of the heart which supplies the lungs may become strained and enlarged. Clubbing of fingers and toes which indicates a chronic lack of oxygen may be present. Staphylococcus infections can easily occur in the lungs since the media is ripe. This causes more thickening of the abnormal secretions, irritates and damages lung tissues and further increases lung obstruction. The time of onset of this disease varies. Symptoms may appear weeks, months, and years after birth. In general, the earlier the onset the more severe the disease. The symptoms range from mild to severe. Any or all symptoms may be present in varying degrees of severity in one individual. The patient develops a chronic cough which may produce vomiting. Dyspnea, wheezing, and cyanosis may occur. He is irritable and tires easily. Gradually, there is a change in physical appearance. X-rays of the chest reveal widespread infection. Evidence of obstructive emphysema, atelectasis, and *fibrosis* of lung tissue may also be present. The prognosis for survival depends on the extent of lung damage. At present, 50 per cent of the patients affected die before the age of ten because of respiratory complications. However, this is only part of the picture, since this disease also affects the pancreas and sweat glands.

PANCREAS INVOLVEMENT. The pancreas lies behind the stomach. Some of its cells secrete *pancreatic juice*. This key digestive juice drains from the pancreatic duct into the duodenum at the same area in which bile enters (see Fig. 56). Changes which occur in the pancreas are due to obstruction by thickened secretions which block the flow of pancreatic

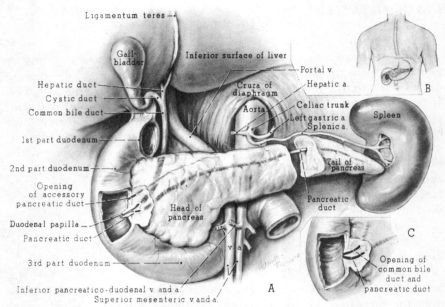

Figure 56. *A*, Relationship of the pancreas to the duodenum, showing the pancreatic and bile ducts joining at the duodenal papilla. A section has been removed from the pancreas to expose the pancreatic duct. *B*, Anatomic position of the pancreas. *C*, Common variation. (From Jacob, S. W., and Francone, C. A.: Structure and Function in Man. W. B. Saunders Co., Philadelphia, 1970.)

digestive enzymes. As a result foodstuffs, particularly fats and proteins, are not properly utilized by the body. In infants the stools may be loose. Gradually, because of impaired digestion and food absorption, the feces of the patient become large, fatty, and foul-smelling. They are usually light in color. The baby does not gain weight in spite of his good appetite. He may look undernourished. The abdomen becomes distended and the buttocks and thighs *atrophy* as fat disappears from the main deposit sites. Laboratory tests show a deficiency of pancreatic enzymes (trypsin, lipase, amylase). A trypsin test is done on the juices which are withdrawn by a tube passed into the duodenum. Absence of this enzyme alone is indicative of cystic fibrosis. This test for tryptic activity can also be done on a stool specimen; however, this is less reliable. A blood *cholesterol* level which is low may indicate poor absorption of fats from the intestine.

An oral pancreatic extract such as Viokase or Cotazym is given to the child with each meal. This replaces the deficient pancreatic enzymes which the child's body cannot produce. This medication is considered specific for the disease since it aids in the digestion and absorption of food, thus improving the condition of the stools. If the child is ill and not eating, the medication is withheld. When meals are erratic, such as during vacations, the mother gives the medication when the largest amount of food will be consumed.

A condition known as *meconium ileus* exists when the intestine of the newborn becomes obstructed with abnormally thick meconium while *in utero*. This is due to the absence of pancreatic enzymes which normally digest proteins in the meconium. The abnormal putty-like stool sticks to the walls of the intestine causing blockage. Rupture with signs of shock may occur. The presenting symptoms develop within hours after birth. Absence of stools, vomiting, and abdominal distention lead one to suspect intestinal obstruction. X-rays confirm the diagnosis. The condition is treated surgically. The death rate is high but more favorable when the obstruction is detected early. Most infants who survive will manifest the disease. Fortunately, the incidence of meconium ileus is rare, because the pancreatic enzyme deficiency is seldom complete. Nevertheless, the practical nurse assigned to the nursery must constantly be on guard for suspicious symptoms.

SWEAT GLANDS. The sweat, tears, and saliva of the patient with cystic fibrosis becomes abnormally "salty." This is due to an increase in the sodium and chloride levels. There is also an increase in the potassium level of sweat glands. The normal amount of chloride in sweat is 1 to 60 mEq. per liter. Higher concentrations are considered specific for the disease. The analysis of sweat is a major aid in the diagnosis of the condition. An agar plate impregnated with silver nitrate is frequently used as a screening device. The child places his hand on the plate; if the salt content is high, the handprint is visible. The more accurate *pilocarpine iontophoresis* technique uses a dilute solution of pilocarpine and a weak direct electric current to stimulate local sweating on the forearm (see Fig. 57). The sweat is collected on a small gauze pad and checked for sodium and chloride levels. Since the patient loses large amounts of salt through perspiration, he must be watched for heat prostration. Liberal amounts of salt should be given with food, and extra fluids and salt provided during the hot weather.

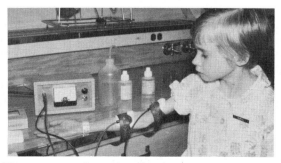

Figure 57. The sweat test, Iontophoresis. (From Kalafatich, A.: Pediatric Nursing. New York, G. P. Putnam's Sons, 1966.)

Complications. Cystic fibrosis is often responsible for rectal prolapse in infants and children. This is partly due to poor muscle tone in the rectal area and the excessively lean buttocks of the patient. However, surgery is almost never required, as the patient obtains relief by taking pancreatic medicine.

As the disease progresses, the liver may become hard, nodular, and enlarged. There may be edema of the extremities. The retina of the eye may hemorrhage, there may be damage to the eye from swelling, and inflammation to part of the optic nerve. *Cor pulmonale* (*cor-* the heart + *pulmon-* lung), heart strain because of improper lung function, is frequently a cause of death. *Osteoporosis* (*osteo-* bone + pore + *osis-* disease) may occur. When caused by cystic fibrosis, the bones become porous due to poor utilization of fat-soluble vitamin D which is necessary for proper calcium metabolism. There is a deficiency of vitamin A, because the child is unable to absorb fats from which this vitamin is obtained.

Treatment and Nursing Care

RESPIRATORY RELIEF. Antibiotics may be given as a preventative measure against respiratory infection; however, this is subject to controversy. Full dosages of antibiotics are given in an acute infection. The doctor determines the particular antibiotic to be used by the results of throat and sputum cultures. The route may be oral, inhaled, or intramuscular. If the medication is being given by injection, the nurse should watch for hardened areas and evidence of trauma. These patients suffer from muscle atrophy, so rotation of injection sites is a must.

Medication by mask or tent is common in cystic fibrosis to relieve dyspnea, to help thin respiratory secretions, and to aid expectoration. The child breathes a fine mist of 10 per cent propylene glycol in water or saline several times a day. This is done by means of a nebulizer powered by compressed air and attached to a mask or mouth tube (see Fig. 58). For humidification the patient sleeps in a mist tent. A dense fog is required. This is usually provided by means of compressed air, but oxygen may be used if necessary. This high humidity may cause condensation within the tent. Proper use of the damper valve will help to reduce this. It should be turned one fourth open, left open for a few minutes and then closed to minimize condensation. Antibiotics may be added to the aerosol solution. This is done by use of a nebulizer on croupettes (see Fig. 59). The nebulizer tubing is connected to a second oxygen source. Oxygen flowing through it will provide a fine mist. Close observation during the first 24 hours of treatment is of particular importance—sudden thinning of secretions may cause the child to raise a great deal of sputum. Fluids are forced as a high fluid intake has a definite expectorant effect. The patient's reaction to therapy, his vital signs, the amount and character of respiratory distress, cough, color and degree of restlessness should be recorded and changes reported. The nurse regularly observes the amount of mist in the tent. She also notes the level of solutions left in nebulizer bottles. All equipment should be washed and

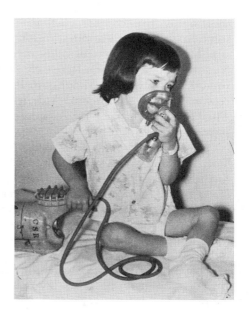

Figure 58. Aerosol therapy. The patient is taking an aerosol treatment with a nebulizer. (From Kalafatich. A.: Pediatric Nursing. Courtesy of National Cystic Fibrosis Research Foundation, New York, New York.)

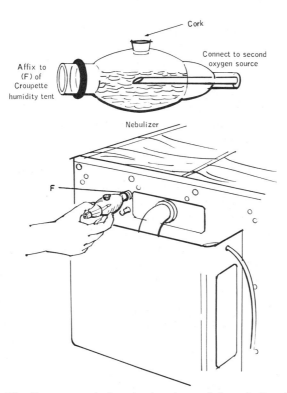

Figure 59. The Croupette nebulizer (top) and use of the nebulizer (bottom). (From Leifer, G.: Principles and Techniques in Pediatric Nursing. Philadelphia, W. B. Saunders Co., 1965.)

thoroughly rinsed after each use to prevent blockage from inhalant solutions and medications. Mist tents, compressors and other needed supplies can be obtained for home use through the local chapter of the National Cystic Fibrosis Research Foundation. They may be purchased, rented, or provided without cost. Parents should be told where to obtain repairs for the equipment. A drug assistance program is also available. This provides partial or complete payment of medicine for a given period of time.

Nebulization may also be given by intermittent positive pressure. This machine inflates the lungs during inspiration, allowing the aerosol medication to penetrate deep into affected areas. Postural drainage, chest clapping, and breathing exercises may be ordered by the doctor. These are performed by the physical therapist during hospitalization. When postural drainage and chest clapping are done properly, the secretions in the chest are moved up and out. During latent periods or in mild cases the patient may not raise sputum. This should be explained to the parents so that they will not discontinue this valuable procedure. Instructions may need to be repeated frequently to encourage full cooperation of the parents and child. These procedures should be done following nebulization and at least one hour after eating. General exercise is good for the patient since it stimulates coughing. Somersaults, headstands, and wheelbarrow play within the child's endurance are therapeutic.

Prevention of respiratory infections is very important. The child is isolated from patients and personnel who may harbor infections, i.e., protective isolation. The period of hospitalization is kept brief if possible to avoid cross-infection. This patient must be given the necessary immunizations against childhood diseases (see page 259). He should receive appropriate boosters so that the immunity obtained is kept up to date.

Diet. The maintenance of adequate nutrition is essential. The diet is high in calories, as much as 50 per cent above normal. There should be increased protein. Fats may be decreased; however, this is subject to controversy. Simple sugars are easy to digest and banana products are particularly good. Skimmed milk may be added to a protein formula during infancy. Fruits, cottage cheese, vegetables, and lean meats which are high in protein and low in fat and starches are recommended. Restrictions on ice cream, peanut butter, butter, french fries, and mayonnaise are advised. Extra salt may be provided by pretzels, salt bread sticks, and saltines. Discrepencies in the diet may be allowed by the doctor to keep meals from becoming drab and to provide a more normal-like setting. At such times the child is allowed to eat what he wishes and is given extra digestive enzymes. Water soluble vitamins are given in large amounts. Salt tablets may be given to the older child during hot weather. The child may be on force fluids since larger amounts of fluid are lost in the stools. The nurse may be asked to weigh the child daily.

The practical nurse feeding the infant with cystic fibrosis must be calm and unhurried. The baby may cough, have difficulty breathing, and vomit. He needs careful burping to avoid abdominal distention. In general the appetite is good. Older children need small amounts of food served attractively and frequently. Food piled high on a child's tray is discouraging. He may have eaten a perfectly good meal for his size, but the nurse who carries the remainder of the tray to the kitchen charts "poor appetite." This patient is on protective precautions and is usually in a private room. Since mealtime is a social time, the nurse should remain with the child if his parents are not with him. While there she must practice a little calculated neglect. It is not necessary to hover over the child to see that he eats every morsel with the proper utensil. Instead, try to make the meal more satisfying by giving good companionship mixed with a little encouragement. The nurse records the fluid intake of the patient following completion. She notes the child's reaction to new foods and any variations in stools resulting from the food. She notes the food refused and the type, character, and amount of vomiting, if any.

General Hygiene. The practical nurse must pay special attention to the skin of the child afflicted with cystic fibrosis. The diaper area is cleansed following each bowel movement. An ointment to protect the skin is advisable because the character of the stool subjects the diaper area to irritation. The buttocks are exposed to air when a rash occurs and light treatment may also be helpful (see page 54). Careful attention to bony areas is necessary in order to prevent decubitus. Because the patient has very little fat and muscle, it is important that his position be changed frequently, especially if he is weak and cannot get out of bed. This will also prevent pneumonia. Be sure that when you change the patient's position he is not left staring into a blank wall. This can easily be remedied by turning the crib around. Soiled diapers are immediately removed from the room to prevent offensive odors. An air deodorant may be advisable. The patient wears light clothing to avoid becoming overheated; it should be loose to allow freedom of movement. Children in mist tents also have to be guarded from chills resulting from damp clothing. The hair of the patient may become sticky from mist solutions. It should be shampooed regularly. Good oral hygiene is necessary since the teeth may be poor due to dietary deficiencies. Mouth care is given after postural drainage as foul mucous may be raised leaving an unpleasant taste in the patient's mouth.

Home Care. Today the child with a lengthy illness spends the majority of his time at home. He is mainly hospitalized for diagnosis, relapses, and complications. This burden which the family willingly assumes is extremely taxing financially, physically, and emotionally. Somehow, the mother must distribute her time and energy within the family, yet give careful attention to her child or, in the case of cystic fibrosis, sometimes children. How does she keep from spoiling the child?

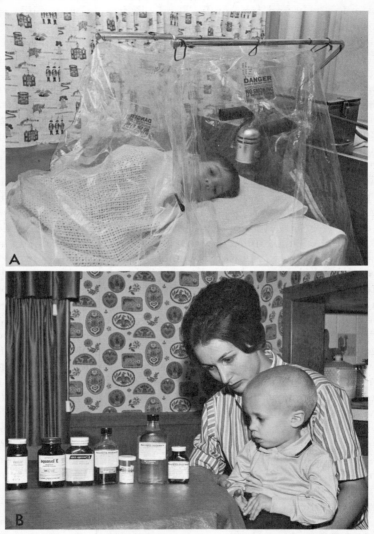

Figure 60. *A*, Boy sleeping in a tent filled with 10 per cent propylene glycol mist. When the tent is in use, the mist is so dense that the patient can scarcely be seen. *B*, Mother and child, who has cystic fibrosis, view an array of bottles which contain a wide assortment of pills. These medications help the boy digest his food and ward off infection. (Courtesy of National Cystic Fibrosis Research Foundation, New York, New York.)

Does she limit the normal activities of the remaining children to spare her sick member? What about birthday parties, camping, Cub Scouts, pets, epidemics at school? What does a trip to the shore or mountains entail? Where do the husband and wife find time for themselves? These seemingly overwhelming problems are being faced daily by many people in every community. Parent groups are helpful in promoting exchange of ideas and in building morale. The National Cystic Fibrosis Research Foundation provides useful information. The practical nurse becomes familiar with the local chapter in her area so that she may guide parents to reliable sources of information.

Parents of these patients need encouragement and reassurance. When the practical nurse meets them in the clinic or hospital, she should be kind and attentive. If a child looks obviously well cared for, mention this to his mother. If you are asked direct questions about the illness you might say, "Doctor Parker is a fine pediatrician. What did he tell you about Bobby's illness?" This encourages the parents to express themselves and will give you an idea of what the patient has been told. The nurse must not contradict or elaborate on what the doctor has said. Nothing is gained by having the patient face a mountain of problems all at once.

Parents need explicit instructions regarding diet, medication, postural drainage, prevention of infection, rest, and continued medical supervision. Many families require the assistance of a social worker to secure funds for equipment and drugs. Parents should be told that help will be available as the need arises. The mother who is most directly involved may benefit from these added hints. (1) She needs rest herself. The family must take over some of the responsibilities of the household. Relatives may care for the child periodically so that she can "get away from it all." It is helpful if she can develop at least one outside interest which is pleasurable. (2) An alarm clock set for medication time will remind her of this task. (3) A downstairs bedroom for the child is preferable. (4) Extra spoons and a pitcher of water on the bedside stand saves steps. (5) The National Red Cross *Home Nursing Textbook* offers many suggestions for improvising hospital equipment in the home, i.e., overbedtable, backrest. Instructions and diagrams are given.

Emotional Support to the Child.   The child who is chronically ill finds it hard to accept restricted activity. The amount and kinds of diversion required vary in cystic fibrosis, because the disease affects children of all ages, with variations in severity. (See page 234 for suitable toys.)

It is felt that the child benefits from simple straightforward answers about his illness. An uninvolved diagram might be helpful. The child who understands why he is being restricted from certain activities will be more cooperative. He should know why he must take medications with each meal, use the nebulizer, and sleep in the mist tent. He should see and handle the equipment before he uses it.

The young child finds it more difficult to be separated from his parents during periods of hospitalization. Even when the prognosis is grave, a child's courage is sustained if his parents are there. Visiting hours for parents must be very flexible. Close contact with school, church, and clubs by way of mail is important in the child of school age. It is helpful for the patient to develop an activity at which he is good, i.e., piano, art. This will increase his feelings of worth and provide outlets for emotions. Consideration must be given to ways of fostering love, acceptance, trust, fair play, security, freedom of choice, creativity, and maintenance of self-identity. The practical nurse must learn the child's likes, dislikes, fears, and interests. She observes him with his family and notes the type of relationship that exists. She forms her own impressions about the child and must not be misled by labels given him by those with lesser understanding. The patient has to be allowed to communicate in a manner which is meaningful to him. Sometimes a child can express his feelings, sometimes he cannot. It is important that the practical nurse be aware of a child's facial expressions, his posture, his eyes, and how he plays. What is he saying to his toys, his playmates? Her observations of the child's behavior are recorded daily in the nurses' notes.

Nurses and parents must not show undue concern for the patient's illness. Do not overindulge the child; this makes him demanding. He may then exaggerate lesser problems. The child's impression of himself and his illness are determined a good deal by how he feels physically, how his family feels about his condition, and how others behave toward him. The actions of the nurse, her interest, or lack of it, speak for themselves.

PHENYLKETONURIA (PKU)

Description. PKU is caused by the faulty metabolism of phenylalanine, an amino acid essential to life and found in all protein foods. The hepatic enzyme, phenylalanine hydroxylase, normally needed to convert phenylalanine into tyrosine is missing. When the baby is placed on milk, either human or cow, phenylalanine begins to accumulate in his blood. It can rise to as high as 20 times the normal amount. Its by-product pheynlpyruvic acid appears in the urine within the first weeks of life. This inborn error of metabolism results in severe retardation which is evidenced in infancy. Early detection and treatment are paramount. Although it is not a common disease and appears only about 1:10,000 births, it is interesting in that this type of mental retardation can be prevented and controlled by proper dietary management. It occurs mainly in children who are blond and blue-eyed. They may show evidence of eczema or other skin conditions, have a peculiar musty odor, or evidence personality disorders. About one-third of the children have epileptic seizures.

Treatment. Several screening tests are used in an effort to prevent or confirm the diagnosis of PKU. These are done on the blood and urine of the newborn. Screening programs for pregnant women have also been advocated to detect elevated phenylalanine levels which could have an effect on the newborn.

BLOOD TEST.   The Guthrie inhibition assay test is now widely used. Many newborn nurseries test the blood from a simple heelprick just before the newborn is discharged. Its advantage lies in early detection before blood levels of phenylalanine become excessive.

URINE TESTS

Ferric Chloride Tests on Urine

1. Place 5 cc. of urine in a test tube. Add 2 to 3 drops of 10 per cent ferric chloride solution. Phenylpyruvic acid is indicated if the urine turns a bluish-green color.
2. Diaper Test. A few drops of 10 per cent ferric chloride solution on a freshly wet diaper will also yield the characteristic color.
3. A phenostix may be dipped in urine or pressed against a wet diaper with the same results.

In many states some type of testing to determine phenylketonuria is mandatory by law.

The treatment consists of close dietary management. Since phenylalanine is found in all natural protein foods, a synthetic food providing enough protein for growth and tissue repair, yet little phenylalanine must be substituted. In the United States, Lofenalac (Mead Johnson) is used. This is a powdered formula which is mixed with water. It may be drank or used in special recipes in place of milk. A table of phenylalanine equivalents is available from Mead Johnson & Company, Evansville, Indiana. The management of the diet is individually based on urine and blood levels and the child's physical and mental response. Once the brain has been damaged, the process cannot be reversed by dietary control. It may nevertheless improve behavior and personality. The approximate age at which the diet can be safely discontinued is subject to close scrutiny. It is felt that if the child remains on the diet until he is four to six years old much of the damage can be averted.

FLUID THERAPY

Oral Fluids.   Whenever possible, fluids are given by mouth. It is the most natural and satisfactory method. The nurse must use her ingenuity to coax the sick child to take enough, because he refuses food and water, and cannot understand their relation to his recovery. Toddlers and infants are not capable of drinking by themselves. The busy nurse must find time to offer fluids, and must be patient and gently persistent. Liquids are offered frequently and in small amounts. Brightly colored containers and drinking straws may be a help. The nurse keeps an accurate record of the patient's intake and output. The doctor cannot determine whether a child requires intravenous fluids with a partially completed chart. *One cannot overemphasize the importance of this particular responsibility on the pediatric ward.*

Parenteral Fluids. Parenteral (*para-* beside or apart from + *enteron* intestine) fluids are those given by some route other than the digestive tract. This is necessary when sickness is accompanied by vomiting or loss of consciousness or when the gastrointestinal system requires rest. It is important in severe cases of vomiting and diarrhea when the loss of excessive water and electrolytes will lead to death if untreated. Solutions given parenterally must be sterile to prevent a general or local infection. The practical nurse must be aware of the importance of parenteral therapy, and the problems that might arise, even though she may not be directly assigned to the patient receiving the treatment.

The infant or child receiving parenteral fluids needs the nurse's warmth and affection. Babies miss being held and are also deprived of the pleasures they receive from sucking. The doctor may recommend that a pacifier he used, if it is not contraindicated. Older children need suitable diversions and company.

SUBCUTANEOUS INFUSION (CLYSIS). Subcutaneous infusion is referred to as *clysis* (from the term hypodermoclysis [*hypo-* under + *dermo-* skin + *clysis* to wash out]). Of the various sites used, the most common are the outer aspect of the thighs and the back. The fluid is absorbed gradually by the subcutaneous tissue; therefore, the particular rate of flow is not ordered as in intravenous therapy. The total amount of solution administered depends on the size and condition of the child.

FLUIDS GIVEN BY VEIN. Intravenous infusion presents certain problems in pediatrics. The procedure is more complicated and dangerous in infants and small children, and is more taxing psychologically. The infant's veins are small and hard to locate. Often the veins of the scalp are used which entails shaving the head. The baby must be effectively restrained to prevent the needle from becoming dislodged. When fluids are given intravenously, regardless of the site the infant must be *closely observed*. Fluids given by vein are passing into a closed space which can only be distended to a certain point without serious difficulties. If the circulation becomes overloaded with fluid that is infused too rapidly, cardiac failure can result. The flow of a solution can become disturbed

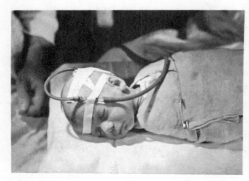

Figure 61. Intravenous feedings are often given to infants through the use of scalp veins. The infant cannot be given oral fluids when he is restrained in this position, because of the danger of choking. Note mummy restraint. (From Gross, R. E.: Surgery of Infancy and Childhood. 1953).

when an infant cries or wiggles. The practical nurse notifies her team leader when she notices an increase in the rate of flow of a solution or swelling at the injection site. She should also report an intravenous infusion that has stopped dripping or is dangerously low in the bottle. An older child may complain of pain at the injection site. A special hourly chart is kept on infants who are being administered fluids by vein. The nurse charts such information as the time, name and amount of the solution, the amount absorbed, the number of drops per minute, and the amount of fluid remaining in the bottle.

Modern adapting devices are now being used to improve the accuracy and safety of intravenous fluids. In the past it was difficult to slow down an intravenous infusion to 4 to 6 drops per minute without stopping the flow completely. The "mini" or "micro" drop decreases the size of the drop and allows the patient to receive 50 to 60 "mini" or "micro" drops per cubic centimeter rather than the usual 15 drops from the standard setup. Another device uses a graduated control chamber which is attached to the intravenous bottle to insure that the child does not receive too much fluid too fast. Such safeguards, nevertheless, do not replace close observation and charting by the nurse.

A surgical cut down into a vein (venous cannulation) may be made when prolonged parenteral therapy is anticipated or when the infant's veins cannot be entered otherwise. A polyethylene tube is inserted and the wound is sutured closed. The sutures are removed at a later date when therapy is no longer necessary. Recently, a special needle has been marketed through which the plastic tubing may be threaded into the vein; the needle is then removed. This eliminates the necessity of cutting into the vein. It is useful in some cases.

The Skin

INFANTILE ECZEMA

Description. Infantile eczema is an inflammation of the baby's skin. The exact cause of this condition is not known. It seems to have a definite familial tendency; emotional factors are often involved. Eczema actually is a symptom rather than a disorder. It indicates that the infant is oversentive to certain substances called *allergens* which enter the body via the digestive tract (food), by inhalation (dust, pollen), by direct contact (wool, soap, strong sunlight), and by injections (insect bites, vaccines). In most cases, the skin heals by the age of two, and the eczema does not occur again.

Symptoms. Although this type of eczema can occur at any age, it is more common during infancy. The baby is usually fat and well nourished. The lesions form vesicles which weep and form a dry crust. They are more severe on the face, but may occur on the entire body, particularly in the skin folds. Eczema is worse in the winter than in the summer and has periods of temporary remission. Foods to which these infants are sensitive include egg white, wheat cereal, cow's milk, and oranges.

The baby scratches because the itching is constant, and he becomes irritable and unable to sleep. The lesions become infected easily, which complicates the condition. Eczema may flair up following baby shots. A smallpox vaccination is not given at this age to affected infants, since a general vaccinia can occur. For this reason, the mother must protect the baby from coming into contact with children who have recently been vaccinated.

Treatment. The treatment is aimed at making the patient more comfortable by relieving his symptoms. Dermatologists vary as to the types of ointments and solutions they consider to be most effective. The patient's reaction to an ointment or solution is the best guide. Frequently, the doctor will apply an ointment to a small area of the skin on a trial basis to determine the sensitivity of the infant to it. If redness and itching occur within a short time, the doctor is notified and the medication removed. Different types of lesions may be on varous parts of the body at the same time. For example, lesions on the face may be of the type that require ointment, while those of the extremities require wet soaks.

An emollient bath is sometimes ordered for its soothing effect on the skin. Oatmeal or a mixture of cornstarch and baking soda are examples of substances prescribed. Shampoos are given using a soap substitute such as pHisoHex. Whenever possible, pateints are treated at home, because of the danger of infection in the hospital.

Corticosteroids may be ordered systemically or locally. Antibiotics are needed if infection is present. A low sodium diet is sometimes used to produce mild dehydration. Medication to help relieve itching is ordered for the patient. A child who is uncomfortable and unable to sleep should receive sedation.

Nursing Care. The practical nurse plays a vital role in the treatment of patients with skin problems. The doctor's prescribed therapy is of little value if ointments and wet soaks are not applied. It is a rewarding experience for the nurse, since she can see the direct results of her efforts more vividly than in other types of nursing.

The infant with eczema is isolated for his own protection when hospitalized, and must therefore receive as much attention as possible. The infant is unhappy and irritable. Little fingers can dig and scratch a week's good treatment to ruins in a matter of minutes. Out of necessity, he is restrained (see Fig. 62). He can tolerate such frustration more easily when he is cuddled frequently in the nurse's lap and his attention is diverted from his problem. This also shows the parents that the nurse

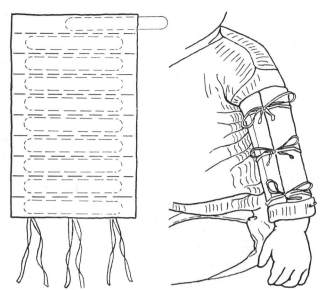

Figure 62. *Left,* elbow cuff restraint. Elbow cuff for use in treatment of eczema. *Right,* elbow cuff applied. (From Blake, F. G., and Wright, F. H.: Essentials of Pediatric Nursing. 7th Ed. J. B. Lippincott Co., 1963.)

is not repulsed by the baby's appearance, and will increase their confidence in the type of care that he will receive.

The kind of restraint used varies with the size and condition of the infant. Combinations of the elbow cuff, abdominal jacket, and ankle restraint are sometimes necessary. The fingernails must be kept short. Cotton socks may be placed over the hands and feet to prevent scratching. The restraints are observed frequently to make sure that they are not interfering with proper circulation. They are removed periodically, one at a time, to enable the baby to move about. His position must also be changed at short intervals to prevent pneumonia.

Medicated baths may be part of the treatment. Obtain towels and needed clothing in advance. Put the prescribed medication into the tube while it is filling and disperse it evenly in the water. Before closing the faucets, run a little cold water into the tub so that the fixtures are not hot in the event that the baby grasps them. The bath should be 95° F. Place the infant in the tub for 15 to 20 minutes. Hot water is not added while the patient is in the tub, for he could be burned. Floating toys amuse the infant. *Remain with the baby at all times while he is in the tub.* Children with eczema should not be overdressed, since undue warmth adds to their discomfort.

Wet soaks are applied to cool the body and in some cases to remove crusts. A gauze bandage is dipped into the prescribed solution, squeezed gently to remove excess fluid, and applied to the involved area. The bandage must cover the entire rash. Soaks are usually ordered continuously, and their effectiveness is measured only in terms of their being *wet*. When they are left on too long and become dried out, itching increases. This type of bandage is *not* covered with towels or rubber sheeting in an effort to protect the bed linens, because the itching is relieved by the cooling effect of the medication and covering the bandage will prevent evaporation.

Wet compresses may also be applied to the face by means of a mask (see Fig. 63), which consists of a square piece of gauze material in which places for the eyes, nose, and mouth have been cut out. It is held in place by strings attached to the four corners. When it is necessary to change wet bandages, they are completely removed, soaked in the solution, and reapplied. Factors for the nurse to chart regarding the application of wet soaks include: time of application, name of solution, strength of solution, area to which it was applied, length of time, general condition of the involved area (changes in the appearance or area of the rash), and condition of the patient following the procedure.

Ointment is usually applied to the skin by hand rather than by a tongue depressor. It is applied evenly, and must be kept constantly on the skin to be effective. Since some of these ointments are expensive, the nurse must not be wasteful in using them. Most hospitals provide special linen for their dermatology patients, since many ointments leave a permanent stain on the sheets. Mattresses with special water-proof covering are preferred, since rubber sheets make the patient perspire. Before the patient is taken to his room, drapes which collect dust are removed from the windows, and the entire room is damp dusted. Wool blankets and feather pillows are removed from the beds.

The doctor may prescribe an elimination diet. A simple diet which is tolerated well by the child is given initially. One new food at a time is added to determine the infant's reaction to it. When the baby is allergic to cow's milk, a substitute such as soybean or goat's milk can be used.

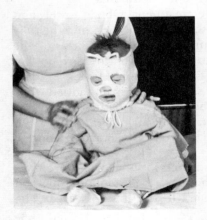

Figure 63. Face mask which can be used on a child with eczema to keep medication in close contact with the skin. (From Marlow, D.: Textbook of Pediatric Nursing. 1969.)

Vitamin supplements are needed, particularly if the infant is not taking enough of the prescribed fruits and vegetables. The nurse charts the kind and amount of food taken at each meal, and any allergic reactions that may have occurred. She plans her time so that treatments do not interfere with mealtime. Elbow restraints are removed from the toddler who is able to feed himself. The nurse assists with the patient's meals and prevents him from scratching irritated skin.

Infants are held and loved during feedings, as an emotional climate which prevents tension is very important to the recovery of this patient.

The practical nurse tries to establish a good working relationship with the parents. They need encouragement, as the course of eczema is unstable and much of the care is given by them to the infant in the home. She should listen to make sure that they understand the doctor's instructions and should clarify matters with the proper authorities as needed.

NUTRITIONAL DEFICIENCIES

Description. Because the infant is in a period of rapid growth, poor nutrition is particularly dangerous at this time. Severe vitamin deficiencies are rare in prosperous countries; those that do occur are caused by poverty, ignorance, or neglect. Severe malnutrition is still rampant in many undeveloped countries and in India and China. Every person must be concerned with the plight of the starving child. Sometimes the baby's body is unable to utilize food, even though his diet is adequate. An example of this is celiac disease, in which the intestines are unable to handle fats and starches. Another condition commonly called "Failure to Thrive" is seen in infants with severe malnutrition due to a faulty relationship between mother and child.

Iron Deficiency Anemia

The most common nutritional deficiency of children in the United States today is anemia due to insufficient amounts of iron in the body. Anemia (*an-* without + *-emia* blood) is a condition in which there is a reduction in the amount and size of the red blood cells, or in the amount of hemoglobin, or both. Iron is needed for the manufacture of red blood cells. This condition may be caused by severe hemorrhage as well as an inadequate diet.

The prevention of iron deficiency anemias begins with good prenatal care to ensure that the mother has a suitable intake of iron during pregnancy. The newborn relies on iron, which is stored in his system during fetal life, for the first few months following birth. Prematures may be deprived of a sufficient supply, since it is obtained late in the prenatal period.

The highest incidence of this type of anemia occurs from the ninth to the twenty-fourth month. During this rapid growth period, the baby outgrows the limited reserve that was in his body. Poorly planned meals or feeding problems contribute to this deficiency. The mother may sometimes rely too much on bottle feedings to avoid conflict at meals. Unfortunately milk contains very little iron. Instead, the amounts of solid food should be increased, and the milk decreased. Boiled egg yolk and meat are good sources of iron. Some cereals prepared especially for babies also contain it. Cookies, bread and crackers are not to be given in place of a well balanced diet (see Table 8–1).

Symptoms. The symptoms are pallor, irritability, anorexia, and a decrease in activity. Blood tests show a low hemoglobin level. Sometimes a slight heart murmur is heard. The spleen may be enlarged. Untreated iron deficiency anemias progress slowly, and in severe cases the heart muscle becomes too weak to function, and heart failure occurs.

Treatment. This disease responds well to treatment. The doctor must first differentiate it from other types of anemias. Iron is given orally two or three times a day between meals. Therapy usually lasts from six to eight weeks. Liquid preparations are taken through a straw to prevent temporary discoloration of the teeth. Recent iron preparations do not have this disadvantage. The mother should understand that the baby's stools will be dark or black because of the iron preparation. Blood transfusions are seldom necessary. The parents need explicit instructions as to the proper foods for the infant. Complex socioeconomic factors are frequently involved; therefore, the services of the public health nurse may be required. The intake of milk may need to be reduced. Behavior problems at mealtime should also be discussed with the doctor.

THALASSEMIA (MEDITERRANEAN ANEMIA, COOLEY'S ANEMIA)

Description. Thalassemia is a hereditary blood disorder in which the patient's body cannot produce sufficient hemoglobin. The red blood cells are abnormal in size and shape and are destroyed rapidly. This results in a chronic anemia. It occurs mainly in persons of Mediterranean origin, e.g., Greeks, Syrians, Sicilians, and their descendants elsewhere. It is seen in both minor and major forms. The symptoms in the minor condition are minimal—the patient is pale and his spleen may be enlarged. The person may lead a normal life, with the illness going undetected.

Symptoms of Thalassemia Major. This variety of the disease is very serious, as a progressive severe anemia becomes evident within the first few months of life. It occurs when both parents have *thalassemia minor*. The patient is pale, his appetite is poor, and he may have a fever. Jaundice, which at first is mild, progresses to a muddy, bronze color.

The liver enlarges and the spleen increases in size enormously. There is a great deal of abdominal distention which causes pressure on the organs of the chest. Cardiac failure is a constant threat. Changes in the facial bones give the child a characteristic look. The teeth protrude due to an overgrowth of the upper jaw bone. The diagnosis is aided by the family history of thalassemia, bone growth studies through x-rays, and blood tests. The prognosis is poor. Death may be due to cardiac failure, severe anemia, or a secondary infection.

Treatment and Nursing Care. The mainstay of treatment in this disease consists of frequent blood transfusions in an attempt to maintain the hemoglobin level above 40 per cent (6 gm. per 100 ml.) of the normal amount. As a result of repeated blood transfusions, excessive deposits of iron may be stored in the tissues. Research is now being done on drugs which will eliminate this by increasing its excretion through the kidneys. Splenectomy may make the patient more comfortable, increase his ability to move about, and allow for more normal growth.

Nursing care adheres to the principles of long term care. The observation of the patient during a blood transfusion are discussed on page 244. Whenever possible the same nurse should care for the patient to provide security for him during transfusion, blood tests, and other unpleasant procedures. This patient has very little energy and should not be disturbed needlessly. He will need encouragement to eat and is given small frequent feedings. It may help if he rests before meals. Good body alignment is necessary to prevent contractures. A change of position will also prevent bed sores. Since the child's muscles are tender and painful, the nurse must move him carefully. The patient should have a warm sponge bath and be clean and dry before retiring to avoid insomnia. Oral hygiene is given. Light-weight covers are more comfortable. Lights should be dimmed and the door of the room adjusted so that corridor lights and confusion do not disturb the child's rest. The room should be adequately ventilated. The emotional health of the child and his parents needs special consideration by the practical nurse. Every attempt to ease the strain of this prolonged illness must be made. Further suggestions applicable to the care of the chronically ill child are discussed throughout the text.

PROTEIN MALNUTRITION (KWASHIORKOR)

Description. In many parts of the world children still starve to death. There are no well-planned maternal and child health programs to elevate health standards. In some areas superstition and ignorance prevent children from utilizing nutritious foods found in their environment. Kwashiorkor, also known by various other names depending on the country in which it is found, is caused by a severe deficiency of protein in the diet, yet the amount of calories consumed may be nearly

Table 8-1.   *Foods to Meet the Needs of Children and Their Families*

Type of Food	Each Day

MILK GROUP

Milk ....3-4 cups (there will be times when a child may take less).

Cheese and ice cream
Cottage cheese ....Occasionally in addition to milk.
Creamed foods

VEGETABLE FRUIT GROUP

One source of vitamin C...One or more servings.

Grapefruit, orange, tomato (whole or in juice); raw cabbage, green or sweet red pepper, broccoli, fresh strawberries, guava, mango, papaya.

One source of vitamin A ....One or more servings.

You can judge fairly well by color—dark green and deep yellow: apricots, broccoli, cantaloupe, carrots, greens, pumpkin, sweet potatoes, winter squash.

Others, including potatoes ....One or more servings.

MEAT GROUP

Meat, poultry, fish ....One or more servings.

Dry beans, peas, peanut butter ....Occasionally in place of meat.

Eggs ....One a day.

BREAD AND CEREAL GROUP

Whole grain, enriched or restored bread and cereals ...4 or more servings daily.

Grits, macaroni, spaghetti, and rice.

OTHER FOODS

Butter or fortified margarine (contains vitamin A) and other fats ....Some each day.

Vitamin D in some form...400 units daily.

Sugars and sweets...Small amount occasionally.

United States Department of Health, Education, and Welfare: *Your Child From One to Six.* Children's Bureau Publication No. 30, 1962, p. 67.

adequate. It is the most serious and prevalent form of malnutrition in the world today. It occurs in children from four months to five years who have been weaned from the breast. The child fails to grow normally. Muscles become weak and wasted. There is edema of the abdomen which may also become generalized. Diarrhea, skin infections, irritability, anorexia, and vomiting may be present. The hair becomes thin and dry. The child looks pathetic and miserable. The treatment is mainly preventative. Although hunger may never be completely erased in the world, many private, public, and world health agencies sponsor programs in an effort to alleviate such suffering (see page 3). Early dietary treatment in established cases may prevent more serious growth retardation.

RICKETS

Rickets is a disease of infancy and childhood caused by deficient amounts of vitamin D. Vitamin D is necessary for the proper absorption and metabolism of calcium and phosphorus, which are needed for normal growth of bones. The classic symptoms of rickets are bowed legs, knock knee, and improper formation of the teeth. Good sources of vitamin D are fish liver oils, sunlight, and vitamin D enriched milk. It is a stable vitamin in heat and during storage. The recommended daily allowance is 400 I.U. for all persons up to 20 years of age.

SCURVY

Scurvy is a disease caused by insufficient fruits, vegetables, and vitamin C in the diet. The symptoms of scurvy include joint pains, bleeding gums, loose teeth, and lack of energy. Good sources of vitamin C are citrus fruits and raw, leafy vegetables. Vitamin C is easily destroyed by heat and exposure to air. Small amounts of water should be used for cooking vegetables to prevent it from being destroyed since it is also water soluble. It is generally given to infants in the form of orange juice, which should not be boiled. The daily requirement for infants is 30 mg. starting at two to four weeks (one or two ounces of orange juice every day.) Older children require more.

ABUSED OR BATTERED CHILD SYNDROME

The term battered-child syndrome refers to a clinical condition in which a child has been seriously abused by an adult, usually a parent. These abused children, often under the age of three, come from wide background variations. Victims who survive are seen in hospital emergency rooms and clinics with burns, fractures, bruises, lacerations, and

brain injuries. Passive neglect, such as lack of medical attention, malnutrition, failure to thrive, and other forms of emotional, physical, and
moral neglect, is seen. The history of the patient is usually vague and the
parents often disappear shortly after admission. X-ray examinations may
reveal several old fractures in various stages of healing. The abused child
is insecure in that he has no one to look to for protection. He may be
withdrawn and apprehensive of adults.

The parents of these children have varied personalities. All are
immature and obviously in need of help in order to become responsible
guardians. Although the laws on child abuse differ from state to state,
most states now require mandatory reporting by the physician of suspicious cases. If the situation cannot be altered, it may be necessary to
remove the child from the home. The services of the social worker are
invaluable. She may serve as a liaison between other agencies.

The child in the hospital needs a great deal of "TLC." A careful
record of his behavior and progress are kept. The nurse must be noncrit-
ical of the parents, even though she may feel otherwise.

STUDY QUESTIONS

1. What measures can the practical nurse take to prevent the spread of
   the common cold in the home? In the hospital?
2. How does the nurse recognize an earache in the infant?
3. Tommy, age nine months, has returned from the recovery room
   following a herniorrhaphy. Discuss his postoperative nursing care.
4. Define hydrocele, umbilical hernia.
5. What is the danger of giving a smallpox vaccination to the infant
   with eczema?
6. How do allergens enter the body?
7. Discuss the nursing care of the infant with eczema. What factors
   must the practical nurse chart in regards to this condition?
8. You are working the evening shift with Mrs. Green, a registered
   nurse, who is assisting the doctor in the treatment room. Baby Lee,
   two years old, has an intravenous infusion running. What would you
   observe about the baby and the intravenous infusion set as you
   made your rounds in the ward?
9. List the symptoms of pyloric stenosis.
10. Why must infants with pyloric stenosis be fed so carefully?
11. What parts of the body does cystic fibrosis affect?
12. In what ways can you as a practical nurse contribute to the emo-
    tional support of the long term patient and his family?
13. Prepare a day's menu for an 11 month old baby.
14. Define anemia. What foods are rich in iron?
15. Four year old Jimmy has a head cold. How would you instruct him
    to blow his nose?

BIBLIOGRAPHY

Anthony, C.: Structure and Function of the Body. 2nd Ed. St. Louis, C. V. Mosby Co., 1968.

Benz, G. S.: Pediatric Nursing. 5th Ed. St. Louis, C. V. Mosby Co., 1964.

Blake, F.: The Child, His Parents and the Nurse. Philadelphia, J. B. Lippincott Co., 1954.

Blake, F., and Wright, F. H.: Essentials of Pediatric Nursing. 7th Ed. Philadelphia, J. B. Lippincott Co., 1963.

Broadribb, V.: Foundations of Pediatric Nursing. Philadelphia, J. B. Lippincott Co., 1967.

Howe, P.: Nutrition for Practical Nurses. 4th Ed. Philadelphia. W. B. Saunders Co., 1967.

Harmer, B., and Henderson, V.: Textbook of the Principles and Practice of Nursing. 5th Ed. New York, The Macmillan Co., 1957.

Ingalls, A.: Maternal and Child Health Nursing. St. Louis, C. V. Mosby Co., 1967.

Kalafatich, A.: Pediatric Nursing. New York, G. P. Putnam's Sons, 1966.

Latham, H., and Heckel, R.: Pediatric Nursing. St. Louis, C. V. Mosby Co., 1967.

Leifer, G.: Principles and Techniques in Pediatric Nursing. Philadelphia, W. B. Saunders Co., 1965.

Marlow, D.: Textbook of Pediatric Nursing. 3rd Ed. Philadelphia, W. B. Saunders Co., 1969.

Mason, M.: Basic Medical-Surgical Nursing. New York, The Macmillan Co., 1959.

Milio, N.: Family Centered Care for Cystic Fibrosis. Nursing Outlook. *11*:718-720, 1963.

Mowry, L.: Basic Nutrition and Diet Therapy for Nurses. 3rd Ed. St. Louis, The C. V. Mosby Co., 1966.

National Cystic Fibrosis Research Foundation: Cystic Fibrosis for Nurses. New York, 1967.

National Cystic Fibrosis Research Foundation: National Cystic Fibrosis News Bulletin, New York, 1966.

Nelson, W. E. (Ed.): Textbook of Pediatrics. 9th Ed. Philadelphia, W. B. Saunders Co., 1969.

Schwab, L., et al.: Cystic Fibrosis. Amer. J. Nurs. *63*:62-69, 1963.

Spock, B.: Baby and Child Care. Rev. Ed. New York, Duell, Sloan and Pearce, Inc., 1968.

United States Department of Health Education and Welfare: Your Child from One to Six. Children's Bureau Publication No. 30, 1962.

Chapter 9

THE TODDLER

VOCABULARY

Acceptable	Fear
Afraid	Hazard
Behavior	Negative
Communicate	Posture
Defecate	Supervision
Explore	Temperament

GENERAL CHARACTERISTICS

The child between the ages of one and three is referred to as a toddler. He is able to get about under his own powers, and is no longer a completely dependent person. By this time he has generally tripled his birth weight and gained control of his head, hands, and feet. The remarkably rapid period of growth and development that took place during infancy begins to slow down. The toddler period presents different challenges for the parents and the child. This chapter deals with what he is like as a person, and ways in which adults can help him to master some of the obstacles he must face.

The toddler is a curious explorer who gets into everything (see Fig. 65). He gains more control of his body as each month passes. Soon he is walking, running, jumping, and climbing. He enjoys repeating these new skills, and with practice becomes less clumsy and awkward. His desires to touch, taste, smell, and smear, lead him into difficulties. He quickly discovers that much of his conduct is alarming to his parents. They no longer accept his actions willingly and without question, as they did in infancy. Since he cannot understand the need for restrictions, he revolts. Temper tantrums are common and behavior is not consistent. He is negative and unreasonable, and says "no" frequently.

Guides to Toddler Care

1-1/2 YEARS

Physical Development

Abdomen protrudes. Climbs stairs and upon furniture.

156

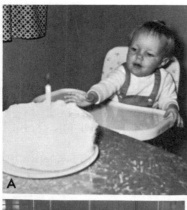
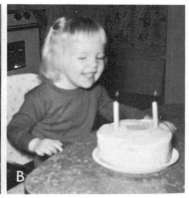
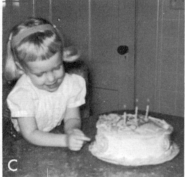

Figure 64. Note the physical changes in Charla on her first, second, and third birthdays. Discuss the emotional development of the child during the toddler period.

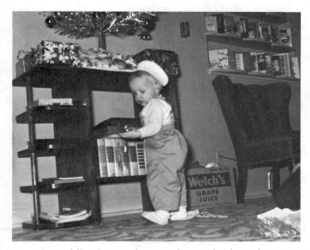

Figure 65. The toddler is a curious explorer who investigates everything.

Social Behavior

Gets into everything. Speaks about 10 words. Rapid shifts of attention. Temper tantrums may occur.

Care and Guidance

Sleep. May stay awake in crib after being put to bed.
Eating Habits. Drinks well from cup. Holds and fills spoon; spills contents. Likes to play in food.
Immunization. DPT booster. Oral polio vaccine (Trivalent OPV).
May begin to signal for potty.
If temper tantrum occurs, remove child from focus of attention. Keep comments brief. Divert child's attention. Avoid punishment and overattention.

2 YEARS

Physical Development

Weighs 26 to 28 pounds. Height about 33 inches. Pulse 90 to 120 per minute. Respiration 20 to 35 per minute. 16 baby teeth.

Social Behavior

Talks in short sentences. Dawdles. Enjoys stories and music. Imitative play. Has trouble sharing.

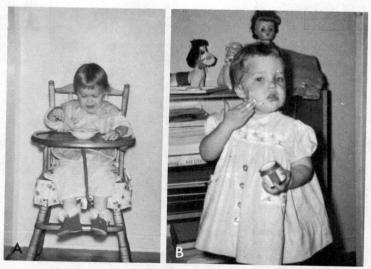

Figure 66. *A,* at two years Tina feeds herself well. *B.* This age delights in imitative play.

Care and Guidance

Sleep. Has a nighttime ritual. Tries to postpone bedtime. May climb out of crib.

Eating Habits. Feeds himself quite well. Appetite fluctuates.

Exercise. Enjoys outdoor play. Needs fenced-in area or constant supervision. Setting limits on behavior will increase his security.

Immunization. Mumps vaccine.

2-1/2 YEARS

Physical Development

Has all deciduous teeth.

Throws a ball. Builds a tower of blocks. Jumps and prances about.

He can make a O.

Social Behavior

Balky—cannot make up his mind. More fearful. Stuttering common.

Mother can leave for a short period.

Care and Guidance

Sleep. May awake during night. Needs reassurance.

Eating Habits. Dawdles at table. Easily distracted.

Exercise. Plays actively. Overtires if left to his own designs.

Immunization. German measles vaccine (Rubella) may be given anytime after one year of age. Indicated for boys and girls, from age one until puberty.

Has a special toy or something.

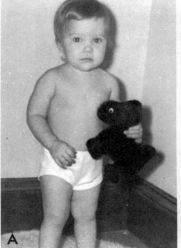 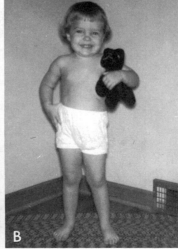

Figure 67. Compare the growth and development of the child of 20 months (*A*) and the child of two and one-half years (*B*).

GUIDING THE TODDLER

The toddler's emotions fluctuate greatly. He loves his mother one minute and hates her the next. He'll cry, kick and slap when he has decided to play outdoors longer, then turns around and kisses Mother for giving him a drink of water. There is no perfect way to manage such inconsistencies; parents are human and bound to make errors. Parents and nurse must not expect too much from the toddler or themselves.

One of the objectives in the management of the toddler is to help him to establish controls for himself and to find socially acceptable outlets for his behavior. (See Fig. 69.) Parents who direct all their child's activities cannot expect him to develop self-confidence in his own abilities. Many activities that are fun, such as writing on the walls, are not socially acceptable. On the other hand, finger painting in nursery school is equally as much fun, and approved by adults.

The toddler needs a certain amount of discipline. He gets into many situations that he does not know how to get out of. When adults make a firm decision for him, the problem is resolved, at least for the time being. The child feels secure because you have helped him to escape from his own primitive nature. A spanking once in a while is helpful. If, however, the parents are constantly punishing a child, they should look further into the situation. Spankings really do not settle anything, but demonstrate to the child that you are bigger and stronger than he is. Adults hit children because they cannot at the moment think of a more democratic way to handle the situation.

Children, like adults, seek approval. It is effective and helps to increase their self-confidence. Take the positive approach as much as you

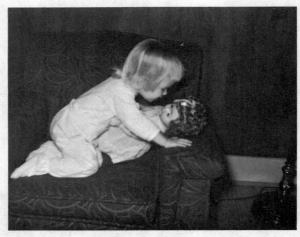

Figure 68. The degree of affection which a child shows depends on the amount he has received from others, especially during the early years of life.

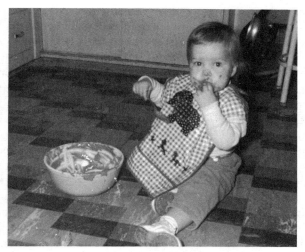

Figure 69. Adults need to assist the toddler to find socially acceptable outlets for behavior.

can. Presume that the toddler is going to be good rather than bad. "Thank you, Johnny, for giving me the matches," will make them arrive in your hand more quickly than "Give me those matches right now," said in a threatening tone.

Fear is a valuable emotion to the child if it does not become too intense. Unfortunately, most children fear many situations that are not in themselves dangerous, sometimes depriving themselves from activities that otherwise would be enjoyable. The physical and mental health of the child at the time of a fear provoking experience will determine the extent of his reaction. Also, if he is alone, his fear may be greater than if he is with someone such as his mother or nurse. Once a fear has been learned, it is hard to eliminate. Persons should attempt to control their own fears in the presence of young children.

SPEECH DEVELOPMENT

At about the end of the first year the baby begins to make noises that sound like "bye-bye," "ma-ma," and "da-da." When he sees the happy response to these sounds he repeats them. This is true throughout the toddler period. In order for small children to want to learn to talk they must have an appreciative audience.

At first, children refer to animals by the sound the animal makes. For example, before saying "dog," the toddler repeats "bow-wow." Soon he can say short phrases such as "daddy gone car." Toddlers respond also to tone of voice and facial expression. If an adult sounds threatening, the toddler may answer "no," and then "no" again in a louder voice. It is well to remember that toddlers who talk remarkably well still cannot comprehend much of adult conversation. Sometimes when adults forget this, they scold the child merely for being too little to understand what is requested of him. Imagine yourself being punished in a foreign country because you could not speak or comprehend the language well enough to defend yourself. Adults who show empathy to small children can help minimize their frustrations.

The toddler who has just learned to walk may practically give up repeating words because he is so overjoyed at being able to get about independently. As soon as his initial fascination becomes less pronounced, he takes up speech again. Delayed speech does not necessarily indicate that the child is mentally slow. The temperament and personality of the child and his family play an important role. No two toddlers have the same vocabulary at the same age. If a mother is concerned with her child's delayed speech, she can discuss it with her doctor during one of the child's routine physical examinations so that it can be evaluated in the light of total physical growth and development. Many late talkers are perfectly normal children who prefer listening to active participation.

DAILY CARE

Adults must keep their everyday conversation with a small child simple. Offering him too many choices will confuse him. When talking to the toddler, the adult should position himself so that he is at eye level with the child. In this way, he will seem less overwhelming to the child. Thus, nurses on the pediatric unit should conduct their conversation with the toddler at his eye level.

By the time the child becomes a toddler, mothers usually have found it easier to bathe him every evening rather than midmorning. A flexible schedule organized about the needs of the entire household is best. The toddler needs a consistent routine, but it does differ during the summer months, when outdoor water play may make a tub bath optional.

About the age of two the toddler begins to imitate adults in his desire to brush his teeth. This is a good time for him to have a small toothbrush of his very own. Toddlers are fascinated by the tube of toothpaste, and delight in putting the paste on their brush. This procedure is fun and is socially acceptable. He enjoys brushing with Mommy after meals and at bedtime. Of course his efforts at first are not very satisfactory. Adults should not try to force him in regard to technique. When he is *ready* to do a better job, a little encouragement and a good example are sufficient. One dental hygienist teaches children to "brush the teeth the way they grow," which is a simple explanation for the young child.

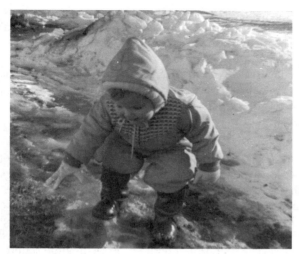

Figure 70. Tina needs security, but she also needs opportunities to explore her world. She must be dressed suitably for the weather.

The clothing of the toddler should be simple and easy for him to put on and take off. Slacks with elastic waists are convenient for him to pull down when he goes to the toilet. All clothing must be fairly loose to provide freedom of movement for jumping and other strenuous activities. In the summer months a light shirt may be needed to protect the toddler, and a bright swim suit is easy to spot on a crowded beach. Head protection is needed for play in the noonday sun. In the winter months, the child needs outdoor clothing that will protect him from the stormy weather. These must be changed when they become wet with snow. (See Fig. 70.)

The toddler wears shoes with firm soles. They should fit the shape of his foot, and be one-half inch longer and one-fourth inch wider than the foot. The heels must fit securely. Since shoes are outgrown quickly, it is best to buy inexpensive ones which can be changed frequently. If expensive shoes are bought, parents are tempted to make the child wear them longer, or at any rate they hesitate to buy new ones because of the expense involved. The child should wear his old shoes when he is taken to the doctor for a periodic checkup, because they show how the shoe has been worn, which indicates to the doctor how the child uses his body.

Whenever possible, the toddler may go barefoot since this strengthens his foot muscles. Stockings must be large enough so that they do not flex the toes. The child is taught to pull his stockings free from his toes before putting his shoes on.

Good posture is the result of proper nutrition, plenty of fresh air and exercise, and sufficient rest. The toddler's mattress must be firm. His chair and play table are adapted to his size. In some cases this can be easily accomplished by placing a few magazines in the seat of the chair.

A small stool placed in the bathroom will bring him to the proper height for brushing his teeth. As in all areas of learning, the child's posture is greatly influenced by that of other members of the family. The toddler who is happy and allowed graded independence will develop a sense of security which will be reflected in his posture. Slouching is sometimes seen in children who are insecure and lack self-confidence.

MEALTIMES

The toddler's need for food is not as great as that of the infant because he is not growing as rapidly. Mothers need not become alarmed because their two year old is inconsistent in his eating habits. It is well to remember that no one likes to eat the same kind and amount of food at each meal. The toddler's refusal to eat may be due to fatigue or to the fact that he is not particularly hungry. He will eat one food with vigor one week and refuse it completely the next. A flexible schedule designed to meet the needs of the toddler and the rest of the family must be worked out by the individual family. Forcing the toddler to eat only creates further difficulties. He is quick to sense frustration on the part of his parents, and may then use mealtime as a tool to obtain attention by behaving poorly and refusing to eat. Discipline and arguments during mealtime only upset everyone's digestion.

The toddler is fond of ritual. This is frequently seen at mealtime. He wants a particular dish, glass, and bib. It is best to go along with his wishes, as long as they do not become too pronounced. It gives him a sense of security, and in the long run saves time and energy for the adult.

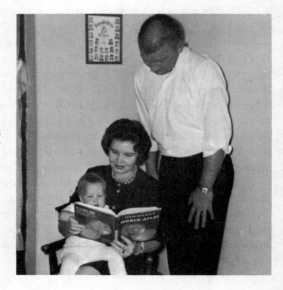

Figure 71. The toddler is fond of ritual. This is frequently seen at meals and bedtime.

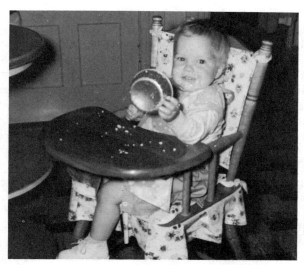

Figure 72. One cannot expect much in table manners from the 15 month old toddler. Note plastic bib and unbreakable dish.

The toddler has a brief span of attention. He may desire to stand in his high chair or wander away from the table. If he has eaten a fair amount of his meal, excuse him, otherwise distraction of some type is necessary. The toddler who feeds himself regularly may enjoy being helped by Mommy. Some restaurants that cater to families provide a pencil and special placemat to keep the small child occupied until adults finish their dinner.

The toddler's food is chopped into fine pieces. The portion should be small and separated. Offer a variety of foods and try to plan contrast in colors and textures. Toddlers like finger foods such as carrot sticks, crisp bacon, or a lettuce wedge. Foods are served at moderate temperatures. Candy, cake, and soda between meals are to be avoided. Nutritious food from the basic four include milk, milk products, eggs, butter or fortified margarine; vegetables and fruits; meat, fish, and poultry; enriched breads and cereals.

Children like colorful dishes, which must be made of an unbreakable substance. Washable plastic bibs and placemats are convenient. Protect the floor around the high chair with newspapers. Silverware should be small enough so that it can be handled easily. Adjust seating equipment so that the child is comfortable and maintains good posture.

TOILET TRAINING

Harsh toilet training can damage a child's later personality. Often, it is the child's first encounter with discipline, and one's initial learning experience is particularly significant. The child may begin to see his mother as a threat to rather than as a provider of security. This negative perception can be carried over into other areas. The child may develop a low opinion of himself when he is constantly scolded and told that he is bad. Anxiety over toilet training can be transmitted into anxiety over sex, since the organs are so closely connected; toilet training is believed to be a forerunner of various sexual problems in adulthood. Training given too early or too rigidly may also result in behavior problems in the child when he shows his frustration by direct or indirect forms of aggression. Likewise, these acts may become part of one's adult personality.

There is no set way to toilet train the toddler. A lot depends on the temperament of the individual child and the person training him. Readiness is important. Some mothers find that toilet training progresses more rapidly if it is not attempted until 18 or 20 months of age. The toddler at this age seeks approval, and likes to imitate the actions of his parents. He wanders into the bathroom and is curious about what is taking place there. If a mother feels that her child will respond to training at this time, she must first put him in training pants. These can be removed quickly and easily, and the child becomes more aware of being wet.

The use of a child's pot chair or a fixture that attaches to an adult seat is a matter of personal preference. A pot chair may make the toddler feel more secure, for it is his very own size. It should support the back and arms of the child. His feet should touch the floor. The toilet

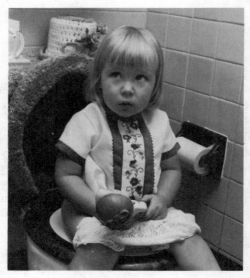

Figure 73. Harsh toilet training can be damaging to the child.

seat type must have a belt to strap the toddler in as a safety measure. The child needs time to become accustomed to his new piece of equipment. He may want to climb in and out of it and drag it about before he actually tries to use it.

Bowel training is generally attempted first; however, some toddlers become bladder trained during the day because they enjoy listening to the "tinkle" in the potty. If the toddler has his bowel movements at the same time each day he may progress fairly rapidly. Do not leave him on the pot chair for more than five minutes at a time.

If the child's bowel movements are not regular, it might be well to delay training for a while, since he will resent being constantly interrupted from play and taken to the bathroom. Toddlers generally enjoy having their mothers remain with them during the procedure. Most mothers find some phase of toilet training discouraging. Perhaps it is because we work at it too hard, thinking it an obstacle we've got to hurdle, rather than a normal process that the toddler will easily master when he's ready. Spankings and threats do more damage than good. Life is smoother for all if mother remains patient and keeps this new adventure pleasant.

Bladder training is begun when the toddler stays dry for about two hours at a time. One morning Mother may discover that Junior has gone the entire night without wetting. It is then logical to put him on the pot chair, and to praise his success. Bladder training varies widely, particularly during the night. Restricting fluids before bedtime may help. Getting the baby up half asleep and putting him on the pot chair accomplishes little.

Most children continue to have occasional accidents until the age of

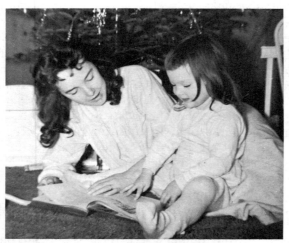

Figure 74.   The toddler needs someone she can depend on to accept her good and bad days.

three. If the toddler has a mishap, parents should accept it matter of
factly and merely change his clothes. When adults show continuous
affection to the child and accept his bad as well as his good days, he
surely benefits from it. (See Fig. 74.)

The word which toddlers use to signal defecation or urination
should be one that is recognized by others besides the immediate family.
Sometimes, a parent may forget to inform the baby sitter or nursery
school teacher of the word the child uses. This causes the child unnecessary frustration, because those about him cannot understand what he is
trying to tell them.

The toddler who is toilet trained at home should continue to use the
potty in the hospital setting. He may literally be embarrassed at wetting
the crib. Nurses regularly consult children's habit and care sheets (see
pp. 20 and 21) in order to make them feel more at home. The attentive
nurse responds quickly to the toddler's plea, and asks herself, "Does he
need to urinate?" Although regression of bowel and bladder training is
common during hospitalization, personnel often contribute to this
regression by not taking the time to investigate the child's needs.

THE TODDLER'S PLAY

The toddler spends much of his day playing. In this way he exercises his muscles, which contributes to his physical well-being. Play also
contributes to his mental health by bringing relief from emotional tension. The toddler enjoys "parallel play" at first, i.e., he plays near other
children but not with them. This is the beginning of socialization.
Gradually as he learns to communicate more easily and becomes more
skilled in handling toys, cooperative play takes place. He learns to give
and take, and begins to sense moral values of right and wrong. Play is
also of educational value. Learning is continuous as he explores and
delights in many new play experiences.

It takes time for the small child to learn to share. He clutches his
toys shouting "Mine." Once in a while he will voluntarily offer a toy to a
playmate. Parents should not force the toddler to share his possessions.
This comes at a later stage of development. If he is constantly corrected
for hoarding, he may eventually give up his toys when he is supervised, but seldom shares when he is left to his own designs.

Toddlers need adult supervision during play, especially when other
children are involved. If he is the oldest in the group he must be
distracted from pushing and hugging, and from directing the play of
others. The youngest child needs protection from being bullied. Toddlers feel secure when they know they will be rescued from alarming
experiences. It is unfair to expect them to rise up to situations that are
beyond their capabilities.

The type of toy the toddler selects for play depends on his age. The
15 month old is content with pots and pans from mother's kitchen, and

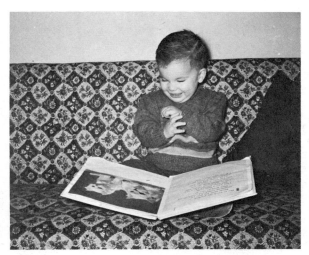

Figure 75. At 21 months, Dougie enjoys looking at the same pictures over and over again.

enjoys repeating acts such as removing clothespins from a bucket and replacing them. The toddler likes certain books and looks at the same pictures over and over again (see Fig. 75). Some children become very attached to a certain stuffed toy or blanket. The two year old likes to unlace his shoes, and removes them frequently. He is fond of water play, and may resent being removed from the tub. He enjoys playing in a sand box, scribbling with a crayon and paper, and prancing to rhythmic music. It is not long before the toddler discovers the stairs. Most small children start up them on all fours. As the child becomes more accomplished in walking upright, he shifts to the method of placing one foot on the stairs and drawing the other foot up to it, supporting himself by the hand rail. Eventually, he can climb the stairs by using the feet alternately as in walking.

Toys that can be pedaled, such as a bicycle, are adapted to the size of the child (see Fig. 76). Wind-up toys as a rule cannot be fully enjoyed by the toddler since he cannot manipulate them alone. Objects that can be pushed or pulled delight the small child. Toys with small, removable parts are dangerous.

ACCIDENT PREVENTION

Accidents kill and cripple more children than any disease known to man and are the *leading* cause of death in childhood. Unfortunately, we do not have a preventive for this, but we do have a defensive weapon. This weapon is knowledge. If parents understand their child's activities at certain ages, they can prevent many serious injuries by taking necessary

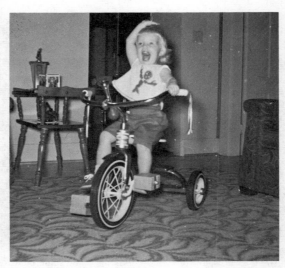

Figure 76.   Play contributes to good mental health by bringing relief from emotional tensions. Note blocks on pedals of bicycle.

precautions. Likewise, when statistics indicate that poisonings or burns are particularly prevalent at a specific age, we can guard against them.

The majority of accidents occur in or near the home. The toddler is particularly vulnerable, because he has a natural curiosity for investigating his environment. Parents must allow him some natural experiences, which teach him to look out for his own safety. They should also strive to teach him what is safe and what is not.

The practical nurse demonstrates safety measures to her patients and their families. This is done most effectively by good example. Measures pertinent to the pediatric unit are discussed on page 14. The nurse in her private life can often contribute indirectly to the welfare of others by the example she sets and by being aware of emergency medical facilities available in her community.

Automobile Accidents

The chief hazard to children is the automobile, because automobile accidents are the leading cause of death and crippling of children. The following is a list of safety measures applicable to this type of threat. Parents should:

1. Teach children to look both ways before crossing the street; the meaning of "red," "yellow," and "green" lights; not to run from behind parked cars or snowbanks; to cross on crosswalks; to sit down when riding in the car; areas that are safe for sliding, bicycles, and so forth; respect for school patrol leaders.

2. Hold the toddler's hand when crossing the street.
3. Not allow children to play in the car or leave them alone in it at any time.
4. Use seat belts. Vest types are available.
5. Not allow children to ride in the back of open trucks.
6. Watch the child under three constantly, or fence in a play yard.
7. Know where the child is before backing from the driveway.

Burns

Children are fascinated by fire. The following measures taken by parents will aid in the prevention of serious burns.

1. Teach the child the meaning of "hot." One mother did this effectively by allowing her toddler to step on beach sand warmed by the sun. This provided a safe learning experience.
2. Put matches and cigarettes out of reach and sight.
3. Turn handles of cooking utensils to the back of the stove.
4. Do not leave the bathroom when hot water is being drawn or after the tub has filled.
5. Beware of hot coffee. Cups should not be left on tables that are within the reach of the toddler.
6. Cover electrical outlets.
7. Test heated foods before putting them in front of the toddler.
8. When selecting a stove, consider safety factors. Built-in wall ovens are less accessible to toddlers. New stoves have temperature dials near the back rather than across the front where small children can reach them.
9. Screen fireplaces.
10. Keep a small fire extinguisher available in your home.
11. Practice what to do in case of fire in your home.

Falls

Children experience a great number of falls in the process of growing up. Fortunately, most of them are harmless. It is best to expect a child to do more than anticipated, because many falls occur after the baby has begun to show some caution. He has to be allowed a certain amount of freedom, as climbing is natural and a useful activity. However, he must be kept safe from situations that can result in severe bodily harm. Parents should:

1. Teach children how to go up and come down stairs when they show a readiness for this task.
2. Fasten cribsides securely, and keep them up at all times while the baby is in the crib.
3. Lock doors leading to cellar stairs.
4. Use gates to guard stairways.
5. Mop spilled water from the floor immediately. Do not wax floors when the toddler is first learning to walk.
6. Use side rails on a large bed when the child first graduates from his crib.
7. Secure the infant to the bathinette or table at all times.
8. Place screens on all windows.
9. Keep scissors and other pointed objects away from the toddler's reach.

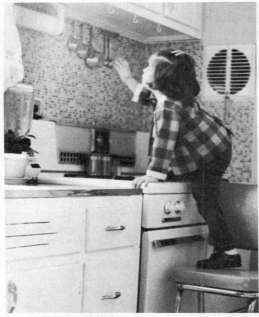

Figure 77. What hazards do you see for this curious toddler?

Suffocation and Choking

The toddler loves to put objects into his mouth. The following safety measures guard against suffocation and choking:

1. Remove small objects such as coins, buttons, and pins from the baby's reach. Substitute something safe for him to chew on such as a rubber teething ring or washcloth.
2. Do not allow small children to play with deflated balloons, as they can be sucked into the windpipe.
3. Do not feed popcorn, nuts, and small candies to the toddler.
4. Remove small bones from fish and chicken.
5. Keep plastic bags away from babies and children. They cling to the face and cause suffocation. Never use them for crib mattress covers.
6. Avoid bedclothes with drawstrings about the neck.
7. If a baby vomits, lift his hips slightly to allow the fluid to drain from his mouth. Do not lift him from the crib while he is vomiting.
8. Do not allow the toddler to play with venetian blind cords.

Poisoning

Poisoning is particularly dangerous between the ages of one and four years (see Fig. 78). Children like to taste substances, especially if they are colorful. The following safety measures can be taken by the parents to guard against this danger:

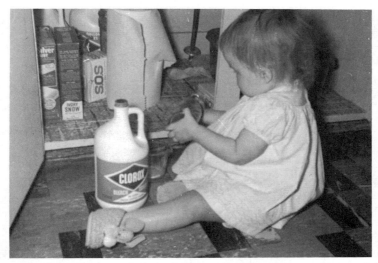

Figure 78. Poisoning is particularly dangerous between the ages of one and four.

1. Store household detergents and other cleaning supplies in a place that is out of the baby's reach. Lock the cabinet if the toddler is particularly fascinated by these items. Do not put chemicals or other potentially harmful substances into food or beverage containers.
2. Keep medicines in a locked cabinet. Put them away immediately after using them. Do not allow one child to give another child medicine. Be sure that all bottles are properly labeled. Follow the doctor's directions when giving medicines to the child. Do not refer to pills as candy. Flush old medicines down the toilet.
3. When painting, use paint marked "for indoor use" or that conforms to American standards z66.1-1955, for use on surfaces that might be chewed by children.
4. Wash fruits and vegetables before eating them.
5. Carry the universal antidote in a first aid kit when camping or traveling.

The child who has taken a poison requires immediate attention. Call a doctor at once. If one is not available, bring the child to the emergency room of the nearest hospital. Take along the container of poison. If it is empty, save the jar; valuable information concerning the contents may be written on the label. If the child vomits spontaneously, save the vomitus, and take it to the hospital where it can be analyzed. Many hospitals today have *Poison Information Centers* which offer telephone consultation services day and night to physicians and parents.

Drowning

Children enjoy playing in the water, which can be hazardous. Parents should:

1. Teach the child to swim when he becomes old enough, and the safety

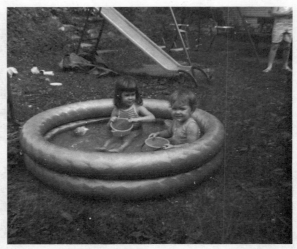

Figure 79. Pam and Tina enjoy water play. Two year olds need continuous supervision for this type of activity.

measures that accompany this sport.
2. Empty wading pools when the child has finished playing.
3. Remain with the toddler at all times when he is in the tub.
4. Not leave basins of water around where they are accessible to the child.
5. Watch the infant and toddler constantly while at the beach and near a pool.
6. Cover cesspools and wells securely.

Mouth-to-Mouth Respiration. Mouth-to-mouth respiration for drowning victims should be commenced as soon as the victim is reached. A 10 second delay may make the difference between life and death.

Method*

1. Place the baby on his back on a table or anywhere, depending on where you happen to be.
2. With your finger, quickly clear the child's mouth and throat of mucus, food, or other obstruction if you can.
3. Tilt his head back, with chin up. Bring his lower jaw forward.
4. Pinch his nose shut.
5. Put your lips to his and blow gently.
6. Release his nostrils and listen for the return of the breath.
7. Take a breath yourself.
8. Repeat the process. Close the child's nostrils, breathe into his mouth, release the nostrils. Count to three slowly and repeat again. Continue at this rate, about 15 to 20 times per minute, until the baby breathes again. Don't give up too soon. Keep your movements slow and gentle.

With a small child, you may be able to seal both mouth and nose with your mouth instead of pinching the nostril shut.

---

*Infant Care, United States Department of Health, Education, and Welfare, p. 86.

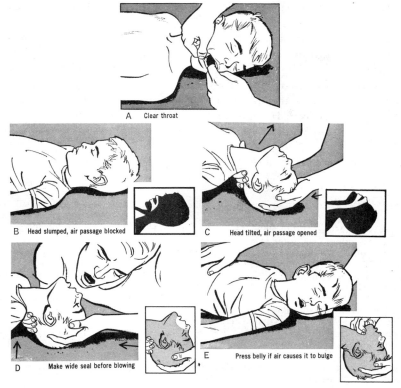

Figure 80. Mouth-to-mouth respiration. (From Rescue Breathing. Health Education Service, Albany, New York.)

SITUATIONS FOR STUDY

1. How can adults meet the emotional needs of the toddler during the "negative" stage?
2. Prepare a day's menu for the toddler. Include between-meal snacks.
3. List several situations that frighten you. What can you do to keep from transmitting these fears to others?
4. Define "parallel play." Of what value is play to the child?
5. What role do adults play in regard to the development of speech in the child?
6. Stevie, age three, has recently had his appendix removed. The doctor has written on his chart that Stevie has had a regression in bowel and bladder control. What does this mean?
7. Mrs. Jones, your neighbor, is discouraged because two year old Billy signals that he needs to go to the toilet after he has soiled his pants. Discuss various ways to cope with this common problem.

8. What factors must be considered when selecting shoes and socks for toddlers?

9. List several factors which contribute to good posture in children.

10. Review your newspaper for one week. Bring to class various accidents which have occurred to children during that week. Be prepared to discuss how they might have been prevented.

11. Make a list of household substances which are potentially poisonous to small children. In what cases would you want to induce vomiting? When would you not want to make a child vomit? (Consult first-aid manual.)

12. Describe mouth-to-mouth respiration.

BIBLIOGRAPHY

Breckenridge, M. E., and Murphy, M. N.: Growth and Development. 8th Ed. Philadelphia, W. B. Saunders Co., 1969.

Gerber Products Company: Recipes for Toddlers. Fremont, Michigan, 1959.

Hurlock, E.: Child Development. 4th Ed. New York, McGraw-Hill Book Co., Inc., 1964.

Kagan, J. and Havemanann, E.: Psychology: An Introduction. New York, Harcourt, Brace, and World, Inc., 1968.

Marlow, D.: Textbook of Pediatric Nursing. 3rd Ed. Philadelphia, W. B. Saunders Co., 1969.

Ross Laboratories: Your Baby Becomes a Toddler. 1962.

Smith, C.: Maternal-Child Nursing. Philadelphia, W. B. Saunders Co., 1963.

Spock, B.: Baby and Child Care. Rev. Ed. New York, Duell, Sloan and Pearce, Inc., 1968.

United States Department of Health, Education, and Welfare: Infant Care. Children's Bureau Publication No. 8, 1963.

United States Department of Health, Education, and Welfare: Your Child from One to Six. Children's Bureau Publication No. 30, 1962.

Chapter 10

DISORDERS OF THE TODDLER

VOCABULARY

Ascites	*Exacerbation*
Asset	*Inhalator*
Contracture	*Immobilize*
Convulsion	*Paracentesis*
Deformity	*Potential*
Disoriented	*Speculum*

The toddler's world is centered around his parents, particularly his mother. Hospitalization is a painful experience for him. He cannot understand why he is separated from his mother and he becomes very distressed. The toddler who has a continuous, secure relationship with his mother reacts more violently to separation because he has more to lose.

Unless the toddler is extremely ill, his grief is obvious. He watches and listens for his mother. His cry is pitiful and continuous until he falls asleep in sheer exhaustion. He calls "Mommy, Mommy" and wonders why she does not come as she always did. Anger may turn to despair. If separated for a long time from his mother, the child may try to deny his need for her by appearing uninterested in her visits. This of course is only a disguise and should not be misinterpreted by the nurse or the mother. It is common for the child to experience changes in behavior upon his return home. He may be demanding and cling to his mother every minute. This is typically expressed by, "he just won't let me out of his sight." The mother should give the toddler extra attention and reassurance until he regains his trust in her.

Nervous System

CEREBRAL PALSY

Description.   Cerebral palsy is a term currently used to refer to a group of nonprogressive disorders that affect the motor centers of the brain. It is not fatal in itself, but at present there is no cure. This disease is caused by many factors, some of which are birth injuries, anoxia, subdural hemorrhage, or infections such as meningitis or encephalitis. Lead poisoning, head injuries, and febrile illness are sometimes responsible during the toddler period. In some cases no single cause can be found. It is estimated that 100 to 600 cases of cerebral palsy occur per 100,000 persons.

Symptoms.   The symptoms of cerebral palsy vary with each child, and may range from mild to severe. Mental retardation sometimes accompanies it; however, many victims have normal intelligence. The disease is suspected during infancy if there are feeding problems, convulsions not associated with high fever, and physical retardation. (The child cannot sit, creep, and so forth at the approximate age level expected.)

There are many types of cerebral palsy. Two of the most common are those marked by *spasticity* or *athetosis* (see Fig. 81), which occur in about 75 per cent of the cases. Spasticity is characterized by tension in certain muscle groups. The stretch reflex is present in the involved muscles. When the child tries to move his voluntary muscles, jerky motions result, and eating, walking, and other coordinated movements are difficult for him to accomplish. The lower extremities are usually involved. The legs cross and the toes point inward. The arms and trunk may also be affected. In athetosis, the patient has involuntary, purpose-

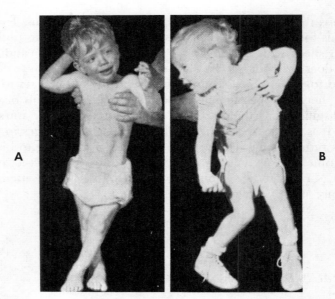

Figure 81.   Cerebral palsy. *A*, spasticity. *B*, athetosis. (From Courville: Cerebral Palsy, San Lucas Press; in Cardwell; Cerebral Palsy—Advances in Understanding and Care. New York, Association for the Aid of Crippled Children.)

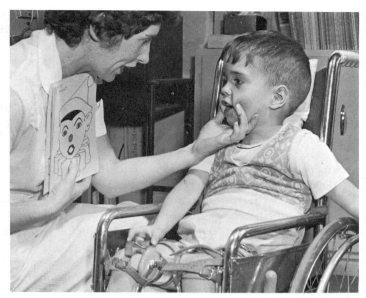

Figure 82. Danny, a victim of cerebral palsy, enjoys his sessions with the speech therapist. (Courtesy of Crotched Mountain Foundation, Greenfield, N.H.)

less movements which interfere with normal motion. Speech, sight, and hearing defects and convulsions may be complications. Emotional problems sometimes present more difficulties than the physical disability.

Treatment and Nursing Care. The objective of treatment is to assist the child to make the most of his assets, and to guide him into becoming a happy, well-adjusted adult performing at his maximum ability.* Both short- and long-term goals must be realistic. The parents need help in accepting the child for what he is, and should not be deceived into expecting miraculous cures from his treatment. The sooner the case is diagnosed, the fewer the physical and emotional problems. Parents must be informed of community resources available to them. The long course of this disability is a financial burden to them. They need to be relieved of the care of the child from time to time, so that they can refresh their own outlook on life. The specific treatment is highly individual, depending on the severity of the disease.

Good skin care is essential for the patient with cerebral palsy. The nurse observes the skin for redness and other evidence of pressure sores while she is rubbing it. The bedclothes are kept clean, dry, and free from wrinkles.

All precautions are taken to prevent the formation of *contractures*, a degeneration or shortening of the muscles due to lack of use. The

*Nelson, p. 1313.

damage may be permanent which results in a loss of function of the part involved, e.g., leg, arm, or finger. A common expression in relation to this is, "What you don't use, you lose." Knowing this, the practical nurse represses her natural desire to help the patient, and encourages him to do as much as he can for himself. When a patient takes his own bath in the morning, he puts his muscles and joints through their normal range of motion. When the nurse gives the bath, she puts *her* muscles through the necessary movements, not the patient's. Of course the nurse must use good judgment as to what activities the patient is capable of performing.

Other measures necessary to prevent deformities include frequent change of position, the use of splints, and passive exercise. The nurse must also assure that the patient maintains good posture while in bed. This is done through the use of footboards and the proper positioning of pillows and other comfort devices. The principles involved in preventing contractures can be applied to the nursing care of all long-term patients. The physical therapist spends many hours with the patient. Her instructions must be carried out by ward personnel to ensure continuity of care.

Braces are frequently used in the treatment of this disability. A brace is a mechanical aid that strengthens or supports weakened muscles or limbs. All braces are checked from time to time for correct alignment, loose or missing parts, and the condition of the straps and buckles.* The child needs assistance to help him adjust to this unfamiliar device. Wheel chairs and crutches are adjusted to the size of the patient.

Orthopedic surgery may be indicated. It may be followed by an extensive period of hospitalization. The nurse must remember that the child is in a continuous state of psychological as well as physical growth during this period. Her interest, or lack of it, may have a decided effect on the personality of the child in later years, particularly if the patient is a toddler. The nursing care of the patient with a cast is discussed on page 87.

The small child may be placed on a *Bradford frame* to facilitate nursing care, especially if he is in a body cast. This special oblong frame that fits into the child's crib is made of one inch pipe covered with canvas strips which run from side to side. These strips can be moved so that the patient can defecate or urinate without changing position. With training, the incontinent child can work out a schedule so that he can urinate or defecate with regularity, and therefore he saved from the embarrassment of incontinence. This type of training is not attempted in the hospital, but is instigated as his condition improves by those in charge of his total rehabilitation program.

Feeding problems can lead to nutritional deficiencies. During in-

*Price, p. 825.

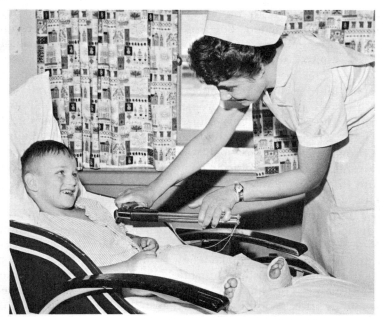

Figure 83. The practical nurse student and the long-term patient become good friends. (Courtesy of Hanover School of Practical Nursing. Hanover, N.H.)

fancy, swallowing and sucking may be difficult. Vomiting is frequent because the gag reflex is overactive. The entire body may become tense. The nurse must be especially careful to feed the child slowly to prevent aspiration. It is difficult for these infants to adjust to solid foods, and takes a great deal of patience on the part of parents and nurses to help them adapt to this new experience. As the child grows, he can be taught to manage special feeding equipment so that he is able to eat independently. He is also taught such activities as dressing and combing his hair.

The handicapped child needs opportunities to play alone and with other children. Games suited to his abilities, such as finger painting, are fun and allow him freedom of expression. Activities that require the use of fine muscular movements of the hand cause frustration in the child whose arms and hands are affected by the disease. The nurse can learn a great deal from the parents in regard to types of play enjoyed by the child.

The child with cerebral palsy tires easily, but finds it difficult to relax. He is under a constant strain to accomplish the simplest of tasks. The nurse must see that he takes frequent naps in a quiet room. He should not become overexcited before bedtime.

Educational opportunities geared to the patient's abilities are essential. Today, special schools are available which are prepared to deal with his physical and emotional handicap. Here physiotherapy and muscle reeducation coincide with numerous other activities required for the total well-being of the child. The patient's mental capacity is determined, not just in the light of I.Q. itself, but also by the potential of the individual. Mental ability is difficult to evaluate because this type of brain injury interferes with both verbal and motor expression.

If the child has a mild case of cerebral palsy, he can attend a regular school. In large cities, special programs for handicapped children are held within the school systems. Nursery schools are also available. Summer camps for exceptional children are becoming more numerous. These programs vary in the quality and the extent of services provided. The parents need the physician's aid in determining the best type of program for their child.

The child with cerebral palsy may appear to be emotionally unstable. This is not surprising when one considers the number of activities he is denied that are associated with normal growth and development. Take for instance the task of tying a shoe. The well child becomes frustrated when he cannot make a bow from the laces. He tries over and over again. When he masters this simple task it is a source of pride and accomplishment. The handicapped child finds the same procedure overwhelming. It is a continuous source of failure. Success breeds happiness; failure, despair. The cerebral palsy team works to bring satisfaction to these patients by making it possible for them to succeed. The amount of confidence and self-respect a handicapped person has depends a great deal on his environment. Though some instability generally accompanies disorders of the nervous system, a great deal of it results from the kind of guidance the person has had, particularly during the formative years.

The requirements for good mental health in the handicapped child do not differ greatly from those for all persons. He needs to have his basic human drives satisfied, and people who are genuinely interested in him. (See Fig. 84.) As the child grows, he needs social experiences with both sexes to help him adjust to adolescence. A child's handicap then takes on new proportions when he is unable to participate in such activities as dancing and sports. If he has not been helped to accept the reality of his disability before this time, complicated problems arise. Choosing a career and finding one's place in life are difficult at best when one has good physical and mental health. Nevertheless, many of us do not take advantage of our health. Perhaps this is why so many people who have handicaps find success. Unlike others, they have learned to make good use of what they have, or perhaps even more important, they learn to be happy within their capabilities.

Attitude of the Practical Nurse.   The inexperienced nurse may find that she is not immediately attracted to children with this affliction. She feels inadequate, and does not know how to approach or assist them. Fear of the unknown is natural. We focus our attention on the abnormalities of the child rather than what he is as a person. The nurse's first

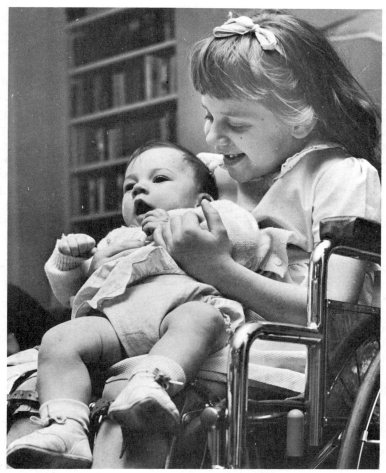

Figure 84. The kind of acceptance which the handicapped child receives as part of the family unit is important. (Courtesy of Crotched Mountain Foundation, Greenfield, N.H.)

problem may be to think of what to say to the child. The best advice is the easiest: be natural and treat the child in a natural manner. Do not be overly kind and solicitous, for this increases his dependency. Let the child do as much for himself as he can. Be there to assist if necessary but do not wait on him hand and foot. The child is happier without pity. Even a patient with the most serious defects can grow up to be happy and self-reliant if we accept him for what he is and encourage him to perform the task he is capable of doing. Expect him to be polite and considerate within reason. He will find security in your firmness. The handicapped child wants to be treated like other children of his age and to be loved for what he is.

Skeletal System

FRACTURES

A fracture is a break in a bone, and is caused mainly by accidents. It is characterized by pain, tenderness on movement, and swelling. Discoloration and numbness may also occur. In a *simple fracture* the bone is broken, but the skin over the area is not. In a *compound fracture* a wound in the skin leads to the broken bone, and there is the added danger of infection. *Greenstick fractures* are common in children because their bones are soft, flexible, and more apt to splinter. This is an incomplete fracture in which one side of the bone is broken and the other is bent. In a *complete fracture* the bone is entirely broken across.

If a fracture is suspected, do not allow the child to use the limb or part, and do not move it yourself. If the child is in a safe place, leave him where he is, keep him warm, and call a doctor. When the fracture is compound, cover the injury lightly with a sterile dressing. If it is necessary to move the child, apply a splint. The joints above and below the break are immobilized by a rolled newspaper or bath towels and tied with handkerchiefs beyond the injury. If the arm is injured, keep it elevated by a sling to reduce swelling and hemorrhage. If a back or neck injury is evident, do not move the child unless it is a dire necessity. Call the doctor immediately.

Fractures of the Femur

The femur, the thigh bone, is the largest and strongest bone of the body. Children may fracture this bone by a severe fall or in an automobile accident. It is one of the most prevalent serious breaks that occur during early childhood. The child complains of pain and tenderness when the leg is moved, and cannot bear weight on it. Clothes are gently removed, starting at the good side and proceeding to the injured side. It may be necessary to cut the clothes. X-rays confirm the diagnosis. Skin traction is used to reduce the fracture, to keep the bones in proper place, and to immobilize both legs. The type commonly utilized is called *Bryant* traction, which uses weights and pulleys to extend the limb as in *Buck's* extension; however, the legs are suspended vertically. (See Fig. 85.)

The nurse observes the traction ropes to be sure that they are in the wheel grooves of the pulleys and that the child's body is in good position. The legs should be at right angles to the body, and the buttocks raised sufficiently to clear the bed. A restraint jacket is used to keep the child from turning from side to side. Do not remove the weights once they have been applied. Continuous traction is necessary. The weights must hang free, and the pull of the weights must not be obstructed by bedroom furnishings such as a chair. The weights are *not* supported when

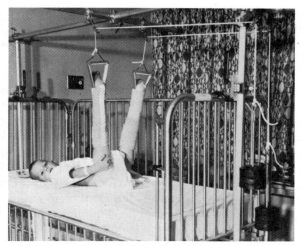

Figure 85. Bryant traction is used for the young child who has a fractured femur. Sufficient weights are used to elevate the child's pelvis from the bed. (Courtesy of H. Armstrong Roberts.)

the bed is moved. The nurse checks the child's toes frequently to see that they are warm and pink. Cyanosis, numbness, or irritation from attachments is reported immediately to the nurse in charge. The child is bathed daily, and his back is rubbed frequently to prevent ulceration. The nurse reaches under the patient's body when she rubs his back and buttocks. The sheets are pulled taut, and are kept free from crumbs. The jacket restraint is changed when it is soiled.

The child is encouraged to drink lots of fluids, and to eat foods that are high in roughage content to prevent constipation due to lack of exercise. Diversional therapy is important, as hospitalization lasts for a month or longer. The child's crib is taken to the playroom when possible, so that he may take part in the excitement of the activities there. Records, stories, and other forms of entertainment are essential to his total nursing care plan. Parents are encouraged to visit the patient as often as possible. The prognosis of this condition is good under proper treatment.

Skull Fractures

The toddler is famous for the number of blows he receives to his head. Fortunately, most are not serious, but they are alarming to parents. A *concussion* is a temporary disturbance of the brain which may result in headache, vomiting, and brief loss of consciousness. A *skull fracture* can result from a severe head injury. In this condition the cranium is actually broken. Bleeding and pressure may be exerted on the brain.

If the child stops crying shortly after he has received a blow to his head, maintains good color, and does not vomit, there is little chance that he has injured his brain. A lump may occur due to broken blood vessels beneath the skin, but this is not meaningful if no other symptoms are present.

Sometimes a child who has suffered a head blow is brought into the hospital for observation overnight. He may have all or some of the following symptoms: headache, drowsiness, anorexia, blurred vision, vomiting or he may be completely unconscious. The nurse observes the patient for signs of increased pressure on the brain. The pulse, respiration, and blood pressure are taken frequently. A rise in blood pressure and a fall in pulse and respiration are dangerous signs. The nurse also observes the patient's eyes; the pupils should remain equal. She arouses the patient periodically to be sure that he is not in coma. The doctor may order skull x-rays.

Digestive System

PINWORMS

Description. Of the several varieties of worms that affect humans, the most common is the pinworm. It is seen more often in toddlers but can develop in older children and adults. Pinworms are not a disgrace, but they do need to be treated. The pinworm looks like a white thread about a third of an inch long. It lives in the lower intestine, but comes out of the anus to lay its eggs, generally during the night. These eggs become infective a few hours after they have been deposited. This type of parasite spreads from one person to another, particularly where large groups of children are in close contact. The child infects himself by handling contaminated toys or soiled linen. The route of entry is the mouth. Reinfection takes place by way of the rectum to the fingers to the mouth, or by way of the rectum to the clothing to the fingers to the mouth.

Symptoms. The most noticeable symptom is itching in the anal area. The child may become irritable and restless. Weight loss, poor appetite, and fretfulness during the night may develop. The rectal area may become irritated from scratching. Worms may be seen on the surface of stools or around the anus. A tongue blade covered with cellophane tape, sticky side out, may be placed against the anal region in an attempt to obtain pinworm eggs. This may also be accomplished by the use of special pinworm diagnostic tapes. This is done early in the morning. The tape is then put on a glass slide and examined under a microscope. Eggs are typical and microscopic.

Treatment and Nursing Care. Several effective anthelmintics are available. Antepar, a pleasant-tasting, fruit-colored syrup, is currently popular. Povan suspension, a one-dose treatment, or Terramycin is also effective. The doctor may prescribe an enema.

METHOD FOR ADMINISTERING AN ENEMA

Equipment. Irrigating can, glass connector and clamp (or funnel and pitcher), No. 10 to 12 French catheter, saline solution (1 teaspoon salt to 1 pint of water), lubricant, toilet paper, rubber sheet, incontinent pad, bedpan with cover, extra diapers.

Procedure

1. Assemble the equipment and take it to the bedside.
2. Place the rubber sheet and incontinent pad beneath child.
3. Pad the bedpan with a diaper. Place the child's pillow under his head and back.
4. Place child on the bedpan. Restrain the legs by a diaper brought under the bedpan and pinned over the legs (see Fig. 86).
5. Allow the solution to run through the tubing to warm it and to expel air.
6. Insert the tube only 2 to 4 inches into the rectum. Do not give more than 300 cc. of solution unless the doctor specifies more. The solution should be from 100° to 105° F.
7. Hold the irrigating can not more than 18 inches above the level of the child's hips. The solution should run slowly without pressure. Clamp the tubing at intervals.
8. Remain with the child while the enema is being expelled.
9. Remove the bedpan and pillow. Cleanse the buttocks.
10. Remove the rubber sheet and incontinent pad.
11. Apply a clean diaper. Check to see if a stool specimen is desired.

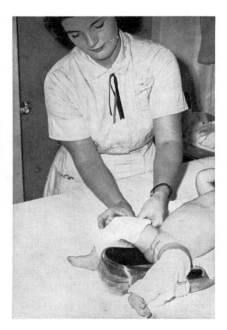

Figure 86. Positioning the infant for an enema. A pillow is under the infant's head and back. The buttocks are placed upon the bedpan, which has been covered with folded diaper to protect the infant's back. The legs are restrained in position with a diaper brought under the bedpan and pinned over the legs. (From Marlow, D: Textbook of Pediatric Nursing, 1969.)

12. Chart: time of procedure; name, amount, and temperature of solution used; amount and character of results; untoward reactions.

Aftercare of Equipment.   Empty and sterilize the bedpan. Autoclave the irrigating can, glass connector, and clamp after washing them thoroughly. Soak the rubber tubing in disinfectant after it has been properly cleansed.

When giving an oil retention enema, use 75 to 100 cc. of oil at 100° F. Apply gentle pressure over the anal area to prevent the oil from being expelled. A cleansing enema generally follows within one-half to three-quarters of an hour.

If it is determined that a hospitalized child has pinworms, linen and stool precautions are taken. His bedpan is sterilized following each use. The child must be taught to wash his hands well following bowel movements. The child's fingernails are kept short. A soothing ointment is applied to the rectal area.

All other members of the family should be treated for this condition to prevent reinfection. In the home, the toilet seat is scrubbed daily. Diapers and bed linens are boiled. The mother should be taught the danger of anthelmintic overdosage.

Respiratory System

CROUP

Description.   Respiratory infections are common in pediatric patients, especially in children under five years of age. Children have smaller air passages and experience greater respiratory distress than adults. Acute infections of the larynx are common in the toddler. Involvement of other parts of the respiratory tract is frequent. The infections are caused by a variety of organisms. The patient's history is valuable in diagnosis, and a *laryngoscopy*, an examination of the interior of the larynx, is sometimes necessary. Croup is sometimes called spasmodic laryngitis.

Symptoms.   Croup is characterized by a hoarse cough and dyspnea. It occurs suddenly during the night, often without earlier symptoms of a cold. Cold air may precipitate an attack in a susceptible child. The child sits up in bed frightened and struggles to get his breath. Inspiration is difficult and is accompanied by *stridor,* a harsh, high-pitched sound. Expiration is normal. The spasms last for a few hours and may recur later in the night. They may return again on the second and third night, but are less severe. Croup is alarming because the child is distressed. Nevertheless, it is not as dangerous as it looks, and is seldom fatal. Croup is not considered a communicable disease.

Treatment and Nursing Care. The treatment is directed toward reducing laryngeal spasm. An emetic such as syrup of ipecac is sometimes prescribed for this purpose. It causes the child to vomit, which helps to reduce the spasm of the muscles of the larynx. A dose of 2 to 4 cc. is generally enough to produce vomiting in the patient two to four years of age. This dose should not be repeated more than once or twice. Phenobarbital, a sedative, may be given after the child has vomited.

The patient is placed in an atmosphere of high humidity to aid in liquefying secretions of the throat and to reduce spasm. An electric steam inhalator is used in the hospital for this purpose. It is employed in connection with a croup tent for the toddler, but may also be used by itself for the older child who has a respiratory infection. (See Fig. 71.) Directions for its use are generally found on the base of the machine.

PREPARATION AND USE OF THE STEAM INHALATOR

Equipment. Steam inhalator, warm water, medication if ordered (generally tincture of benzoin).

Method
1. Fill the inhalator with warm water.
2. If medication is ordered, it is placed in cup of the machine.
3. Invert the bottle and lock it in place with ring bar.
4. Take the inhalator to the patient's bedside and explain its use.
5. Plug the inhalator into a wall socket and turn the switch to high until steam is produced through the extended spout. It can later be turned to medium or low, depending on the amount of moisture desired.
6. Close the doors and windows, and make the patient comfortable. The patient may be in semi-sitting position unless contraindicated.
7. Place the nozzle 18 to 24 inches from the patient to prevent burning him. Caution the older child not to touch or place his face close to the nozzle. Steam should surround the patient's head so that he breathes the medicated vapor.
8. Refill with water whenever necessary. (Steam may be used continuously or for 20 minutes three or four times a day.)
9. Time the treatment when steam begins to flow.
10. Chart: time and length of treatment, medication used, if any, how the patient tolerated the procedure, and the amount of relief obtained.

Aftercare of Equipment. Empty the water jug, wash in warm water, and dry. Wash cup containing medicine. Return machine to proper area.

CROUP TENT. A croup tent in the hospital can be made as follows:

Equipment. Sheet, cotton blanket, steam inhalator, screen or piece of wire, safety pins.

Method
1. Place a sheet and cotton blanket over half the crib so that they form a top and cover the sides. The blanket forms the inside layer to absorb the moisture and keep the hot, condensed steam from falling on the patient.
2. Pin them securely in place. Pins are placed on the outside of the blanket away from the patient's reach. The other half of the crib is left uncovered to provide sufficient ventilation.
3. Place the steam inhalator next to the crib. Place the spout of the inhalator forward inside the head of the tent.

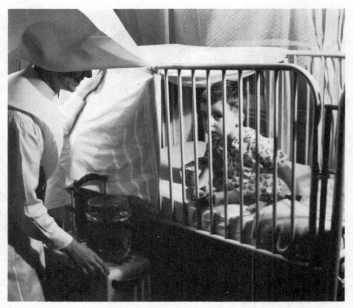

Figure 87. Warm moist air can be provided for the child when a vaporizer and a croup tent are used. (William M. Rittase.)

4. Fasten a screen or piece of wire between the spout and patient to protect him from being burned.
5. Observe the patient frequently. Refill the steam inhalator whenever necessary.
6. Chart: time, amount of relief obtained, rate and nature of respirations, color of child, degree of restlessness, untoward reactions.

In the home, a kettle of water placed on an electric plate can substitute for the steam inhalator. The steam is directed toward the patient with a lead-in pipe of cardboard. Be sure that the hot plate is not close to bedclothes. Remain with the child until the spasm has ceased. An electric plate left unattended is a fire hazard.

A simpler method is to take the child into the bathroom and turn on the hot water in the shower and sink. Let him inhale the moist air. Commercial electric vaporizors are also available. Buy a large one that turns off automatically when the water supply is low.

The toddler admitted to the hospital with respiratory distress is anxious and fatigued. The nurse remains calm while she prepares the croup tent. She can begin to acquaint the child with it. Children enjoy special hideaways, and this thought may appeal to the patient. The nurse also directs attention to the mother, who needs reassurance. As the mother becomes more relaxed, the patient also becomes less apprehensive. Constant attendance is desirable in such cases. Restraining a child who has respiratory distress keeps him in one position too long, and complications can develop more easily.

If an emetic is given, the nurse remains with the child until vomiting has occurred. The patient's hands and face are washed following, and clean linen is applied to the bed if necessary. The nurse gives the child sips of clear water to rinse his mouth. The patient is settled quickly, so that he will not become too exhausted.

Symptoms the nurse observes and records include temperature, pulse, and respiration, and blood pressure if ordered. Particular attention is given to the nature and rate of respirations. The child's color and the amount of restlessness and anxiety are also observed. Respiratory distress should begin to diminish as the child remains in the tent. An increase in respiratory distress is reported immediately, for complications may arise that necessitate a *tracheotomy* (trachea + *-tomy* incision of). Specific nursing care is indicated in such cases.

CROUPETTE.   A Croupette is often used in the case of patients with respiratory infections and other conditions of the respiratory tract treated with cool, moist air (see Fig. 88). This apparatus makes it easier for the child to breathe because it liquefies the secretions of the bronchioles. It also has the advantage of reducing the patient's temperature.

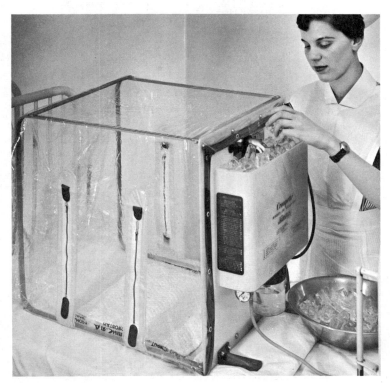

Figure 88.   Croupette. The trough at the back of the Croupette is filled with ice and tap water to the level indicated. (From Air-Shields, Inc., Hatboro, Pa.)

Oxygen may be used to provide pressure for the cool mist, or if the child does not require oxygen, air under pressure may be used for this purpose.

Although the practical nurse student would not be requested to prepare the Croupette initially, she does assist with the care of the patient as his condition improves. It is necessary therefore, that she understand the principles of how it works (see Fig. 89). Once she understands how to use the Croupette, she is able to concentrate her efforts on the needs of the individual child. The following is a list of factors that the practical nurse may find helpful in caring for the child in a Croupette.

1. A rubber sheet and cotton blanket are placed on the crib beneath the croupette. The rubber sheet prevents oxygen from escaping, since oxygen is heavier than air. The cotton blanket absorbs moisture from the water vapor.
2. Secure the metal frame of the tent to the bedspring with gauze.
3. The trough at the back of the Croupette is kept filled with tap water and ice to the level indicated (about 10 inches).
4. The canopy is tucked securely under the frame on both sides. It is sealed at

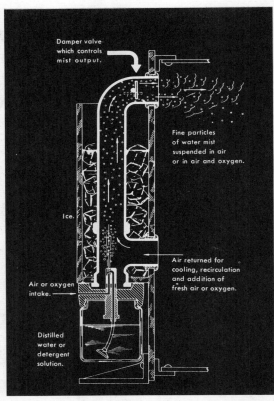

Figure 89. "How the Croupette Works." (From Air-Shields, Inc., Hatboro, Pa.)

the front with a folded cotton blanket or sheet which is tucked loosely under the mattress at the sides to allow carbon dioxide to escape.

5. The jar into which oxygen or air under pressure flows is filled three quarters full with *distilled* water. This is the source of water vapor. It is refilled every eight hours. Rotate the jar to unscrew it from the cap.

6. The damper valve is turned one-fourth open, left open for a few minutes, and then closed to minimize condensation.

7. The excess water from the melting ice is drained into a bucket from time to time through the drainage tube at the side of the Croupette trough. When the tube is not in use, it is kept elevated in the notch provided.

8. Be sure that pillows placed in the Croupette do not block the lower opening of the recirculation pipe for this will cause the tent to become warm.

9. Flush the tent with oxygen before placing the child in the unit.

10. Keep the child comfortable. Change his clothes when they become damp to prevent chilling. Organize necessary articles so that you will not have to be opening zippered portholes more than necessary. Allow the child to rest undisturbed as much as possible.

11. Charting includes date, time that the child was put in and taken out, his color, respirations, degree of restlessness, and his response to therapy.

12. When ending therapy it is desirable to reduce the oxygen concentration gradually by loosening the canopy or opening the side zippers for a short time to check the patient's response to normal atmosphere.

13. Aftercare of equipment. Empty the distilled water jar; wash it and wipe it dry. Drain ice and water from the trough and wash it with warm water and soap. Do not use alcohol. Clean the canopy with mild soap and warm water. Fold neatly. Return to designated area on the ward.

NOTE: The usual precautions used with oxygen therapy are employed when oxygen is used with the Croupette, i.e., no smoking, proper posting of signs, do not use grease, oil, or electrical equipment about the Croupette.

BRONCHIAL CONDITIONS

Description. From your study of the respiratory system, you will recall that the air tubes that lead to the lungs resemble an upside down tree. The trachea is the main trunk, followed by the bronchi, bronchioles, and alveoli. These passages proceed from large to small and are lined with a continuous membrane. If there is an infection of the bronchial tree, it seldom confines itself to one area but more often involves other structures. The physician designates the exact passages involved. The practical nurse may see terms such as acute tracheobronchitis, bronchiolitis, and laryngotracheobronchitis. The more extensive the infection, the more sick the child. The nursing care problems are bascially the same, but the degree of attention required is different. A discussion of acute bronchitis follows; however, the author has extended the nursing care to allow for adaptations by the nurse to patients who have more involved infections.

Acute Bronchitis is an infection of the bronchi. It seldom occurs as a primary infection—it is usually secondary to a cold or communicable disease. It is caused by a variety of organisms. Poor nutrition, allergy, and chronic infection of the respiratory tract may precipitate this condition. Age is an important factor—most patients are under four years of age. The patient may have a family history of acute bronchitis.

Symptoms.   The most noticeable symptom is a dry cough which becomes looser as the disease advances. Large amounts of sputum develop. This may be raised by the older child but is frequently swallowed by the infant and sometimes aspirated into the trachea and bronchi. Vomiting may occur. The child has a moderate fever, not usually over 102°. Older children may complain of a dry throat and sore chest.

Treatment and Nursing Care.   Uncomplicated acute bronchitis can usually be treated at home if the child is healthy. The patient must rest, drink plenty of fluids, and take the prescribed medications. Aspirin is used to relieve discomfort and quiet the child. Increased humidity is necessary, and the use of cool air humidifiers is especially helpful. A warm moist washcloth placed over the sinus area may help to loosen the secretions. Post nasal drip may precipitate coughing at night. Sometimes, relief may be obtained by placing the child on his abdomen. Nosedrops may be prescribed by the physician especially before feedings. Instruct the mother to purchase a small bottle and to discard it after the illness. The family dropper bottle is a hazard for this child because it probably is contaminated and will lead to a further spread of infection. Cold air irritates the respiratory tract; therefore, the child must remain indoors during inclement weather. Pneumonia is seldom a complication since the advent of the newer antibacterial drugs. The acute symptoms last for about a week, but a cough and expectoration remain for another week or two. The child who suffers from repeated attacks of bronchitis should be thoroughly examined so that the possibility of infected tonsils and adenoids, cystic fibrosis, allergy, tuberculosis, and other disorders may be ruled out.

More Extensive Infections.   The patient who is admitted to the hospital requires more extensive observation and care. Infants' respiratory passages are smaller than adults'; therefore, when they swell real respiratory distress occurs. In addition, a little child's cough reflex is not too effective in raising sputum, his immune mechanism may be poorly developed, and his wide straight eustachian tubes invite ear infection. The nurse must organize her work so that she does not disturb the patient unnecessarily. Sometimes coughing is reduced by giving him sips of water. When the patient has a coughing spell, the nurse places him in a sitting position and supports his chest and back with her hands. If persistent coughing disturbs the patient's sleep, the doctor should be notified.

The baby breathes more easily if he is sitting up. In this position the organs of the abdomen do not press against the diaphragm. The infant in an Isolette can be raised to a sitting position by elevating one end of the mattress. Babies in large cribs benefit from the use of an infant seat.

This is supported by a pillow at the back and secured to the crib. Supporting a baby with an infant seat is better than propping him with pillows, because the baby does not have a tendency to slump. The infant seat can be placed in a Croupette if necessary. The Croupette, mistifier, or similar apparatus is used to provide the necessary increase in humidity (see page 191). The nurse notes the date and time in which the infant is put in and taken out of the apparatus. Babies who suck their thumb become frustrated since they cannot suck and breathe at the same time. Mucus should be cleansed from the nose as circumstances may require, and aqueous nosedrops administered.

Solid foods may be refused. Such foods as custard, gelatin, cream soups, and ice cream may be offered. Fluids are forced and the intake and output are recorded. A good urinary output is necessary for the excretion of aspirin. Give water or milk with aspirin to reduce gastric irritation. Parenteral fluids may be indicated. Medications and fluids are given slowly. The nose is cleansed prior to bottle feedings, because the baby cannot suck and breathe at the same time. He sucks briefly, pulls away, and cries in frustration. Offer frequent small feedings; do not hurry the patient.

Careful observation and charting are paramount. The practical nurse watches for signs of dyspnea such as mouth breathing, flaring of the nostrils, sternal retractions, and stridor. She should note whether the difficulty occurs on inspiration, expiration, or on both. She should observe the skin, mucous membranes, and fingernails of the patient to determine his color, i.e., pink, white, gray, blue. In the Negro child, the palms of the hands, soles of the feet, and the lower lid of the eye may be observed for signs of pallor and anoxia. Restlessness, an indication of air hunger, should be reported and charted. The general behavior of the child is significant and should be recorded in the nurses' notes, i.e., cranky, listless, irritable, content.

The psychological factors involved in caring for the infant and small child are closely intwined with the physical care which the nurse administers. When the nurse takes a real interest in her patient, it is reflected in every procedure that she does for him. Her kind and gentle ways in giving the morning bath, her sense of humor, her eagerness to help produce feelings of security, belonging, and love. On the contrary, lack of warmth and attention by the nurse creates feelings of hostility, depression, and a negative attitude on the part of the patient. If his condition permits, the child should be removed from the Croupette at least once during every shift to be played with, rocked, and cuddled. When this is contraindicated, the nurse should visit her patient and pat or touch him in a loving way and provide toys for his diversion. The child with respiratory distress is very apprehensive; therefore, the presence of the nurse is reassuring. This is true even in the very youngest of children. The parents of the child need continuous reassurance, also. Nothing is more frightening than to see your child gasping for every

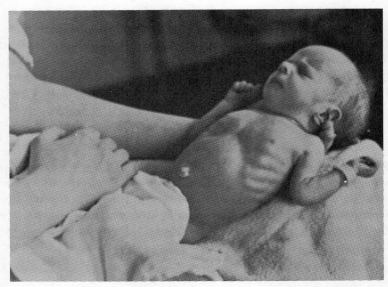

Figure 90.   Sternal retractions. Note the triangular indentation over the sternal area of the chest which indicates marked retraction during inspiration. Intercostal retractions are also evidenced. The infant is inactive. All of his energy is being used to breathe. (From Kalafatich, A.: Pediatric Nursing. New York, G. P. Putnam's Sons, 1966.)

breath of air. The nurse must direct her attention to the mother during visiting hours, listen to her, and, in general, treat her with as much consideration as time allows.

PNEUMONIA

Description.   Pneumonia or pneumonitis is an inflammation of the lungs in which the *alveoli*, or air sacs, become filled with exudate. The affected portion of the lung does not receive enough air. Breathing is shallow. As a result, the blood stream is denied sufficient oxygen.

There are many types of pneumonia. A text may classify them according to the causative organism, i.e., bacterial or viral; or by the part of the respiratory system involved, i.e., lobar or bronchial; or by various other methods. The *pneumococcus* was the chief causative organism among infants and children before the advent of antibiotics and sulfonamides. Today, *staphylococcal pneumonia* is particularly dangerous since strong strains of this organism do not respond to antibiotic therapy. It may begin as a skin infection in the newborn nursery, pediatric unit, or at home. The patient may then carry the germs in his nasal passages until a later date when he or someone close to him contracts the disease.

Some types occur primarily in certain age groups. Pneumonia in the newborn may be directly connected with the birth process, i.e., aspiration of infected amniotic fluid, or may result from exposure to infected personnel. It is responsible for about 10 per cent of neonatal deaths. *Lipoid pneumonia* occurs mainly during infancy. The baby inhales an oily substance into his airways. Oily medication such as cod liver oil is never forced upon the crying toddler for this reason. Nose drops with an oil base are dangerous. The toddler who drinks kerosene may also develop a type of pneumonia. *Hypostatic pneumonia* occurs in older patients who have poor circulation in their lungs, and who remain in one position too long. The child recovering from anesthesia also needs to be turned frequently to stimulate the circulation through his lungs.

Pneumonia may occur as the initial *or primary* disease, or it may complicate another illness in which case it is termed *secondary* pneumonia. Secondary pneumonia can accompany various communicable diseases or it may follow surgery. It is more serious than primary pneumonia since the patient is already weak and debilitated.

Symptoms. The symptoms of pneumonia vary with the age of the patient and the causative organism. They may develop suddenly or be preceded by an upper respiratory infection. The cough is dry at first, but gradually becomes productive. Fever rises as high as 103° to 104° F., and may fluctuate widely during a 24 hour period. The respiration rate may increase to 40 to 80 times per minute in infants, and in older children to 30 to 50 times per minute. Respirations are shallow in an attempt to reduce the amount of chest pain. Sternal retraction may be seen as the assisting muscles of respiration are brought into use. Flaring of the nostrils may appear. The child is listless and has a poor appetite. The patient tends to lie on his affected side.

Treatment. The patient is given a complete physical examination. The doctor gives particular attention to the examination of the child's chest. X-rays will confirm the diagnosis and determine whether there are complications. Blood specimens show a marked increase in the number of white blood cells (16,000 to 40,000 per cubic millimeter). The number of red blood cells and the amount of hemoglobin may be slightly reduced. The urine is dark amber in color, and there is a decrease in the amount voided. The specific gravity is high. Cultures are taken from the nose and throat to attempt to isolate the causative organism.

Antibiotics or sulfonamides are begun early in the disease to prevent it from obtaining a foothold. This is continued for four or five days after the temperature drops. Aspirin may be given to reduce fever. When indicated, oxygen is given for dyspnea or cyanosis. When treatment is begun early, the child is less restless and does not require as many sedatives or drugs to relieve pain. Since drug therapy has become so effective, many uncomplicated cases can be treated effectively at home.

Complications are not common under proper treatment. Abdominal distention due to a paralysis of a portion of the ileum is a serious difficulty, but occurs mainly in patients who have not received proper treatment.

If it is necessary for the patient to be admitted to the hospital, he is placed in isolation.

Nursing Care.   Nursing care in all types of pneumonia is basically the same. The age of the patient determines the nurse's approach and the type of equipment used. (The infant receives oxygen in the Isolette, whereas the older child requires a Croupette.)

Rest is an important part of the treatment of this disease. The nurse must organize her work so that she does not disturb the child unnecessarily.

The practical nurse checks the vital signs at regular intervals. During the acute stages, the temperature may rise as high as 103° to 104° F.* The nurse may be asked to give the child tepid sponge baths to help reduce this fever. Tepid water is used for children unless alcohol is specifically ordered. The nurse offers the older patient the bedpan before the procedure is begun.

SPONGE BATH PROCEDURE

Equipment.   Basin of tepid water, three facecloths, towel, two bath blankets, rubber sheet, icebag, hot water bottle.

Method
 1. Assemble the equipment at the bedside. Explain the procedure to the patient.
 2. Screen the child. Take and record temperature, pulse and respiration.
 3. Cover the patient with a bath blanket. Fanfold bedclothes to the foot of the bed. Place a rubber sheet and bath blanket beneath the patient.
 4. Remove the pillow from the bed. Remove patient's gown.
 5. Apply brief friction to the skin with a dry facecloth to stimulate it and to prevent chilling.
 6. Wash the patient's face and neck with tepid water.
 7. Lift the corner of the bath blanket and bathe the child's body, part by part. Use long strokes.
 8. Place moist, folded cloths over blood vessels that lie close to the skin (underarms and groin).
 9. Turn the patient and repeat the procedure, beginning with the neck, shoulder, back, and so forth.
10. Check color and pulse to be sure that the child is tolerating the procedure well.
11. When the bath is completed, pat the skin dry and cover the patient with only a sheet.
12. Remove the rubber sheet and blanket. Reapply the hospital gown.
13. Arrange pillows and bedding for the patient's comfort.
14. Take the patient's temperature within 30 minutes of the time the procedure ended, and record. If the temperature has not started to go down, check to see if the procedure should be repeated. Note: The temperature is not expected to drop to normal, but merely to a more reasonable level.
15. Chart: time procedure began, solution used, length of time administered, untoward reactions, patient's temperature before and after procedure.

---

*When a child is flushed with fever, *remove heavy clothing and blankets.*

The infant may merely be placed on a large turkish towel. He is covered by a receiving blanket. Older children may have an icebag placed on their head and a warm water bottle placed at their feet. This is not practical with the toddler.

The nurse encourages the child to take fluids. Small sips of water are offered frequently. If vomiting persists, parenteral fluids are given. It is important to provide an adequate fluid intake to avoid kidney complications when sulfonamides are used, and to maintain normal specific gravity of the urine. This also helps the body to excrete toxic substances via the urinary tract. The appetite of the child improves as his condition does.

The patient is turned *regularly*. Although this is painful, it is paramount to total recovery. The doctor will prescribe an analgesic to increase the patient's comfort.

The child is placed in isolation until otherwise ordered. A paper bag is pinned to his bed for the disposal of paper tissues, which are discarded according to hospital procedure.

The nurse observes the patient for unfavorable symptoms such as a weak, rapid pulse, cyanosis, distention, constipation, and disorientation. Although recovery from uncomplicated pneumonia is dramatic today, recuperation takes time.

Urinary System

NEPHROSIS

Description. Nephrosis is a kidney disease that is peculiar to young children (average age: two and one-half years). It is more common in boys than in girls, and the cause is not known. Children who suffer from nephrosis are unusually susceptible to other infections; many died from meningitis or peritonitis before modern drugs were discovered. Today, complications are rare. If a child can be carried through threats of infection, he has an even chance of surviving with a complete cure or of developing a chronic form of the disease which is fatal.

Symptoms. The characteristic symptom of nephrosis is *edema*. This occurs slowly; the child does not appear to be sick. It is noticed at first about the eyes and ankles, but later becomes generalized. The edema shifts with the position of the child during sleep. The patient gains weight because of the accumulation of this fluid. The abdomen may become so distended that *striae,* or stretch marks similar to those that appear on the skin of a pregnant woman, may occur. The child is pale, irritable, and listless, and has a poor appetite. Urine examination reveals albumin. The *glomeruli,* the working units of the kidneys which filter the blood, become damaged and allow albumin and blood cells to enter the

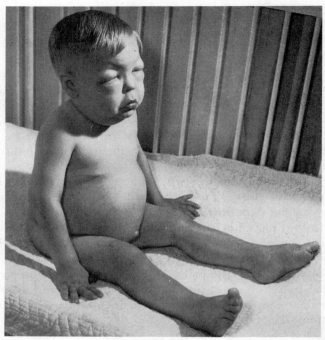

Figure 91. Nephrosis. (From Benz, G.: Pediatric Nursing. St. Louis, C. V. Mosby Co., 1967.)

urine. There is a fall in the level of protein in the blood, and a rise in cholesterol content. Vomiting and diarrhea may also be present.

Treatment

CONTROL OF EDEMA.   The child with nephrosis is given medications designed to increase the output of urine. Hormonal therapy is currently used for this purpose. Corticotropin is given parenterally. Prednisone, given when the condition is first recognized, has also proved valuable. The symptoms of this disease generally disappear when it is given daily for one month. Intermittent doses may be ordered between exacerbations. The therapy is carried out over a prolonged period of time. Since hormones mask the signs of infection, the patient must be watched closely for more subtle symptoms of illness. Prompt antibacterial therapy is begun when an acute infection is recognized. Diuretics have not generally been effective in reducing nephrotic edema.

DIET.   A well balanced diet high in protein is desirable, because protein is constantly being lost in the urine. The carbohydrate and fat content of the diet should be high enough to prevent protein from being used for energy. If either dietary protein or body protein is used for energy, the waste product urea is excreted through the kidneys, which increases their work load.* Salt-free diets may be ordered for short periods during the course of the disease, but they are generally not

*Mowry, Basic Nutrition and Diet Therapy for Nurses, 1966.

appealing to the child. Normal amounts of water are given unless otherwise ordered.

ASCITES.   Ascites, an abnormal collection of fluid in the peritoneal cavity, is seen in advanced cases of nephrosis. This fluid causes pressure on the heart and organs of respiration. The doctor removes some of this fluid by a procedure known as an *abdominal paracentesis* (*para-* beside + *centesis* puncture). Fluid may also accumulate in the chest. This is termed hydrothorax (*hydro-* water + *thorax-* chest).

MENTAL HYGIENE.   The doctor gives supportive care to the parents and child through the long course of this disease. Whenever possible the child is treated at home and brought to the hospital for special therapy only. Parents are instructed to keep a daily record of the child's weight, urinary proteins, and medications. Signs of infection, weight gain, and increased protein in the urine must be reported promptly. The child is allowed up and about after the acute stage of the illness subsides, so that he may participate in normal childhood activities.

Nursing Care.   The nursing care of the patient with nephrosis is of the greatest significance, because the nature of this disease is one that requires long-term therapy. The patient is admitted periodically and becomes a familiar personality to hospital personnel. The following factors are important in determining nursing care plans for the individual child.

CARE OF THE SKIN.   Good skin care is especially important during periods of marked edema. The skin is bathed daily and whenever necessary. Special attention is given to the neck, under arms, groin, and other moist areas of the body. The patient is handled gently to prevent the skin from being injured. The male genitals may become edematous. They are bathed and dusted with a soothing powder. When necessary, the scrotum is supported with a soft pad held in place by a T binder. Cotton is used to separate the skin surfaces to prevent a rash from forming.

POSITION.   The patient is turned frequently to prevent respiratory infection. A pillow placed between the knees when the patient is lying on his side prevents pressure on edematous organs. The child's head is elevated from time to time during the day to reduce edema of the eyelids, and to make the patient more comfortable. Swelling impairs the circulation of the lacrimal secretions. It may be necessary to bathe the eyes with normal saline to prevent the accumulation of exudate.

DIET.   The appetite of the patient is poor. Serve small quantities, attractively arranged on bright colored dishes. Serve his favorite foods if they are nutritious. Colored straws may also be used. Sit by the patient when feeding him. Relax and allow him plenty of time. If the child is able to feed himself, encourage him to do so. Whenever possible, remain with the patient during meals, for it is more enjoyable for him, particularly if he is in a private room. If the parents are available, the child can enjoy their company during meals.

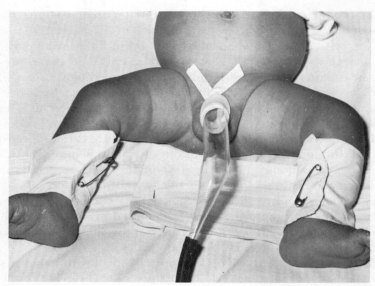

Figure 92. Procedure to be used for the collection of a 24 hour urine specimen from an infant boy. The collecting tube is held in place by adhesive tape. The ankle or extremity restraint is used to restrain the infant's legs. Note how the restraint is pinned in the middle in order to make it smaller. (From Marlow D.: Textbook of Pediatric Nursing, 1969.)

The fluid intake of the child is recorded following each meal. This is the responsibility of his nurse regardless of who feeds him. The nurse must instruct the parents to inform her of how much fluid has been taken. If she does not do this, the visitors may leave the hospital and the fluid balance of the day will not be accurate. The importance of keeping *proper fluid balance sheets* on patients with diseases of the kidneys cannot be overemphasized.

URINE. As stated previously, the patient's urine must be carefully measured. This is difficult with the toddler who is not toilet-trained or who has had a regression in urinary habits. The nurse must often estimate the amount. In such cases a careful check of the number of voidings is of particular value. The character, odor, and color of the urine are also important. If a 24 hour urine collection is ordered, *every* voided specimen within that time must be saved or the test will not be valid. If a specimen is discarded by accident, the nurse notifies her team leader at once. The infant is restrained for this procedure. (See Fig. 92.)

Determining the Specific Gravity of Urine. The practical nurse may be asked to measure the specific gravity of the urine. The normal range is 1.005 to 1.030. This is done in the following manner:

Equipment. Urinometer and Urine specimen.

1. Fill the test tube three-fourths full of urine.
2. Insert the bobbin of the urinometer. Spin it gently to be sure that it is not touching the sides of the container.
3. Take the reading from the bottom of the meniscus.
4. Record results.

Albumin Determination. The practical nurse working in a doctor's office or clinic may also be requested to test urine for albumin, i.e., protein. Normally little or no albumin is found in the urine of a healthy child. Reagent strips especially intended for this purpose are now available. The nurse dips the end of the strip into urine and compares it with a special color chart. Specific instructions accompany test materials.

The *heat and acetic acid method* to determine albumin may also be used:

Equipment. Test tube holder, 2 per cent acetic acid, dropper, urine specimen, Bunsen burner.

1. Fill the test tube two-thirds full of urine.
2. Add three to five drops of dilute acetic acid, 2 per cent.
3. Using a test tube holder, hold the upper portion over a Bunsen burner and bring it to a boil.
4. Add a few more drops of acid.
5. Reheat.
6. If albumin is present, a cloudy precipitate forms after the acid has been added. It helps to examine the test tube against a black background to detect faint clouds.
7. Record results.

The patient is weighed two or three times a week to determine changes in the degree of edema. He is weighed on the same scale each time, and at about the same time of day.

The nurse makes every effort to protect her patient from exposure to upper respiratory infections. She washes her hands carefully before caring for him. The child who is up and about must not be allowed to wander into areas where he would be in danger of contracting an infection.

The vital signs of a patient with nephrosis are taken regularly. Ordinarily, there is no elevation of temperature unless there is an infection present. Blood pressure remains normal. If there is an increase in blood pressure it must be reported. A reading that remains high over a period of time is a grave sign.

Parental guidance and support should be given by all members of the nursing team. Rooming-in is desirable but not always possible. The parents should be allowed to visit the patient as often as they can. The child with nephrosis is kept under close medical supervision over an extended period of time.

The Ear

DEAFNESS

Description. The deaf child presents special challenges to the nursing team. He may be hospitalized for direct evaluation and treatment of his hearing loss, or he may have other medical or surgical problems that may or may not be related to his deafness. The student should have a basic knowledge of the problems that confront the deaf child in order to give him comprehensive nursing care.

The inner ear is fully formed during the first months of prenatal life. If an expectant mother contracts German measles or other virus infections during this period, the child may be born with a hearing loss, which is termed congenital deafness. Deafness can also be acquired. Such infectious diseases as measles, mumps, chicken pox, or meningitis can result in various degrees of hearing loss. The common cold, certain allergies, and ear infections may also be responsible.

The old adage "An ounce of prevention is worth a pound of cure" is particularly applicable to the invisible handicap, deafness. Excessive cleansing of the ear can be damaging, especially if one probes into the canal with such objects as a hairpin. If a foreign object is in the ear, consult a doctor. Persons who try to remove it themselves may cause further damage.

The nurse must stress the importance of proper immunization during childhood to prevent many of the communicable diseases. Vaccines against regular measles (rubeola), mumps, and German measles (rubella) are now available. The child should be taken to the doctor for periodic health examinations. Early diagnosis and treatment of the deaf child is important to prevent adverse physical and mental complications from developing. Members of the health team concerned with the child who is hard of hearing include the physician, otologist, audiologist, speech therapist, specially trained teachers, social worker, psychologist, nurse and the child's family.

The various degrees of deafness range from complete bilateral to so mild that the problem is never discovered. Bilateral deafness is that which affects both ears. If this is complete, the child misses all of the pleasures that sound brings to life, and has difficulty in communication since children learn to talk through imitating what they hear. Behavior problems arise since the child does not understand directions. He may become aggressive to other children in his attempt to communicate with them. If ridiculed by playmates, his personality development will be affected. Unless the child is helped he will become socially isolated. and will be unable to attend school.

Partial bilateral deafness may be responsible for behavior problems and poor progress in school. This may be caused by chronic infections such as otitis media, or by blockage of the eustachian tube. It may be a warning signal of more serious defects in later life. Children who are deaf in one ear are less handicapped, if the hearing in the other ear is normal.

Treatment and Nursing Care. Early diagnosis and prompt treatment are primary requisites, regardless of the patient's age. Complete bilateral deafness is usually discovered during infancy. Partial deafness may be unrecognized until the child begins school. Many hearing problems are detected then by the use of standard hearing tests. A machine called an *audiometer* is used. Each child puts on an earphone which is connected to it. When the audiometer is turned on it makes various noises and pitches of sound. The child raises his hand as he hears the tones. The results of these tests are interpreted by specialists in this field. When a test shows that the child is hard of hearing he is then given a careful examination by an otologist, or ear specialist. School children should be tested every three years.

Children who suffer a severe loss of hearing need more extensive help from special hearing and speech centers. The decision of whether the child should attempt special classes in a regular school or attend a school for the deaf is decided on an individual basis. Some children who spend a few years in a school for the deaf can be advanced to a regular school. These children need to begin their education early, to aid them in catching up on that which they have missed since infancy.

Various methods are used to bring the child into the world of sound. Lip reading, sign language, writing, visual aids, music, and amplified sound are but a few. Today, the deaf child is taught to speak so that others in his environment can comprehend him. This is not accomplished overnight. If a hearing aid is indicated, the child is equipped with one and taught how to use it. The parents are instructed in means of communication which will coincide with that used by the teachers. Unfortunately, the number of good schools with qualified teachers is at a minimum at present.

Role of the Practical Nurse. The practical nurse must be aware of the symptoms of deafness in the child. The infant who makes no verbal attempts by the eighteenth month of life should undergo a complete physical examination. Poor school performance and behavior problems may also be signs of deafness. The nurse should inquire into the facilities that are available in her community for such a patient. Since the prevention of this disease is so important, the practical nurse should take advantage of opportunities to demonstrate and teach proper hygiene of the ears to the child and his family. She must stress the importance of baby shots to parents with newborns. Proper safety measures must be taken to prevent injury to the ears from trauma to the head, especially during the toddler period.

The deaf child in the hospital needs the same opportunities to develop a healthy personality as the child who does not have this handicap. When the nurse approaches the deaf child she should smile. Her

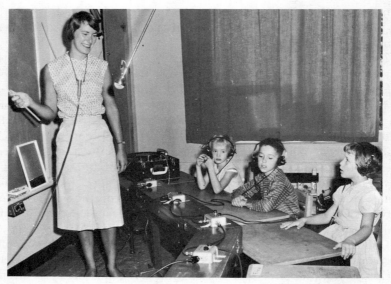

Figure 93. The deaf child is brought out of his silent world through the use of amplified sound and other special techniques. (Courtesy of Crotched Mountain School for the Deaf, Greenfield, N.H.)

manner relates many things to this patient, especially if there is a severe communication problem. Face the child when you speak to him, and position yourself so that you are at his eye level. Use short sentences when you speak, rather than separate words. Speak clearly in a natural tone. It is not necessary to exaggerate speech. The nurse who is relaxed in her manner with the patient will create an atmosphere which others will follow.

If the child is able to write, he can also use this as a means of communication. Have the patient read aloud what he has written. In this way you will become better accustomed to his speech. Regression in speech patterns may occur during hospitalization. Do not assume that because the child is not talking a great deal he does not understand what is being said to him. Repeat or reword certain statements as you would with any child.

Determine whether or not the child fully understands what you ask of him. Deaf people tend to answer "yes" or "no" before they have caught the complete meaning of the question. When you have finished explaining a procedure to the patient, question him to be sure that he understands what is expected of him. This is a good point to bear in mind in relation to all small children who are in the hospital. Children respond to nurses who are interested and patient enough to listen to what they say.

The practical nurse is often called upon to assist the physician in an ear examination. She holds the toddler in her lap with his head pressed against her chest. She places one hand on the child's forehead and the other securely around his body. The head is held still so that the delicate ear canal will not be injured by the *otoscope*. The doctor may need cotton swabs to remove excess secretion from the external ear. The ear *specula* (funnel-shaped devices that come in direct contact with the ear) must be washed and disinfected following each use.

A hearing aid is expensive and invaluable to the patient. See that it is placed in a safe place when it is not in use. When the patient goes to surgery it should be placed in the hospital safe. Check the pockets of hospital gowns before placing them in the laundry chute. Sometimes a patient puts his hearing aid there for convenience. The nurse can gain valuable information concerning the use of the particular hearing aid from the parents of the child.

Poisoning

SALICYLATE POISONING

Description. More children are poisoned by aspirin than by any other drug. It is used in most homes and often is stored carelessly on bedside stands or in mother's purse. This drug acts rapidly but is excreted slowly. Although most cases of aspirin poisoning are of an emergency nature, a child may be unknowingly poisoned by parents who are not aware of its accumulative effect. It is wise, therefore, to administer

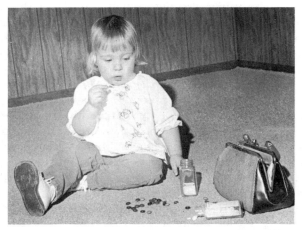

Figure 94. Mother's purse should be kept away from the toddler. It may contain aspirin or other medications.

aspirin sparingly when needed, but it is even better to use it only under the direction of a physician.

Measures are being taken to reduce aspirin poisoning. Children's aspirin must now be packaged with only 36 tablets to a bottle. Safety caps make it more difficult for a toddler to open medicine. Nonetheless, candy-flavored medicine has an appeal to the determined youngster; therefore, safeguards in storage must always be maintained. *Oil of wintergreen* (methyl salicylate) is also extremely hazardous when mistakenly administered as cough medicine or swallowed by the curious child. It is sometimes used as a home remedy for arthritic pains. Even a dosage as small as 1 teaspoon can cause the death of a child.

Symptoms. The symptoms of salicylate poisoning are varied and often individual. In general, the younger the child the more serious the overdose. Mild poisoning may consist of ringing in the ears, dizziness, anorexia, sweating, nausea, vomiting, and diarrhea. Hyperpnea (*hyper-* above + *pnea-* breathing) is an early symptom of more serious trouble. The patient's respirations are increased and deeper than usual, much like the breathing evidenced after one exercises. This is because the respiratory center is stimulated by the drug. Dehydration, acidosis, high fever, convulsions, and coma may follow. Bleeding is sometimes seen since excessive aspirin inhibits the formation of prothrombin necessary for normal blood clotting.

Treatment and Nursing Care. There is no specific antidote for salicylate poisoning; therefore, treatment is aimed at relieving the patient's symptoms. In mild cases of poisoning, the drug is discontinued and fluids are forced. In cases where a child has swallowed an unspecified amount, gastric lavage is performed. A blood sample is taken to detect the level of salicylate poisoning. The doctor may request that the child be admitted to the hospital for observation. A sponge bath may be given to reduce fever. The patient's vital signs are closely observed and recorded. The nurse also determines the pH of the urine. When intravenous fluids are necessary to correct electrolyte imbalance and rid the body of toxins, the child's intake and output of fluid is charted hourly.

Oxygen may be indicated. Vitamin K is administered to control the bleeding. Peritoneal dialysis (*peritoneum-* + *dialysis-* passing of a solute through a membrane) is a therapeutic measure used in acute renal failure. The therapy utilizes the principles of osmosis and diffusion through the semipermeable peritoneal membrane, the purpose being to remove toxic substances from the blood. The artificial kidney is another method used for essentially this purpose. An exchange transfusion may also be given. In severe poisoning cases, the latter procedures are executed in an attempt to save the life of the child.

The practical nurse, realizing the above, must constantly practice and teach safety measures for the prevention of such tragedies. She should also scrutinize treatment, utility rooms, and drug baskets to ensure that nothing poisonous is within reach of ambulatory patients.

LEAD POISONING

Description.   Lead poisoning results when a child repeatedly ingests substances which contain lead. This condition is most common between the ages of one and one half and three. The incidence is increased in tenement areas of large cities. The patient chews on window sills and stair rails. He ingests flakes of paint, putty, or crumbled plaster. This lead can have a lasting effect on the nervous system — mental retardation may occur in severe cases.

Symptoms.   The symptoms occur gradually and range from mild to severe. Because the infant or young child's central nervous system is extremely vulnerable, severe symptoms of encephalitis may follow a relatively short period of exposure. The lead settles in the soft tissues and bones and is excreted in the urine. In the beginning weakness, weight loss, anorexia, palor, irritability, vomiting, abdominal pain, and constipation may be seen. In the later stages signs of anemia and nervous system involvement are evidenced, e.g., muscular incoordination, neuritis, convulsions, encephalitis.

Treatment and Nursing Care.   Blood and urine tests are performed to determine the amount of lead in the system. X-rays of the long bones will also evidence deposits of lead. The history of the patient may reveal *pica*. This is a condition in which the child has a perverted appetite. He will eat a variety of things which most persons consider unpalatable, e.g., sand, grass, wool, glass, plaster, coal, animal droppings, and paint from furniture. This tendency is sometimes seen in neurotic children and is common in the mentally retarded. An underlying nutritional disturbance may also account for it.

Treatment is aimed at reducing the concentration of lead in the tissues and blood and promoting its deposit in the bones. This is done in two ways. First, the child is removed from the source of lead and is closely supervised. Secondly, large amounts of milk are given as milk forms lead salts which are poorly absorbed by the intestine. EDTA (ethylenediamine tetracetic acid) is given to render the lead nontoxic and to increase its excretion in the urine, thus decreasing its level in the blood. It is usually given intravenously. Complete deleading takes several months and retreatment may be necessary when the child has an acute infection or other metabolic disturbance. The prognosis is generally poor. About one-half of the affected infants and children show some signs of encephalitis and the mortality rate of these is about 25 per cent.

Prevention of this condition is foremost. Lead paint should not be used on children's toys or furniture. Instead use paint marked for indoor use or that which conforms to American standards z66.1-1955 for use on surfaces that might be chewed by children. The practical nurse should stress the importance of this to parents of small children. Close observation of children in this age group also acts as a deterrent. The nurse and the mother should provide opportunities for the toddler to suck and chew on safe objects such as a teething ring or wash cloth during the oral stage of development, this will meet the normal sucking and chewing need. Nursing care is symptomatic. Unnecessary handling of the patient is avoided to prevent stimulating the central nervous system. Observation and charting of convulsions are discussed on page 94. Indications of respiratory distress are reported immediately. The services of the public health nurse are valuable in investigating the environment of the child and in continuing the education of the parents.

CORROSIVE STRICTURES

Description.   Children who have ingested such toxic substances as lye, bleach, ammonia, or drain cleaners are frequently seen in hospital emergency rooms. The destruction varies from slight pharyngitis and esophagitis to death in extreme cases.

Symptoms.   The first mouthful that is swallowed is painful and acts as a deterrent to some children; however, the damage is done. Swelling of the lips, chin, tongue, throat, and esophagus occurs. Ulcerations appear on the mucous membranes. The patient is unable to swallow. Edema may interfere with breathing; in this case a tracheotomy is necessary. If the patient survives, an esophageal stricture generally develops within a short period of time. This is evidenced by anorexia and difficult swallowing.

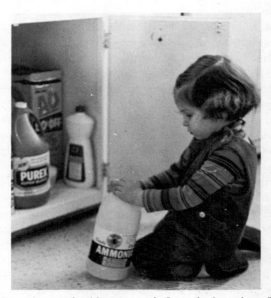

Figure 95.   Corrosive esophagitis may result from the ingestion of lye or ammonia, causing prolonged and intermittent hospitalization.

Treatment.   An antidote for the particular caustic is given immediately. Olive oil is applied to the patient's lips and excoriated areas in an attempt to make him more comfortable. An analgesic is given intramuscularly. Emetics or lavage are not advocated because of the danger of perforating the esophagus or stomach. The patient is given intravenous fluids initially. A gastrostomy may be necessary for continued feedings. To prevent strictures of the esophagus, the physician passes a weighted tube (bougie) into the esophagus. The catheter is passed daily and each time its size is increased (from size 16 French mercury-filled bougie to a number 30 or 32). This is begun 24 to 48 hours after the accident and is continued daily for two weeks. The treatments are gradually reduced; however, the patient may require dilations for several years after the original accident. It is not uncommon to see a 5 year old child in for treatment of a stricture obtained at the age of two. The use of cortisone in conjunction with the dilatation has been found useful in reducing the inflammation and lessening the possibilities of stricture. In severe cases surgical procedures are necessary.

Nursing Care.   The nursing considerations again stress the importance of prevention and education of the public. Toxic substances should never be placed in food containers such as pop bottles or water glasses. Children should not be allowed to play in the family garage unless it has been made "child proof," or unless an adult is closely supervising the activity. The practical nurse should also stress the potential dangers of furniture polish, kerosene, ant traps, insecticides, and toilet bowel cleaners.

A gastrostomy (*gastro-* stomach + *stoma-* opening) is made for the purpose of introducing food directly into the stomach through the abdominal wall. This is done by means of a surgically placed tube. The practical nurse may be asked to administer such feedings.

GASTROSTOMY TUBE FEEDING

Equipment.   Tray with warmed formula, sterile funnel, or asepto syringe without bulb, 15 to 30 cc. of sterile water to flush tube as ordered.

Method
1. Attach syringe to gastrostomy tube. Fill with formula. Remove clamp. (This prevents air from entering the stomach and causing distention.)
2. Elevate asepto syringe. Allow formula to flow slowly by gravity — force should not be used.
3. Continue to add formula to the syringe before it empties completely.
4. Clamp the tube as the final formula or water is passing through the lower part of the syringe. (Note: In infants some physicians may prefer that the gastrostomy tube remain open at all times to produce a safety valve in the event that the baby vomits. In such cases the tube is elevated above the patient's body with the asepto syringe barrel attached.
5. Whenever possible hold the patient quietly after feeding.
6. Record the type (gastrostomy feeding), the amount given, and how the patient tolerated the procedure. If the patient is on measured fluids record on intake and output sheet.

Good oral hygiene is essential. It is administered gently to prevent injury to damaged tissues. The skin around the gastrostomy tube must be kept clean and dry in order to prevent excoriations. The psychological needs of the child are important since he is not receiving satisfactory sucking and ingesting of foods in the normal manner. He should be given additional attention and love by cuddling and other forms of contact whenever feasible.

STUDY QUESTIONS

1. What measures can the practical nurse take to prevent contractures from developing in the bedridden patient?
2. Define the following: Bradford frame, Croupette, brace, steam inhalator.
3. What facilities are available in your community for the following handicaps: cerebral palsy, deafness, blindness, and mental retardation?
4. Johnny, age two, fell from your front steps and struck his head on the pavement. He is crying loudly but you cannot see any visible cuts. What would you do immediately in this situation? Later on?
5. Ann, age four, suffered a fractured femur in a fall from a tree. She has been hospitalized for three weeks in Bryant traction. What factors would you consider in planning her daily care?
6. Frank, age two and a half, was admitted with a diagnosis of nephrosis. He has little interest in food. Discuss measures that would be effective in encouraging him to eat.
7. List the symptoms of croup. What is the purpose of the Croupette?
8. Define primary and secondary pneumonia. Discuss the nursing care of patients with pneumonia.
9. Your are assigned to a child with a fatal illness. What responsibilities do you have to the child? His parents? Yourself? Be prepared to discuss your answer in class.
10. Anthony, age seven, is admitted for an appendectomy. You notice he is wearing a hearing aid. What additional information should you obtain from his parents to make his adjustment to the hospital a satisfactory one?
11. What measures can be taken to reduce aspirin poisoning in the home?
12. Define the following terms: bougie, gastrostomy, pica.

BIBLIOGRAPHY

Air-Shields, Inc.: The Croupette. Hatboro, Pa.
Benz, G.: Pediatric Nursing. St. Louis, C. V. Mosby Co., 1964.
Blake, F., and Wright, F. H.: Essentials of Pediatric Nursing. 7th Ed. Philadelphia, J. B. Lippincott Co., 1963.

Broadribb, V.: Foundations of Pediatric Nursing. Philadelphia, J. B. Lippincott Co., 1967.
Canfield, N.: Save Your Child's Hearing. Better Hearing, Zenith Radio Corporation, 1958.
Geis, D., and Lambertz, S.: Acute Respiratory Infections in Young Children, Amer. J. Nurs. 68:294-295, 1968.
Latham, H., and Heckel, R.: Pediatric Nursing. St. Louis, C. V. Mosby Co., 1967.
Leifer, G.: Principles and Techniques in Pediatric Nursing. Philadelphia, W. B. Saunders Co., 1965.
Marlow, D.: Textbook of Pediatric Nursing. 3rd Ed. Philadelphia, W. B. Saunders Co. 1969.
Mason, M.: Basic Medical-Surgical Nursing. New York, The Macmillan Co., 1959.
Mowry, L.: Basic Nutrition and Diet Therapy for Nurses. 3rd Ed. St. Louis, The C. V. Mosby Co., 1966.
Nelson, W. (Editor): Textbook of Pediatrics. 9th Ed. Philadelphia, W. B. Saunders Co., 1969.
Pratt, G.: Oral Education for Deaf Children. Volta Bureau, Washington 7, D. C.
Price, A.: The Art, Science and Spirit of Nursing. 3rd Ed. Philadelphia, W. B. Saunders Co., 1965.
Rapier, D., et al.: Practical Nursing, 3rd Ed. St. Louis, The C. V. Mosby Co., 1966.
Spock, B.: Baby and Child Care. Rev. Ed. New York, Duell, Sloan and Pearce, Inc., 1968.
United States Department of Health, Education, and Welfare: The Child Who Is Hard of Hearing. United States Government Printing Office, 1953.

Chapter 11

THE PRESCHOOL CHILD

VOCABULARY

Aggressive	*Guidance*
Angry	*Imaginative*
Cooperate	*Independent*
Curious	*Relax*
Discipline	*Social*
Gait	*Strange*

GENERAL CHARACTERISTICS

The child from three to six is often referred to as the preschool child. This period is marked by a slowing down of the growth process. The infant who tripled his birth weight at one year, has only doubled his one year weight by the age of six. For instance, the baby who weighs 20 pounds on his first birthday will probably weigh about 40 pounds by his sixth. The child between three and six grows taller and loses the chubbiness seen during the toddler period. Appetite fluctuates widely. The normal pulse rate is 90 to 110. The rate of respirations during relaxation is about 20 per minute. The systolic blood pressure is about 85 to 90 mm. Hg; the diastolic is about 60 mm. Hg.

The preschool child has good control of his muscles and participates in vigorous play activities. He becomes more adept at using old skills as each year passes. He can swing and jump higher. His gait resembles that of an adult. He is quicker and has more confidence in himself than he did as a toddler.

While the preschool age may seem more or less quiet and steady in respect to physical development, certain difficulties stem from increased independence, life in a social world, and the beginning consciousness of what is right and wrong.

PHYSICAL, MENTAL, EMOTIONAL AND SOCIAL DEVELOPMENT

The Trusting Three's

The three year old is a delight to his parents. He is helpful and can partake in simple household chores (see Fig. 96). He obtains articles

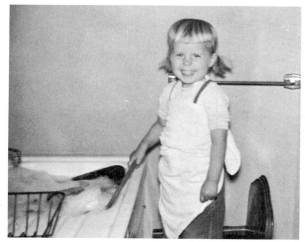

Figure 96.   Becky, age three, enjoys helping Mom.

when directed, and returns them to the proper place. The three year old comes very close to the ideal picture that parents have in mind of their child. He is a living example that their guidance during the terrible two's has been rewarded. Temper tantrums are less frequent, and in general he is a pretty good guy (see Fig. 97). Of course, he still is his individual self, but he seems to be able to direct his primitive instincts better than previously. He can help to dress and undress himself, uses the toilet, and washes his hands. He eats independently, and his table manners have improved.

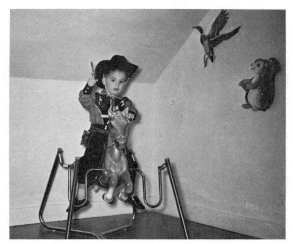

Figure 97.   The three year old is "the good guy." His play is imaginative.

Two year old girl	Three year old girl
The rug	Hey, I found Captain Kangaroo
The pretty rug	Mummy?
Table	Can I have this?
Dish	What shall I fix with this?
Doggy tired	What did you found?
The book fall down	Won't it be fun to play with these?
Want hankie	I show you how to play animals
Other side	Hey, this is my dollie
Oh, other side	And then now I will line all mine up like this

Figure 98. In language, what a difference a year makes. The above list contains the verbatim comments of two small girls, both of whom were playing with toys in the presence of their mothers and other adults. Note the much greater language skill of the three year old, including her ability to ask questions. (From Psychology: An Introduction. By Kagan and Havemann, Harcourt, Brace and World, New York, 1968, and The First Two Years. Institute of Child Welfare Monograph No. 7. By Mary M. Shirley, University of Minnesota Press, Minneapolis. Copyright 1933 by University of Minnesota.)

The three year old talks in longer sentences and can express his thoughts: "What are you doing?" "Where is Daddy?" He is more company to his parents because he can verbally share his experiences with them. He is imaginative and talks to his toys, and imitates what he sees about him. Soon he begins to make friends outside of the immediate family. Since he can now converse with playmates, he finds satisfaction in joining their activities. The three year old does not play cooperatively for long periods of time, but at least it's a start. Much of his play still consists of watching others, but now he can offer verbal advice, should he feel the need. He can ask others to "come out and play." If the three year old is placed in a strange situation with children he does not know, he commonly reverts to "parallel play" because it is more comfortable to him.

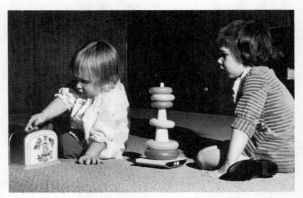

Figure 99. Much of the play of the three year old consists of watching others.

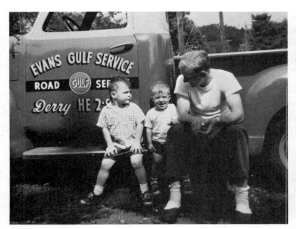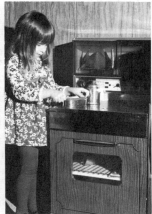

Figure 100. *A,* the child identifies himself with the parent of the same sex. *B,* little girl at stove.

At this time, there is a change in the relationship of the child and his family. He begins to find enjoyment away from Mom and Dad, although he wants them to be right there when needed. He begins to lose some of his interest in Mother, who up to this time has been more or less his total world. Father's prestige begins to increase. Romantic attachment to the parent of the opposite sex is seen during this period. Johnny wants "to marry Mommy" when he grows up. The child also begins to identify himself with the parent of the same sex (see Fig. 100 *A* and *B*).

The preschool child has more fears than the infant or older child. Some of the many causes of this are increased intelligence which enables him to recognize potential dangers, the development of memory, and graded independence which brings him in contact with many new situations. The toddler is not afraid of walking in the street because he does not know any better. The preschool child realizes that trucks can injure him, and therefore he worries about crossing the street. This type of fear is grounded, but many others are not. The fear of bodily harm is particularly peculiar to this stage. The little boy who discovers that baby sister is made differently worries that perhaps she has been injured. He wonders if this will happen to him. Masturbation is common during this stage as the child attempts to reassure himself that he is all right. Other common fears include fear of animals, fear of the dark, and fear of strangers. A little night wanderer is typical of this age group.

The preschool child becomes angry when others attempt to take his possessions. He grabs, slaps, and hangs on to them for dear life. He becomes very distraught if toys do not work the way they should. Being disturbed from play is resented. He is sensitive, and his feelings are easily hurt. It is well to bear in mind that much of the unpleasant social behavior seen during this time is normal and necessary to the child's total pattern of development.

The Frustrating Fours

Four years is a stormy age. The child is not as eager and willing as he was at three, is more aggressive, and likes to show off. He is eager to let others known he is superior, and is prone to pick on his playmates, often taking sides and making life difficult for the child who does not measure up to his standards. The child of four is boisterous, tattles on others and may begin to swear if he is around children or adults who use profanity. Personal family activities are repeated with an amazing sense of recall, but where his bicycle has been left is forgotten. At this age the child becomes very interested in how old he is, and wants to know the exact age of each playmate. It bolsters his ego to known that he is older than someone else in the group. He also becomes interested in the relationship of one person to another: Timmy is his brother, but also Daddy's son and so forth.

The four year old can use scissors with success. He can lace his shoes. Vocabulary has increased to about 1500 words. He runs simple errands, and can play for longer periods of time with others. Many feats are done for a purpose. For instance, he no longer runs just for the sake of running. Instead, he runs to get some place or see something. He is imaginative and likes to pretend he's a fireman or cowboy. He is beginning to enjoy playing with friends of the same sex better than those of the opposite sex.

The preschool child enjoys simple toys. Raw materials are more appealing than toys that are ready made and complete in themselves (see Fig. 102). An old cardboard box which can be moved about and climbed into is more fun than a doll house with tiny furniture. A box of sand or

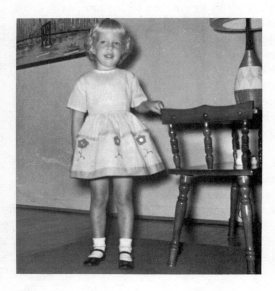

Figure 101. Charla, at four, shows her increased poise.

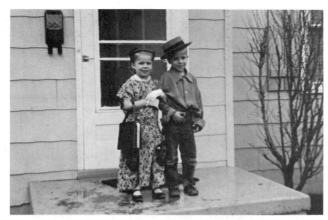

Figure 102. "Let's make believe." Old clothing of adults appeals to the preschool child.

colored pebbles can be made into roads and mountains. A small mirror becomes a lake. On rainy days he can use a piece of soap and write on the window pane. It's harmless and easily removed. In nice weather, he can have some water and a brush to paint the outside of the house. Today, parents tend to shower their children with ready made toys instead of selecting material that is absorbing to the child.

Stories that interest the young child depict his daily experiences. If the story has a simple plot, it must be related to what he understands to hold his interest. He also enjoys music; he likes records he can march around to and simple instruments he can shake or bang. Make up a song about his daily life and watch his reaction.

The child's curiosity concerning sex continues to heighten. If the parents answered his questions simply, they should not be alarmed to find him checking up on them. It is common for children of this age to take down their panties in front of the opposite sex. They discuss their differences with their friend. Older children who are more sensitive about their bodies should be told that this is a natural curiosity seen in small children. This may rid them of guilt feelings which they might harbor, particularly if they participated in similar activities during the preschool period. The child is as matter-of-fact about these investigations as he would be about any other learning experience, and is easily distracted to more socially acceptable forms of behavior.

Between three and four, the child begins to wonder about death and dying. He may be the cowboy who shoots the Indian dead, or he may witness a situation in which an animal is killed. His questions are very direct. "What is dead? Will I die?" There are no set answers to these inquiries. The religion of the family plays an important role as to the interpretations of this complex phenomenon.

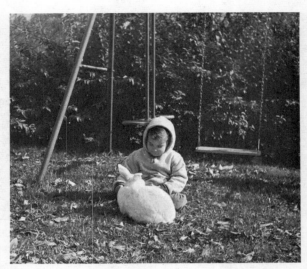

Figure 103.   The preschool child's knowledge of reproduction can be augmented by observing nature's creatures.

Perhaps the child can be acquainted with death through objects that are not of particular significance to him. For instance, the flower dies at the end of summer. It doesn't bloom any more. It no longer needs sunshine or water, for it is not alive. Usually the young child realizes that others die, but he does not relate it to himself. If he continues to pursue the question of whether or not he will die, parents should be casual and reassure him that people do not generally die until they have lived a long and happy life. Of course, as he grows older he will discover that sometimes children do die. The underlying idea nevertheless is to encourage questions as they appear and gradually help him to accept the truth without undue fear. Reality is often unpleasant, but children must be prepared to accept it.

The Fascinating Five's

Five is a comfortable age. The child is more responsible, enjoys doing what is expected of him, has more patience, and likes to finish what he has started. The five year old is serious about what he can and cannot do. He talks constantly, and is inquisitive about his environment. He wants to do things right, and seeks answers to his questions from those whom he considers "know" the answers. The five year old can play games governed by rules. He is less fearful because he feels his environment is controlled by authorities. The worries that he does have are not as profound as they were at an earlier age.

The physical growth of the five year old is not particularly outstanding. His height may increase two to three inches, and he may gain three to six pounds. The variations in height and weight of a group of five year olds is remarkable. The child may begin to lose his deciduous teeth at this time. He can run and play games simultaneously, can jump three or four steps at once, and can tell a penny from a nickel or a dime. He can name the days of the week, and understands what a week-long vacation is. The child of five can usually print his first name.

The five year old can ride a tricycle around the playground with speed and dexterity. He can use a hammer to pound nails. Adults should encourage him to develop motor skills and not be continually reminding him to "be careful." (See Fig. 104.) The practice that he gets will enable him to compete with others during the school age period, and will increase his confidence in his own abilities. As at any age level, he should not be scorned for failure to measure up to adult standards. Overdirection by solicitous adults is damaging. The child has to learn to do the task himself in order for the experience to be satisfying.

The amount and type of television programs that parents allow the preschool child to watch is a topic of current discussion. Although the child enjoyed it at three or four, it was usually for short periods of time. He could not understand much of what was going on. The five year old has better comprehension, and may spend a great deal of time before it. The plan of management differs with each family. Whatever is decided needs to be discussed with the child. Television should not be allowed to interfere with good health habits of the child, e.g., sleep, meals, physical activity. Most parents find that children do not insist on watching television if there is something better to do.

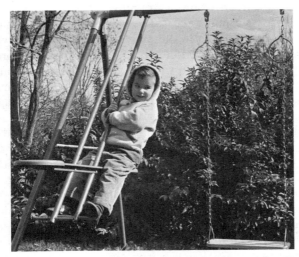

Figure 104. The preschool child has good control of his muscles. He becomes more self-confident as his motor skills increase.

GUIDING THE PRESCHOOL CHILD

Discipline

Much has been written on the subject of discipline, and it has changed considerably with the passing of time. Today, authorities place a great deal of importance on development of a continuous, warm relationship between the child and his parents. This they feel prevents many problems. Nevertheless, situations do occur which require attention. The following is a brief discussion of some of the underlying factors to be considered.

One of the most important things for parents to keep in mind is that the penalty must be directed to the *seriousness* of the act and *not* the child. The child must feel that his parents love him *always*, but that they do not always love *what* he does. How often have you heard, "Mommy won't love you if you do such and such." Instead, a mother should say, "Jimmy, Mommy loves you but you must not bring the sand into the house," and so forth. Then naturally if he cannot bring the sand in on Monday, it can't be brought in on Tuesday, or Wednesday, or any other day. Being consistent is one of the hardest things for adults to do.

Also, one should not expect more of the child when others are around. A child is sometimes punished because of fear that others will pass judgment on the parents if they do not. For instance, there is the old problem of jumping on the beds. Johnny perhaps gets in a few jumps without alarming anyone, until Grandma arrives on the scene. Then mother feels pressured to prohibit the act which she would otherwise allow. This does not mean that children should be allowed to jump on beds; it is merely an example for illustration.

Spankings for the most part are not effective. The child associates the fury of the parents with the pain rather than the wrong deed, because anger is the most predominant factor in the situation. Thus, the real value of the spanking is lost. Bodily punishment administered by a parent as a release for his own pent-up emotions is not desirable. To be effective, discipline must be given at the time the incident occurs.

Rewarding the child for good deeds is a positive and effective method of discipline. This is done by the use of praise, and should not be confused with bribery. It can always be tied in with the act: "Thank you, Susy, for picking up your toys." As the child understands more, privileges can be withheld, but the child must know what it is all about. Standard punishment cannot be used in all situations; it is easier, but is not as effective as suiting the penalty to the individual misdemeanor. Parents should take a middle-of-the road stand: not too strict or too lenient. This sounds difficult, but it is aided by the natural bond of love and friendship that exists between the child and his parents.

Bad Language

Parents express astonishment at the words that flow from the mouths of their sweet little children during the preschool period. This is inevitable. The practical nurse should suppress her first desire to emphatically shout her disapproval. The small child delights in attention, and it does not matter, unfortunately, whether this attention is good or bad. Swearing at this time is not particularly meaningful, since the child is merely imitating what he hears, and it does not have any real significance to him. He uses it as a way of identifying himself with the older children in the neighborhood, and to shock adults. One mother dealt with this problem in the following way: "Johnny, Mommy doesn't mind if you hear or know what that word means, but we don't use it in our home anymore than you would think of going outdoors without your clothes on." Johnny felt free to discuss what he heard with his mother, and shortly thereafter his interest was taken up by other subjects.

Jealousy

Jealousy is a normal response to actual, supposed, or threatened loss of affection.* The child or adult feels insecure in his relationship with the person he loves. The closer a child is to his mother, the greater his fear of losing her. The only child envies the new baby. He loves him, but at the same time resents his presence. He cannot understand the turmoil that is taking place within himself (see Fig. 105). Jealously of a new baby is strongest in children under five, and is shown in various ways. The child may be aggressive, and bite, pinch, and so forth, or he may be rather discreet and hug and kiss the baby with a determined look on his face. Another common situation occurs when the child attempts to identify himself with the baby. He reverts to wetting the bed or wants to be powdered after he urinates. Some four year olds even try the bottle, but it is usually a big disappointment to them.

The preschool child may be jealous of the attention that his mother gives to his father. He may also envy the children he plays with, if they have bigger and better toys than he has. The school age child is more often jealous of those who are more athletic or popular. There is less jealousy in an only child, since he is the center of attention, and has only a minimum of rivals. Children of varied ages in one family are apt to feel that the younger ones are "pets," or, in reverse, that the older ones have more special privileges.

Parents can help to eliminate jealousy by the proper management of the individual occurrence. Preparing the young child for the arrival of the new baby will lessen the blow. He should not be made to think that he is being crowded. If the new baby is going to occupy his crib, it is best

---

*Hurlock, p. 242.

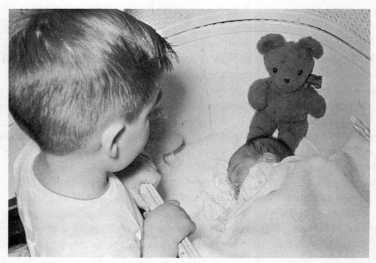

Figure 105.   Dougie, age four, has mixed emotions about the arrival of his new sister.

to get the older child happily settled in a large bed before the baby is born. The child should feel that he is helping with the care of the infant. Parents can inflate his ego from time to time by reminding him of the many activities that he can do which the new baby cannot. If it is convenient, the new baby is given his bath or one of his feedings while junior is asleep. In this way he will miss out on one of the occasions in which the mother shows the newborn affection for a relatively long period of time. Some persons feel that giving the child a pet to care for at this time helps. The mother of quintuplets recently expressed her delight that each of the five children at home would have a baby to care for. Unfortunately most people are not that lucky.

If the child intends to hit the baby or another child, they must be separated, but the one who has caused or is about to cause the injury needs as much if not more attention than the victim. Aggressiveness similar to this is seen when the child is made to share his toys. It is even more difficult for him to learn to share his mother, so he must be given time to adjust to new situations. The child should be assured that he is loved, but also told that he cannot injure others.

NURSERY SCHOOL

The change from home to nursery school is a big step toward independence. At this age the child is adjusting to the outside world as well as to the family group. Some children have the complicating factor of a new baby in the house. The child also finds at this time that his

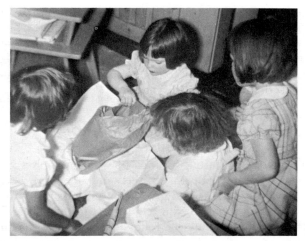

Figure 106. Socialization is an important phase of the preschool period. Children begin to understand the meaning of friendship.

parents are beginning to expect more of him in regard to neatness and cooperative play with others. This transition period is troublesome.

A good nursery school provides the child with opportunities to get rid of some of his pent-up emotions. There is plenty of room to run and shout. The toys are sturdy, and he can manipulate them because they are his own size. Since they are not his own, he finds them easier to share. The child is not as emotionally involved with his teacher as he is with his parents. He feels more able to express his negative and positive feelings, and the teacher is able to be more objective about them. Rules and regulations are kept at a minimum. The teacher expects the child to decide what materials he will play with, and with whom he wishes to play. He takes responsibility for his own belongings.

Children are accepted into nursery schools between the ages of three and five. Most sessions last about three hours. Parents should not send their child with the expectation that he is going to acquire many new skills. Nursery school is not meant for this purpose. Rather, it is an attempt to acquaint the child with this social world, and in such a way that it will add to his security and increase his independence. Although home is cozier, the child soon discovers that nursery school can also be a lot of fun.

A parent who is considering nursery school for his child should consider the following factors: How many teachers are there? What is their educational background? Are the physical facilities adequate? How many children are there per teacher? What is the cost? Is the child ready for nursery school? Many of these questions can be answered by the local family service agency. Parents will also want to visit the school and talk directly with the person in charge.

The student practical nurse may have the opportunity to visit a nursery school during her studies of the well child. This can be a rewarding experience if she uses her powers of observation. When observing an individual child, she should compare him to *others* of his own age group and not merely to one other child. The following outline may aid the student in her observations:

Observing the Individual Child

Aim: To give the student an idea of what nursery school teachers are working to accomplish, to supplement her knowledge of child growth and development, and to give her an opportunity to observe the preschool child and the behavior characteristic of this particular age group. Watch for and evaluate the following in terms of a child's security and independence:

Physical Development

Ability to
    walk, run, jump, use equipment, tricycles, swings, and so forth.
General health. Easily fatigued. Give examples.

Emotional Development

Easily excited.
Whines. Cries frequently.
Evidence of temper tantrum.
Persistence in a task.
Aggressive.
Shy.
Reaction to failure.

Social Development

Talkative.
Quiet.
Plays with others.
Plays near others.
Special friendships.
Tends to lead. Give examples.
Tends to follow. Give examples.
Degree of friendliness with children, with adults.
Ability to share.
Ability to take turns.
Behavior when he desires an object or the attention of the teacher.

Degree of Independence

Removing coat, hat, boots, putting them away.
Attending to toilet needs.

Getting a drink.
Amount of time getting from one activity to another.
Dependence on adult suggestion and help.

Relaxation

Relaxes during rest period.
Sits and listens to stories.
Restlessness. Give examples.

Specific Routines

Music period
    Sings.
    Plays games.
Snack
    Eats his lunch.
    Takes that of others.
    Wanders about.
    Disturbs those around him.
    Plays with food.
Free play period
    Toys preferred.
    Amount of skill using hands.
    Span of interest.
    Evidence of destructive play.
    Plays with others or alone.
    Imaginary friends. Give example.

DAILY CARE

The child between three and six does not require the extensive physical care given to a baby. He still needs a bath each day (more than ever), and a shampoo at least once a week. It is best to keep hair styles simple. A little girl fares the worst in this area, particularly if mother expects her to sit still for an elaborate coiffure.

The child needs to visit a dentist regularly, at least every six months. The deciduous teeth are important for the proper formation of the permanent teeth, and should not be neglected. The first visit may be merely for an examination. In this way the child becomes acquainted with the dentist and the appearance of the office. When calling for the appointment, the mother should tell the receptionist that this is Johnny's first visit. It will also help to tell Johnny a little in advance that he is going, and that the dentist will look into his mouth. Too much detail may frighten the imaginative preschool child. The child's diet should continue to emphasize milk, vegetables, and fruits. Excess sweets which contribute to dental decay are restricted. He must be reminded to brush his teeth regularly.

The preschool child likes to do things for himself. Simple clothes make it easy for him to dress. A hook nailed on the door within his reach is helpful. He should dress and undress himself as much as he can. His mother can assist him but not take over. He must be reminded to use the toilet from time to time. Some three year olds may still need assistance to get up onto the seat. There are occasional spills which embarrass the preschool child, and he usually rushes to get a mop. A stool kept next to the bathroom sink enables him to wash his hands.

The child needs simple, nourishing meals (see Table 8-1, p. 152). His appetite fluctuates, and he should not be bribed, scolded, and coaxed. Mealtimes should be happy. When parents use good manners, before long they will be delighted with the way the child responds. The milk glass must be unbreakable and not filled completely. A waterproof tablecloth is useful. The child is included in the conversations, but not allowed to take over. A nourishing dessert such as a custard pudding eases the apprehension about what has been left on the child's plate.

The child needs periods of active play both in and out of doors. His clothes should be loose enough to prevent restriction of movement. A parent who sees that the child is having a particularly good time, should ask himself if it is necessary to interrupt him right at this moment. When there are verbal arguments, a parent should avoid rushing in to defend the child. No one ever said that growing up was easy, and each child has to be allowed to do it in his own way.

The sleep habits at this time vary. Toward the end of this stage the child may balk at taking a nap. Instead of insisting that he sleep, the mother should see that he engages in something interesting, but restful. She may read him a story or let him play with a simple puzzle. He needs an opportunity to relax. The child may also awake during the night frightened. The parent should attend to his needs, and reassure him that he is safe, and that the parents are close by. If he persists in awaking, and is usually frightened, this is discussed with the doctor during one of his checkups. Children of this age should have a complete physical examination each year. Booster injections of the various immunizations are given when required. The child has a repeat of his smallpox vaccination before entering school.

Accidents are still a major threat during the years from three to five. At this age the child may suffer an injury from a bad fall. The preschool child hurries up and down stairs. He climbs trees and stands up on swings. He plays hard with his toys, particularly those that he can mount. Stairways must be kept free from clutter. Shoes should have rubber soles, and new ones are bought when the tread becomes smooth. When buying toys, parents must be sure they are sturdy and can take a beating. The preschool child is never asked to do anything that is potentially dangerous, e.g., to carry a glass container or knife to the kitchen sink.

Automobiles continue to be a threat. The child should be taught where he can safely ride his tricycle and where he can play ball, and should not be allowed to use his sled on streets that are not blocked off for this purpose. He must not play in or around the car.

Burns that occur at this age are frequently due to the child's experimentation with matches. Children are also intrigued by fancy cigarette lighters. Both such items are kept well out of reach and their dangers are explained to the child.

Poisoning is still a danger. The child tries to imitate adults, and is apt to sample pills, especially if they smell good. His increased freedom brings him into contact with many interesting containers in the garage or basement.

The preschool child is also taught the dangers of talking to or accepting rides from strangers. If he is stopped and asked directions to a certain street, he should not approach the car but should give the necessary information from the sidewalk. Mothers should make it clear to the child in nursery school that they will never send a stranger to call for him. Children must know the dangers of playing in lonely places and of accepting gifts from strangers. The child should always know where he is to go if his mother cannot be found. The preschool child still requires a good deal of unnoticed supervision to protect him from dangers which he may confront owing to his immature judgment, or social environment.

OVERVIEW OF PLAY IN HEALTH AND DISEASE

Value of Play

It has often been said that play is the business of children. Recent investigations stress the importance of play to both the well and sick child's physical, mental, emotional, and social development. The child climbing on a jungle gym develops coordination of his muscles and exercises all parts of his body. He uses up energy and develops feelings of self-confidence. His imagination may take him to the jungle where he is swinging from limb to limb. He mentally faces fears and solves problems which would be much more trying if not impossible in reality. He communicates with the other children and advances a further step in his development of moral values, i.e., taking one's turn, consideration of others. Other types of play help the child to learn colors, shapes, sizes, and textures, and teach him to be creative. This natural and readily available outlet must be tapped by institutional personnel. The child may be unfamiliar with every facet of the hospital, but he knows how to play and this is a good way for the practical nurse to come in contact with him.

Practical Nurse's Role

Some hospitals have well-established play programs supervised by play therapists known as "Play Ladies" to the children. Play experience may be included during the nurse's training period. It is not necessary to be an expert in manual dexterity, art, or music. To be of assistance one must be able to understand the needs of the child. Play is not just the responsibility of those who are assigned to it, nor is it confined to certain times or shifts. Broadribb states, "One frequently sees the student nurse out at the desk after her morning cares are done. Certainly she needs to read her patient's chart, and to obtain all the information she can about the patients in the department, but it sometimes is an indication that she feels insecure and inadequate with the child after his physical care is completed. She is apt to take refuge in some activity that takes her away from him. She feels sorry for the child, but she does not know what to do for him, and so she frequently finds herself busy elsewhere. She is also apt to feel guilty because of her withdrawal from the child, and the pediatric experience becomes less of a fulfillment for her."*

There are a lot of factors involved in providing suitable play for children of various ages in the hospital. The patient's state of health has to be considered. This will determine the amount of activity in which he can participate. The nurse can provide many activities which will relieve stress and provide enjoyment for the patient on bedrest. Overstimulation, nevertheless, would be hazardous for the severely ill child, e.g., the child with a heart disorder, who needs to conserve his strength. The nurse should always be on guard for signs of fatigue in her patient and use her judgment accordingly.

Basically, toys should be safe, durable, and suited to the child's developmental level. Toys should not be sharp, nor have parts which are easily removed and swallowed. Too many toys at one time are confusing to the child. Complicated toys are frustrating and disappointing to the child. Well-selected toys, e.g., balls, blocks, dolls, are useful throughout the years (see Fig. 107). Each child needs sufficient time to complete the activity. In general, quiet play should precede meals and bedtime for both the well and sick child. Investigations have shown that the toys which are enjoyed by both boys and girls are more similar than dissimilar.

The nurse can entertain the child during routine procedures by nursery rhymes, stories, nonsense games, songs, finger play. Often the other children in the ward can be included for "I'm thinking of something blue, red, green," and so forth. Simple crafts are fun. The nurse may find various instructions from children's magazines or the local public library. Scrapbooks are entertaining. The child may even want to make a storybook about his hospital experience. The older practical nurse who is a veteran den mother can make a definite contribution. A younger student may have helped out at a summer camp, babysat, or assisted at Sunday School. Surprise boxes in which a gift is

---

*Broadribb, V., *Foundations of Pediatric Nursing.* (Philadelphia: J. B. Lippincott Co., 1967), p. 32.

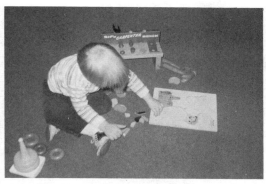

Figure 107. Basically toys should be safe, durable, and suited to the child's developmental level.

opened every day provide anticipation for the patient. Collections of scrap material containing bright ribbons, bits of string, old popsicle sticks, coat hangers, pipe cleaners, paper bags, newspapers, or bits of cotton can be started in the classroom. Since the turnover of patients is fairly rapid, many projects can simply be repeated with different children.

Good music is provided by the radio, phonograph, and piano. Special children's recordings are available. Drawings, finger paints, and modeling clay foster creativity. They require merely a flat surface, such as the overbed table, and the particular medium. The bedridden child can participate in messy projects, too. Merely protect the bed with rubber sheets. Children in cribs need adequate back support for such projects. This is done by elevating the mattress or through the use of pillows.

Storing Toys

The playroom may house many of the toys. Toys should be available for all shifts and not be locked up at the end of the day. Each child may have a durable, washable bag tied to his bed for his own possessions. Closets, open shelves, toy chests, cupboards, and bins on rollers may be utilized in the hospital or home. Pegboards for hanging items frequently used are effective. Sturdy boxes, plastic ice cream containers, laundry baskets, are other suggestions for housing articles of various size and shape. Children need to be taught how to care for toys following play. If the child is to open and close drawers he should use the handles so that his fingers will not get pinched.

Playmates

Children need playmates to promote social development. The one year old plays near other children. The two year old grabs, pushes, and

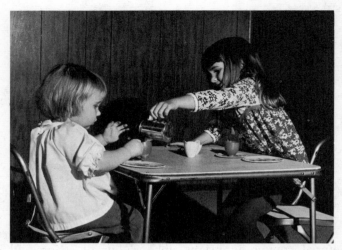

Figure 108.   Playmates promote social development.

cannot share but in his own way acknowledges other children. The older preschool child shows a beginning readiness for cooperative play. The ability to play with others increases during the school years and in late elementary years girls prefer to play with girls and boys prefer to play with boys. This preference to play with the someone of the same sex changes during adolescence. Playmates can be provided in the hospital playroom or in wards. Children who are ambulatory can visit and play table games with the bedridden patients. Of course the type of illness which each child has must be considered for their protection. If there is a question as to the advisability ask your head nurse to obtain permission from the physician.

Factors which would be applicable to the healthy child at home should also be considered during hospitalization. Occasional play with younger children offers relief from competition with his peers. Continuous association with younger children tends to make a child immature in his interest and behavior. Eventually he would fall behind his peers in physical skills and language. On the other hand, the child who is in the constant company of older children tends to feel inferior. This sets the pattern of submission to others. Older children tend to dominate and interfere with the friendships of younger children which leads to bickering and disruption of play. When this is pronounced the young child will lose his friends and is unable to develop effective relationships with his peers.

There are also potential dangers created by adults through domination, indifference, and overconcern for the child. The nurse or parent who directs all of the child's activities, chooses his friends, and plans and thinks for him is doing the child a grave injustice. If one is indifferent to the social needs of the child, he will be lonely in the hospital, avoid his

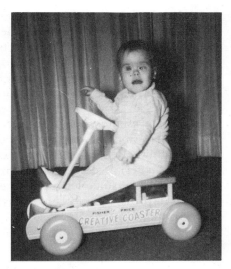

Figure 109. The practical nurse must consider the mental age rather than the chronological age when selecting toys for the mentally retarded child.

peers, and remain friendless. Overconcerned adults cannot bear to have the child mistreated in any way during the normal give and take of childhood play. They scold the supposed offender and separate the children. This eventually isolates the child, making it impossible for him to make the necessary social relationships needed for a healthy personality.

Play and the Retarded Child

The child who is mentally retarded is in more need of stimulation through play than the normal patient. The nurse must consider the mental age of the child rather than his chronological age when selecting

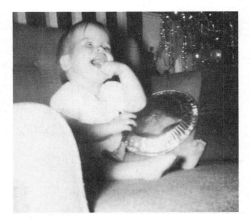

Figure 110. Improvised games and songs amuse Kelly.

toys. Bright colored objects should be strung across the crib for the infant. The environment should be as colorful and gay as possible. The child may be introduced to objects of various sizes and textures. Play with other children must be supervised, because the poor judgment of the retarded child gets him into difficulty. He tends to be aggressive and does not realize his own strength. Adequate space in which to run is necessary. He should be brought into group play gradually. Materials should be presented one at a time. The retarded child has to be taught how to play since he has not had the preschool play experience of the normal child. Repetition of play experiences is necessary. Equipment and play materials need to be altered to accommodate the child's larger size and yet be suitable for his mental age. The nurse or teacher will need to improvise games and songs in order to meet the special needs of this group.

Table 11-1. Choosing Toys

Age	Toys	General Considerations
Infant	Soft stuffed animals and dolls Cradle gym Soft balls Bath toys Rattles Pots and pans	Baby likes to pat and hug. Toys should be brightly colored, of different textures, washable. Large enough so that they can't be aspirated. Smooth edges. Infant's attention span is short. He looks at, reaches, grabs, chews.
Toddler	Nest of blocks Push-pull toys Dolls Telephone Rocking horse or chair Wooden pegs and hammer Clothbooks Pots and pans Ball	May have favorite toy. Enjoys exploring drawers and closets. Likes to place things in containers and dump them out. Parallel play. May injure others.
Preschool	Crayons Simple puzzles Paints with large brushes Finger paints Dolls Dishes, housekeeping equipment Sand box, playground equipment Floating boats for water play Trucks Horns, drums, simple musical instruments Books about familiar circumstances Records	Shifts from solitary to parallel to beginning cooperative play. Exchanges ideas with others. Active play—climbs, runs, and hammers. Imitative play—fireman, teacher. Imaginative play—let's pretend. Creative and dramatic play. Toys that do not require fine hand coordination. Games which teach safety in everyday life.

Other Aspects

Play and toys can be of therapeutic value in the retraining of muscles, in the improvement of eye-hand coordination, and in helping children to crawl and walk, i.e., push-pull toys. An instrument such as the clarinet promotes flexion and extension of the fingers. Blowing is an excellent prerequisite for speech therapy. The physical therapist supervises such activities. She gives specific instructions to the head nurse if she wishes her work reinforced on the ward.

The nurse may also hear the term *play therapy* used. This technique is used for the emotionally disturbed child. A well-equipped playroom is provided. The child is free to play with whatever articles he chooses. A psychiatrist may be in the room observing and talking with the child, or the child may be observed through a one way glass window. By using these as well as other methods the therapist obtains a better under-

Table 11-1. *Choosing Toys* (Continued)

Age	Toys	General Considerations
School	Dolls Doll house Toy housewares Handicrafts Jump rope Skates Construction sets Trains Dressup materials Table games Books for self-reading Bicycles Puppets Music	Attention span increases. Play is more organized, more competitive. Interested in hobbies or collections of things.
The convalescent child	Ball on string that can be dropped from bed and returned Telephone Easy puzzles Large beads to string Record player close to bed Gold fish bowl Miniature autos, trains, dolls, farm animals Stick 'ems, paper dolls Hand puppets Lap blackboard Alphabet boards Cutouts (Many toys previously listed are also applicable.)	Play should not require a great expenditure of energy. Offer a wide variety because the child's interest span is decreased. Consider bed limitation. Toys should not require long continuous focusing of eyes. Consider toys that will be a little easier than those he likes when well. Pay attention to special interests of individual child.

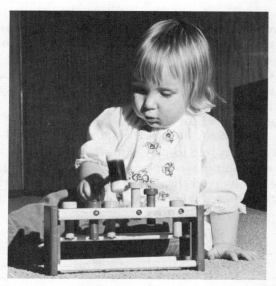

Figure 111. Wooden pegs and hammer appeal to the toddler.

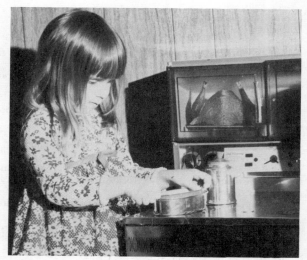

Figure 112. Susan, a preschooler, enjoys her housekeeping toys.

standing of the patient's likes, dislikes, fears, resentments, and feelings toward himself and others. When the child acts out his feelings through *dramatic play*, they are brought out into the open where they can be dealt with more readily. The interpretation of child behavior is not in the realm of practical nursing as it requires a great deal of time and study before it can be fully understood.

The nurse who is with the child daily can describe his behavior. It is important to describe good as well as poor behavior, conversations which you may feel are pertinent, and the child's relationships with other children on the ward. What is the child's approach to play? Does he join in freely or linger outside the group? Does he prefer active or quiet activities? Does he seem to be able to tolerate frustrations? Can he talk with his playmates and get his ideas across? What type of attention span does he have? This type of charting is much more meaningful than "A.M.—care given," and it should be used to describe the activities of pediatric patients.

STUDY QUESTIONS

1. In what ways do the needs of the preschool child differ from those of the infant? The toddler?
2. Debbie, age three, has a new baby brother. Discuss how you would prepare her for this situation.
3. What is meant by the term discipline? How do you feel about bodily punishment? Be prepared to discuss your answer in class.
4. Mrs. Welsh is wondering what to do with four year old Freddie. She states, "Lately he just never bothers to come into the house to urinate." What do you think would be the most effective way to handle this situation?
5. How do you feel the preschool child would react to hospitalization. Give reasons for your answer.
6. Henry is five years old. His father died unexpectedly. What special problems would this present to the preschool child?
7. What is a nursery school?
8. You have been observing nursery school children during the past week. How will this experience help you during your assignment to the pediatric ward?
9. Sandy, age three, and Joan, age two, are playing in the living room. There is a squabble, and when you appear Sandy is snatching a book from Joan. Joan starts to cry. What would you do?
10. What is the role of the practical nurse in guiding parents of preschool children?
11. What accidents is the preschool child subject to in particular?
12. Discuss the fears of a child of three, four, and five. What measures can adults take to prevent them?
13. Define the following: play therapy, dramatic play, chronological age.

BIBLIOGRAPHY

Benz, G. S.: Pediatric Nursing. 5th Ed. St. Louis, C. V. Mosby Co., 1964.

Blake, F.: The Child, His Parents and the Nurse. Philadelphia, J. B. Lippincott Co., 1954.

Blake, F., and Wright, F. H.: Essentials of Pediatric Nursing. 7th Ed. Philadelphia, J. B. Lippincott Co., 1963.

Brigley, C.: Pediatrics for the Practical Nurse. Albany, Delmar Publishers. Inc., 1965.

Broadribb, V.: Foundations of Pediatric Nursing. Philadelphia, J. B. Lippincott Co., 1967.

Cleaverdon, D.: A Work-Play Program for the Trainable Mental Deficient. Reprinted from the Amer. J. Ment. Defic. Vol. 60, 1955.

Cleaverdon, D.: Why—Play in a Hospital. How—. New York, The Play Schools Association.

Hurlock, E.: Child Development. 3rd Ed. New York, McGraw-Hill Book Co., Inc., 1956.

Langdon, G.: How to Choose Toys. New York, American Toys Institute, Inc.

Langdon, G.: How to Choose Toys for Convalescent Children. New York, American Toys Institute, Inc.

Langdon, G.: Make Room for Toys. New York, American Toys Institute, Inc.

Leifer, G.: Principles and Techniques in Pediatric Nursing. Philadelphia, W. B. Saunders Co., 1965.

Marlow, D.: Textbook of Pediatric Nursing. 3rd Ed. Philadelphia, W. B. Saunders Co., 1969.

Metropolitan Life Insurance Company: A Formula for Child Safety. New York.

Nelson, W. (Editor): Textbook of Pediatrics. 9th Ed. Philadelphia. W. B. Saunders Co., 1969.

Smith, C.: Maternal-Child Nursing. Philadelphia, W. B. Saunders Co., 1963.

Spock, B.: Baby and Child Care. Rev. Ed. New York, Duell, Sloan and Pearce, Inc., 1968.

United States Dept. of Health, Education, and Welfare: Your Child from One to Six. Children's Bureau Publication No. 30, 1962.

Verville, E.: Behavior Problems of Children. Philadelphia, W. B. Saunders Co., 1967.

Wolf, A.: Helping Your Child to Understand Death. New York, Child Study Association of America, 1958.

Chapter 12

DISORDERS OF THE PRESCHOOL CHILD

VOCABULARY

Acute	Infiltration
Chronic	Isolation
Contaminated	Serum
Facilitate	Synthetic
Headache	Vaccine
Immune	Weak

Hospitalization is not as threatening to the preschool child as it is to the toddler, and is easier for patients who have had more outside contact such as nursery school and kindergarten than for those who have been with their parents constantly. Since the child of this age understands more, he can be better prepared for what will occur. He should be made to realize that hospitalization is not a punishment for something he has done wrong. Some parents make the mistake of threatening that the child will become sick if he does such and such. When illness actually strikes, the child may feel guilty, particularly if an accident happens because of some mischief on his part, as in the case of burns or falls.

The preschool child is distressed when his mother prepares to leave him, but, unlike the toddler, he can understand "tonight" and "tomorrow." The nurse and the parents must not tell the child that they will return unless they intend to.

Rivalry within a ward or in the playroom is common because the ages of the children are so varied. The younger child may wish to have the games or privileges that are allotted to the older children. He should be made to understand that certain rights come with age. The nurse deals with each child according to his needs. Some require more emotional support than others.

At this age, the child is afraid of bodily harm. He worries about other children in the ward who have physical deformities, and wonders if this will happen to him. His questions concerning other children should not be ignored. The nurse listens to him and assures him that his fears are groundless. The child relieves his tension through play. Tongue depressors, bandaids, and other materials related to everday hospital life are relished by the sick child.

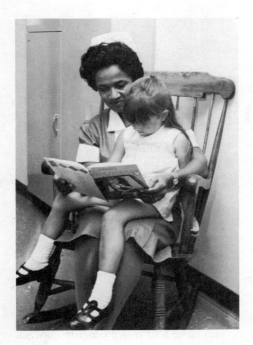

Figure 113. "T.L.C." is a vital ingredient of pediatric nursing. (Courtesy of St. Barnabas Medical Center, School of Practical Nursing, Livingston, N.J.)

The parents are faced with a disrupted home life throughout the child's hospitalization. The mother cannot cope with her everyday tasks when she is lonesome and worried about her child. The frequent trips to the hospital interfere with her daily routine and may be resented by other children in the family. When the child is finally discharged, he may be demanding and irritable. The mother needs the kind support of hospital personnel to enable her to meet these added strains. She should be reassured that the child will settle into his rightful place in the family, and that she can gradually give him less attention and expect a reasonable code of behavior.

The Blood

LEUKEMIA

Description. Leukemia (*leuko-* white + *-emia* blood) is a disease of the blood-forming organs of the body that results in uncontrolled growth of white blood cells. The normal white blood cell count is 5000 to 10,000 per cubic millimeter (a tiny drop) of blood. In leukemia the count may rise as high as 50,000 per cubic millimeter.

There are several types of white blood cells. Some are produced in the red marrow of the bone; others are produced in the spleen and lymph nodes. When the specific diseased white blood cells are isolated, the doctor will designate it in his diagnosis, e.g., lymphocytic leukemia or monocytic leukemia. This disease is also classified according to its rate of development, i.e., acute, or chronic. The characteristic white blood cell of leukemia is immature and not capable of carrying out its normal functions.

Cancer, the second highest cause of death in children, is preceded only by accidents. Leukemia is the principle type of cancer in children; its incidence is highest between three and eight years of age. The cause and cure of this disease is unknown. Current research on the relationship of viruses to this disease is underway. All tissues of the body are affected either by direct infiltration of cancer cells or by the changes in the blood which is carried to them. There is a reduction in the number of red blood cells, which produces anemia. The platelet count is also reduced, and since platelets are essential for the clotting of blood, hemorrhage occurs. Intracranial bleeding is a common, immediate cause of death. Hemorrhage from other vital organs may occur.

Symptoms. The most common symptoms during the initial phase of the illness are low grade fever, pallor, tendency to bruise, leg and joint pain, listlessness, and enlargement of lymph nodes. These symptoms may develop gradually or be sudden in onset. As the disease progresses, the liver and spleen become enlarged. *Petechiae,* or pinpoint hemorrhagic spots beneath the skin, may be seen. Anorexia, vomiting, weight loss, and dyspnea are also common. If the kidneys are affected, hematuria may result.

Because the white blood cells are not functioning normally, bacteria easily invade the body. Ulcerations develop about the mucous membranes of the mouth and anal region, and have a tendency to bleed. Anemia becomes severe despite transfusions. The child may die as a direct result of the disease or from secondary infection. The symptoms are the same regardless of the type of white blood cell affected, and vary widely with each patient, depending on the parts of the body involved.

Diagnosis. The diagnosis of leukemia is based on the history and symptoms of the patient and the results of extensive blood tests. A bone marrow aspiration is commonly performed. A piece of the marrow of the bone is removed from the sternum or iliac crest by the use of a special needle. The marrow of the bone is where many white and red blood cells are produced, and it is used for purposes of study. X-rays of the long bones show change in the bones.

Treatment. The treatment is supportive and aimed at relieving the symptoms and thereby making the patient more comfortable. The child's life can seldom be prolonged more than three or four years from the discovery of the disease. Untreated leukemia results in death in about two months. The drugs used for relief of symptoms include cortisone, hydrocortisone, and ACTH. The usual side effects of hormone therapy may be seen. Other drugs such as methotrexate and 6-mercaptopurine act against chemicals vital to the life of the white blood cell. An alkylating agent, cyclophosphamide (Cytoxan), which is given by mouth has been used to induce remissions in acute leukemia. It is a derivative of nitrogen mustard with similar but more prolonged action; however, it is somewhat less toxic than nitrogen mustard. Another drug, vincristine (VCR) is also used. These various drugs may be given in cycles. Antibiotics are administered to prevent or control infection and blood transfusions are given in an attempt to correct anemia. Sedatives necessary for the patient's comfort are also administered.

Nursing Care.   The child suffering from acute leukemia requires extensive nursing care. He is uncomfortable, irritable, and afraid. His parents should be allowed unlimited visiting hours. The mental anguish experienced by the patient and his parents is much more difficult to meet than their physical needs. The practical nurse will not find it easy to care for the dying child. However, some good comes from all tribulation, even though it may not be understood at the time. To the nurse, it provides an opportunity to aid in the suffering of another human being, to grow in gentleness and patience, and to learn through the experience how to deal more effectively with other such problems that she will surely encounter in the hospital, if not in her personal life.

If a nurse avoids the parents of the dying child because she feels she cannot express herself adequately, she may unknowingly contribute to their insecurities. They may feel that she rejects their expressions of grief or is indifferent to their plight. Formal condolences are not necessary, but interest in the child and sympathy are. Grief is displayed in a number of ways. Mothers, in particular, feel the impending loss of a child as such a defeat that strong feelings of dependency surface. The nurse must be prepared to accept the parents' actions even though they may seem inappropriate to her at the time.

The child's anxiety often centers about his symptoms. He fears that the treatments necessary to correct his problems may be painful. His sense of trust in others is in a precarious balance. It is very important that the practical nurse inform him of what she is about to do and why it is necessary. This is done in terms which he will understand. The inevitable question which we all dread, "Am I going to die?" may arise. There are several ways of one answering the question. One may answer the question with a question, such as "Why do you ask that? Do you feel badly today?* This will hopefully encourage the child to verbalize his feelings. On the other hand, the nurse might acknowledge that he does feel rather badly today but end on an encouraging note, such as "We are

---

*Bright, F., and France, Sister M. L., *The Nurse and the Terminally Ill Child.* (Nurs. Outlook, 1967) pp. 39-42.

all working very hard to make you feel better; you can help us by eating your toast and drinking a little of this juice."

Physical care is intense, and whenever possible the parents should be allowed to help with it. The dying child needs someone present at all times, even if he is comatose. If this is impossible, the nurse should be sure that he is in a room close to the nurse's desk, so that he is reassured that someone is close by. The child is handled gently, and his position is changed frequently. The skin is bathed daily and whenever necessary. Careful attention is given to the body creases. The nurse reports any irritations from bed linens and so forth immediately so that proper steps are taken to prevent infection. Good oral hygiene is essential. (See Fig. 114.) The mouth may be rinsed with lukewarm saline and water if the child is conscious. If the child is comatose, a tray for mouth care is kept at the bedside. This contains a small glass of glycerin and lemon juice (or a mild mouth wash), cold cream, and cotton swabs. The nurse gently cleanses the mouth with a swab dipped in the desired solution. Cold cream may be applied to the lips.

The child's hair is combed daily and whenever necessary. Hair loss because of drug therapy may be evidenced. A wig may be obtained which can be worn when the child feels better. The fingernails and toenails are kept short, so that the child cannot scratch himself. The doctor may prescribe special soothing ointments to be applied to the anal region. Sedatives are given as needed. The practical nurse should choose

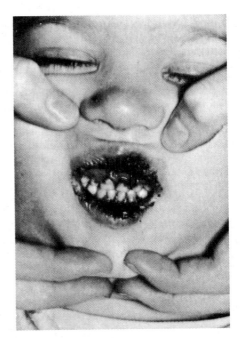

Figure 114. The mouth lesions of leukemia. (From Blake, F., and Wright, F. H.: Essentials of Pediatric Nursing. 7th Ed. J. B. Lippincott Co., 1963.)

diversions that are suited to the general condition of the child. The room is kept neat and cheerful.

The patient is served well balanced meals planned from foods that he likes. Since food is not appealing to the child with leukemia, the individual nurse must use her ingenuity in getting him to eat. Mealtimes are kept pleasant. The nurse should note the patient's likes and dislikes, so that she may discuss them with the dietitian. Food from home may be indicated in some cases. If the parents are present they may enjoy assisting the child. When the child is too tired or irritable, between-meal feedings are given. If the parents understand this, they will be less anxious about what the child takes at one particular meal.

Small amounts of fluid are offered frequently. If the nurse places her fingers over the end of a drinking tube after it is in a glass of water, she will create a suction which will hold water in the tube. She may be able to give the listless child fluids in this way. When parenteral fluids are given, they must be carefully observed (see p. 144). A careful record is kept of all fluid taken.

If the practical nurse is asked to assume responsibility for the child during the time he is receiving a blood transfusion, she requests explicit directions from her team leader or charge nurse. She observes the patient for signs of a transfusion reaction which are: elevation of temperature, chills, itching, rash, and pain in the back or elsewhere. If such reactions occur, the practical nurse clamps off the tubing immediately and reports to the nurse in charge. She does *not* remove the needle unless specifically directed to do so. The patient's temperature is taken before blood is administered so that it may be used as a basis of comparison.

Respiratory System

TONSILLITIS AND ADENOIDITIS

Description. The tonsils and adenoids, located in the pharynx, or throat, are made of lymph tissue and act as part of the body's defense mechanism against infection. The tonsils and adenoids have formerly been blamed for causing many assorted illnesses, and for a time it was thought that having them removed was part of growing up. Today doctors stress that *not all* children need to have them removed. A careful physical examination and an evaluation of the patient's history are made to rule out other diseases. The fact that tonsils are enlarged is not sufficient evidence. These structures are normally larger in early childhood than in later years. More significant symptoms are recurrent or persistent sore throat and obstruction to swallowing or breathing.

Treatment.   The removal of the tonsils and adenoids, referred to as a T and A, is not usually recommended for the child of two or three. It is felt that if surgery is postponed until later, the condition may correct itself, since the tissues become smaller as the child grows. It is also easier for the child to cope with hospitalization when he is older. His fears are not as intense, especially those of bodily harm.

The decision as to whether or not surgery is required is perhaps the most important single factor from a medical standpoint. The tonsils and adenoids are usually removed at the same time, but occasionally surgery is done separately. The use of antibiotics during acute infections has reduced the need for surgery. The patient should be free of symptoms for at least two weeks before an operation is attempted. In cases in which infection is persistent, the child is given sulfonamides or antibiotics a few days before and after surgery. They are also administered to children with a history of a rheumatic fever, regardless of the presence of infection.

Preoperative Care.   The child should be told in advance that he is going to be hospitalized. He is generally admitted a day before surgery so that a complete physical including blood tests and urinalysis may be done. (See Fig. 115.) He is observed for signs of an upper respiratory infection which might prohibit surgery. If the practical nurse suspects that the child has any loose teeth, she reports this to the head nurse. They should be attended to before surgery. Food and fluids are

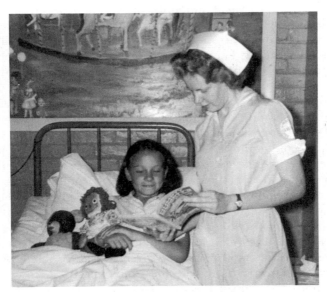

Figure 115. Janie will have her tonsils and adenoids removed in the morning. The practical nurse student helps to make her feel at home. (Courtesy of Exeter School of Practical Nursing. Exeter, N.H.)

withheld before surgery. The child's bed is properly tagged with an N.P.O. sign. In some hospitals a card is attached directly to the child's clothing. Preoperative medication consists of atropine and one of the barbiturates. The nurse checks to see that the child's identification band is securely attached to his wrist. The patient should void before leaving the ward. One hospital employs a simple and effective system. The child and his nurse walk to surgery. Outside of the surgical suite is a playroom where he stays with his nurse until it is time for surgery. Preoperative medication is given in the operating room suite. This method eliminates a number of procedures that are strange to the child, such as being pushed on a stretcher, and the presence of his nurse and other children is reassuring. Another hospital provides a slumber room where preoperative patients await surgery. A special nurse plus students entertain the children in an atmosphere which is free of ward confusion. No treatments other than preoperative medication are allowed here.

Postoperative Care. Immediately following surgery, the child is placed partly on his side and partly on his abdomen with the knee of the uppermost leg flexed to hold him in position. In this way respirations are not hampered by pillows. When he regains consciousness, he may be turned on his back and supported in a semisitting position. The child is watched carefully for evidence of bleeding, i.e., an increase in pulse and respiration, restlessness, frequent swallowing, and vomiting of bright red blood. An ice collar may be applied for comfort. An emesis basin and tissues are provided. The child's face and hands are wiped with a warm face cloth, and his hospital gown and linen are changed whenever necessary. Small amounts of liquids are given when the vomiting has ceased. Synthetic fruit juices are used because they are not as irritating as natural juices. A popsicle may appeal to the child. Milk is also given. The child is kept on bed rest for the remainder of the day. Special effort is made to prevent him from becoming exposed to infections.

Hemorrhage is the most common postoperative complication. The practical nurse should not assume that because surgery is minor it does not involve certain risks. Because bleeding after this type of surgery is concealed, the nurse must watch carefully for evidence of hemorrhage. When bleeding is suspected, packing and sometimes ligation is indicated. Lung abscesses and pneumonia are infrequent complications.

Hospital Discharge. Written instructions are given to the parents when the child is discharged. The child should be kept quiet for a few days and receive nourishing fluids and soft foods. After this he must continue to take a nap or a rest period so that he has a sufficient convalescent period. Aspirin may be given to reduce discomfort in the throat. The child needs to be protected from exposure to infections. The mother is told the signs of bleeding so that she may call the doctor if they occur. Some physicians recommend that a glycerin suppository be given to promote evacuation of the bowels. Earache may follow a T and

A, so this is explained to the mother. It should not, however, be accompanied by fever. A follow-up appointment is made, since the surgeon will wish to observe the operative site after it has healed.

ASTHMA

Description.   The patient suffering from asthma has the unfortunate luck of being allergic to certain substances which are harmless to most people. These substances called *allergens* cause the smooth muscle of the bronchi and bronchioles to go into spasm. This is accompanied by swelling of the mucosa and an increase in mucus which further obstructs the air passages. Many children who suffer from infantile eczema (see page 145) develop asthma as they grow older. It is regrettable that children who are prone to allergies often trade one sensitivity for another. House dust, animal dander, wool, feathers, pollen, mold, and certain foods are some of the frequent offenders. Vigorous physical activity, especially in cold weather, may precipitate an attack. Emotional upsets which affect smooth muscle and vasomotor tone (*vas-* vessel + *motor-* mover, pert. to nerves) are closely intwined with the condition. A strained relationship between the child and his parents may require professional help. A positive family history of allergies is often seen, although the patient may suffer from a different manifestation.

Symptoms.   The symptoms of asthma may begin slowly or abruptly. The patient coughs, wheezes, and has difficulty breathing, particularly during expiration. Signs of air hunger such as flaring of the nostrils, cyanosis, and the use of the accessory muscles of respiration, i.e., chest and abdominal muscles, may be evident. Orthopnea appears. The child is restless, perspires, and sometimes complains of abdominal pain. Vomiting may occur. Pulse and respiration are increased and rales may be heard in the chest. Inflammation of the nose and sinuses may accompany asthma. These attacks often happen during the night and are very frightening for the child and his parents.

Treatment.   The physician obtains the child's history in detail. He must gain the cooperation of the parents and devise a program of treatment to be carried out over a prolonged period of time. Skin tests are administered initially to determine the cause of the allergy. It is then necessary to try to eliminate the offender whether it be food or environmental. Foods which are known to cause an allergic reaction such as cow's milk, eggs, chocolate, oranges, and wheat are to be avoided. The elimination diet and the nurse's role concerning it are discussed on page 148. Care must be taken to assure that the growing child has a well-balanced diet.

If the offending substance cannot be removed from the patient's environment, the doctor may feel that it is advisable to begin a program to *desensitize* the patient. He tries to decrease the patient's sensitivity by giving him extracts from the material causing the problem. The dosage is gradually increased but should not at any time cause symptoms of the allergy. By doing this it is hoped that the patient will build up a tolerance to the allergen. The length of time which this takes varies. Some patients are never able to build up a tolerance.

Another method of treatment is to change the body's response to the allergen. Adequate rest, good health habits, and a generous amount of fluid may prevent an attack. The patient must try to avoid situations which upset him emotionally. Antihistamines and hormones may be prescribed to relieve symptoms. Epinephrine (Adrenalin), a vasoconstrictor, relaxes the smooth muscles of the respiratory tract. Its action is immediate and very effective during acute attacks. Other drugs frequently used are ephedrine and aminophylline. ACTH and cortisone are also used to relieve symptoms. Oxygen will reduce anoxia and improve the patient's color. Increased humidity will help the child to raise sputum. If the child has an infection along with the attack, he is treated with the appropriate antibiotics and an expectorant such as potassium iodide or syrup of hydriodic acid. Sedatives are used sparingly as some decrease the cough reflex, thus preventing the child from clearing his lungs. The services of an allergist and in some cases a child psychologist may prove to be very beneficial. Asthma can generally be brought under satisfactory control so that the child can lead a normal life with modest limitations. This condition sometimes disappears with puberty.

Nursing Care.   The practical nurse may work in an allergy clinic during or after her training period; she may care for the child with asthma in the hospital situation. The environment provided for the child in either case should be one of warmth and pleasantness. Children soon adjust to the frequent inoculations, but their anxieties are certainly heightened in an atmosphere that involves prolonged waiting followed by a flurry of activity and directions. Unfortunately, in many large clinics this is all too often the case. One nurse can do a lot to make this short visit more pleasant simply by her kind interaction with the parent and child.

General control of the environment is explained to the parents by the physician. The practical nurse should be aware of these measures so that she may reinforce knowledge as needed. In doing this it is hoped that the patient will be kept free from symptoms. Certain pleasures must be eliminated—no pets or stuffed toys. The child's bedroom is damp-dusted every day and rugs, upholstered furniture, venetian blinds, and drapes which collect dust must be removed. A foam rubber pillow is substituted for a feather pillow and a plastic covering is placed on the mattress. The furnishings should consist of the necessities—bed, dresser, and wooden chair. The doors and windows to the bedroom are kept shut during the day. An air conditioner is advised during the summer. No woolen clothing is allowed to be worn, and cotton blankets are to be used. Foodstuffs which are detrimental to the child's health are avoided as was previously mentioned. These measures are also instituted during hospitalization.

The child hospitalized for asthma does not usually require intensive physical care. He may be in for lung studies, further evaluation, blood and sputum tests. A condition known as *status asthmaticus* exists in which the attack lasts for several days and nights and in which death could result; however, this is the extreme case and usually the result of neglect. This patient requires the supervision of a registered nurse.

It is necessary for the patient's general health that he receive a well-balanced diet. He should be allowed ample time for meals as his respiratory distress may interfere with eating. He may be more comfortable sitting than lying. The nurse organizes her chores so that the child obtains sufficient rest. She assists the child with the use of his nebulizer if this is required. Asthma attacks when properly treated are not lengthy and the child generally remains free of symptoms between attacks.

Besides assisting with the patient's therapy, the nurse should carefully observe and chart his behavior. How does he act when alone, with other children, with his parents during visiting hours? Many of the points noted on pages 226–237 under Observing the Individual Child are applicable to the hospital situation. *Changes* in behavior are of particular importance. Chart exactly what you see. Compare it to the day before if it seems pertinent. Observations must be done in a discreet manner so that the child does not get the impression that you are hovering over him.

As the child grows older he begins to long for increased activity. This is particularly hard on boys who wish to enter competitive sports. Camping activities are limited for both sexes. The nurse should try to understand the child's disappointment and the parent's anguish when he must be denied pleasures which more healthy children take for granted. The medical team and auxilliary services must work with the parents to direct these children into channels which they are physically capable of handling and which will be intellectually satisfying for them.

The Urinary System

ACUTE GLOMERULONEPHRITIS

Description. Acute glomerulonephritis is a disease which seems to be an allergic reaction to an infection in the body. The infection is generally a group A beta hemolytic streptococcal infection of the throat. It may appear after the patient has had scarlet fever or skin infections. It is the most common form of nephritis in children and occurs most frequently in males between the ages of three and seven. Both kidneys are affected. From a study of the urinary system one may recall that the nephron is the working unit of the kidneys. These nephrons number in the millions. Within the bulb of each nephron lies a cluster of capillaries called the glomerulus. It is these structures which are affected, as the name implies. They become inflamed and sometimes blocked permitting red blood cells and protein which are normally retained to enter the urine. The kidneys become pale and slightly enlarged.

The prognosis is good. Mild cases of the disease may recover within ten to fourteen days. Protracted cases may show urinary changes for as long as a year with complete recovery. Chronic nephritis is seen in a small number of children, death being generally the result of renal or heart failure. These severe complications plus hypertensive changes in the blood supply of the brain necessitate careful observance and care of each individual case.

Symptoms. Symptoms range from mild to severe. From one to three weeks after a streptococcal infection has occurred in the child, the mother may notice that his urine is smoky brown in color or bloody. This is frightening to the mother and child; medical advice is immediately sought. This may be accompanied by swelling about the eyes, fever (high at first but gradually leveling off to about 100° F.), headache, diarrhea, and vomiting. Urinary output is decreased. The specific gravity is high and albumin, red and white blood cells, and casts may be found upon examination. The urea nitrogen level of the blood is elevated along with the erythrocyte sedimentation rate. The patient's blood pressure may fluctuate during the first week but this shortly returns to normal.

Treatment. Although the child may feel well, he is placed on bed rest until gross hematuria subsides. The urine is examined regularly. Every effort is made to prevent the child from becoming overtired, chilled, or exposed to infection. A liquid diet is given initially. This is followed by a soft to full diet as tolerated. When edema is pronounced, a low salt diet may be in order. It may also be necessary to restrict protein intake in complicated cases. Penicillin is given during the acute phase and may be continued orally for a period of time to prevent renewed activity before healing is complete. Second attacks of glomerulonephritis are rare.

Nursing Care. The practical nurse should try to make the period of bed rest as pleasant as possible for the patient by providing quiet diversions to keep him contented. She should protect the child from being chilled during his bed bath and trips to various departments. Sufficient blankets are provided at night. When the child is allowed up, the nurse observes him frequently for signs of fatigue. He should be protected from contact with infectious persons.

The patient's vital signs are taken regularly preferably with the same apparatus. A rise in blood pressure is reported immediately. The systolic blood pressure may be elevated to as high as 200 mm. of mercury and the diastolic pressure to 120 mm. Such elevations indicate vasospasm, and heart failure or brain damage can develop. Between readings the

Table 12-1. *Average Blood Pressures of Children**

AGE	SYSTOLIC	DIASTOLIC
4	85	60
5	87	60
6	90	60
7	92	62
8	95	62
9	98	64
10	100	65
11	105	65
12	108	67
13	110	67
14	112	70
15	115	72
16	118	75

*(From Nelson, W. E. (Editor): Textbook of Pediatrics, 1969, p. 948.)

nurse should be alert for symptoms such as headache, drowsiness, vomiting, and blurring of vision. If any of these are noticed, the child is returned to bed and the cribsides or rails are raised. Since convulsions can occur, someone should remain with the child until medication is given. Hypotensive drugs, such as reserpine and hydralazine hydrochloride (Apresoline), given intramuscularly may be ordered by the physician. These reduce the blood pressure rapidly and the cerebral symptoms subside. If cardiac failure is evidenced by an EKG or chest x-ray, sedation, oxygen, and digitalis may be required.

An *accurate* record is kept of the patient's fluid intake and urine output. Fluids may be restricted especially if the urinary output is scant. The physician will order the oral intake allowed, for example, 650 cc. daily. This must be distributed throughout the 24 hour period. Each shift should know the specific amount of fluids the patient is to receive so that an excess amount is not given. The greater amounts of fluid are allotted to the day and evening shifts when thirst is more pronounced. The individual needs of the child should be observed and incorporated into the day's events. Daily weighing of the patient will also help to de-

Table 12-2. *Average Daily Excretion of Urine**

AGE	FLUIDOUNCES	CUBIC CENTIMETERS
First and second days	1–2	30–60
Third to tenth day	3–10	100–300
Tenth day to 2 months	9–15	250–450
2 months to 1 year	14–17	400–500
1–3 years	17–20	500–600
3–5 years	20–24	600–700
5–8 years	22–34	650–1000
8–14 years	27–47	800–1400

*(From Nelson, W. E. (Editor): Textbook of Pediatrics, 1969, p. 1106.)

termine his progress. Persistent anuria may require dialysis by the artificial kidney.

The practical nurse may be asked to determine the specific gravity or protein level of the urine. These tests are detailed on page 202. An Addis sediment count which determines the condition of the nephron may also be done. This requires special preparation. The nurse observes the procedure outline by the hospital laboratory where she is employed.

Although glomerulonephritis is generally benign, it can be a source of anguish for parents and child. If the patient is treated at home the mother must plan activities to keep the child occupied while he is confined to bedrest. She must understand the importance of continued antibiotic therapy and medical supervision as follow-up urine and blood tests are necessary to ensure that the disease has been eradicated.

MENTAL RETARDATION

Description. The term mental retardation is often misconstrued. One clear definition is that the "mentally retarded are children and adults who as a result of inadequately developed intelligence are significantly impaired in their ability to learn and adapt to the demands of society.* Tests to measure intelligence are numerous. One test which is frequently given to children and adolescents is the Stanford-Binet. Alfred Binet of France was a pioneer in the field of intelligence measurement. His work was modified and revised in America by Lewis Terman of Stanford University. These tests differ somewhat depending on the age of the subject. Intelligence testing of children is difficult to evaluate and is best done on an individual basis. Personality tests such as picture story tests, inkblot tests, drawing tests, and sentence completion tests may also be administered. All such tests have their limitations and, of course, are subject to the abilities of the person interpreting them. The tests, nonetheless, are of definite value when used in conjunction with a thorough study of the child's physical, mental, emotional, and social development.

There are many causes of mental retardation. Some conditions which can develop during the prenatal period are phenylketonuria, cretinism, Down's syndrome, malformations of the brain (such as microcephaly, hydrocephalus, craniostenosis), maternal infections, and anoxia. Birth injuries or anoxia during or shortly after delivery may also cause retardation. Diseases such as meningitis, lead poisoning, neoplasms, and encephalitis can retard a child or adult at any age. Heredity is a factor of mental retardation. It is also possible for a child to live in such a physically and emotionally deprived environment that he becomes mentally retarded.

The diagnosis is determined after a thorough study is made by a

---

*From United States Government Printing Office: A Proposed Program for National Action to Combat Mental Retardation.

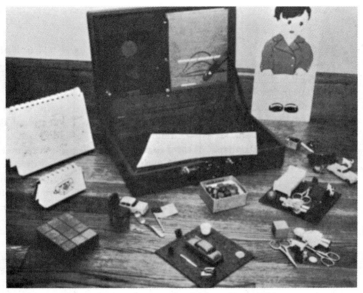

Figure 116. Equipment for the Stanford-Binet Test. These are the props used in administering the Stanford-Binet Scale to young children. (Courtesy of Houghton Mifflin Co.)

team of experts which include a pediatrician, psychologist, psychiatrist, public health nurse, and social worker. Conditions such as epilepsy, cerebral palsy, severe malnutrition, emotional disturbances, blindness, deafness, or speech disorders, must be ruled out. Severe mental retardation may be noticeable at birth. The nursery nurse must be alert for the following symptoms: failure to suck, feeding difficulties, spasticity, listlessness, twitchings or convulsions, vomiting, jaundice, unusual looking stools, unusual odor of urine, enlarged tongue, oriental appearance. Early recognition in certain cases can lessen or prevent brain damage. Other symptoms are associated with landmarks of the growth process. A child who does not smile, sit, climb stairs, stand, or walk within the usual age limits may be suspicious. He may also be slow in speech, in learning to help himself, or in toilet training. Unusual clumsiness and failure to respond to stimuli are early indications. Sometimes this handicap is not discovered until the child enters school.

For purposes of clarification, mental retardation is classified in groups. This is helpful in determining what the child is capable of doing. Each case must be frequently reevaluated according to the child's individual progress. No patient should be kept stagnant merely because he happens to fall within a certain category. The old terms of idiot, imbecile, and moron are now obsolete because they carry such undesirable connotations.

Table 12-3.   *Characteristics of the Mentally Retarded from Birth to Adulthood**

Type	BIRTH THROUGH FIVE	SIX THROUGH TWENTY	OVER TWENTY-ONE
MILD (I.Q. 53–69)	Often not noticed as retarded by casual observer but is slower to walk, feed self, and talk than most children.	Can acquire practical skills and useful reading and arithmetic to a third to sixth grade level with special education. Can be guided toward social conformity.	Can usually achieve social and vocational skills adequate to self-maintenance; may need occasional guidance and support when under unusual social or economic stress.
MODERATE (36–52)	Noticeable delays in motor development, especially in speech; responds to training in various self-help activities.	Can learn simple communication, elementary health and safety habits, and simple manual skills; does not progress in functional reading or arithmetic.	Can perform simple tasks under sheltered conditions; participates in simple recreation; travels alone in familiar places; usually incapable of self-maintenance.
SEVERE (20–35)	Marked delay in motor development; little or no communication skill; may respond to training in elementary self-help—for example, self-feeding.	Usually walks barring specific disability; has some understanding of speech and some response; can profit from systematic habit training.	Can conform to daily routines and repetitive activities; needs continuing direction and supervision in protective environment.
PROFOUND (below 20)	Gross retardation; minimal capacity for functioning in sensorimotor areas; needs nursing care.	Obvious delays in all areas of development; shows basic emotional responses; may respond to skillful training in use of legs, hands, and jaws; needs close supervision.	May walk, need nursing care, have primitive speech; usually benefits from regular physical activity; incapable of self-maintenance.

*(From Kagan, J., and Havermann, E.: Psychology: An Introduction. New York, Harcourt, Brace & World, Inc., p. 515. Courtesy of U. S. President's Panel on Mental Retardation.)

Management and Nursing Goals

In order for the practical nurse to be of substantial help to the retarded child and his family, she must face her own feelings and develop a positive attitude toward the problem. It is not unusual for a person to feel repelled and dismayed when she sees a severely retarded child for the first time. It is helpful for the student to discuss her personal views in a group situation where ideas and feelings can be exchanged. She should realize that the experienced personnel who work with these patients see them in an entirely different way than the casual observer.

The parents of a retarded child need compassion and understanding, not pity, from the nurse. It should be clear to them that the nurse does not regard the child's condition as a disgrace. Usually the problems confronting the parents become greater as the child develops physically and chronologically but still requires constant supervision. The decision to institutionalize the patient is a difficult one. Many things must be taken into consideration, such as the health of the parents, the effect on other children in the family, community services available, the financial status of the family. Even when the decision is made there are long waiting lists in many places. Facilities are overcrowded and the tendency is to take the most severly retarded child first. Thus the number of patients living within the community is increasing. New or expanded programs must be made available to meet this need. It is important that the practical nurse know the resources of her community so that she may direct the family to them. The local chapter of the National Association for Mentally Retarded Children may conduct training centers or nursery classes. The child guidance clinic or the psychological services of a nearby college or hospital may be tapped. The visits of the public health nurse are invaluable in many cases. Patients may also be eligible to obtain help from the local vocational and rehabilitation agency. In some communities parent groups meet to discuss mutual problems. Arrangements for proper dental health must be made as in some cases dental care must be given under total anesthesia.

The training of the retarded child is similar to that of the child with normal intelligence, only slower. He does, however, lack the ability to think abstractly so he cannot transfer learning from one situation to another. He must learn by habit formation which involves routine, repetition, and relaxation. The practical nurse working with these patients must have a good understanding of the growth and development process. It is important that the child show a *readiness* for the task whether it is toilet training, eating, or dressing. The atmosphere should be one of friendliness, and directions should be kept simple. The retarded child has to have limits set on his behavior as do all children. The adult must be firm and consistent. Correction must directly follow the offense. Love, liberal praise, respect, and infinite patience are essential in helping this patient to develop to his fullest capacity.

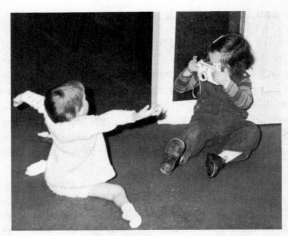

Figure 117. The four year old retarded child with her back to the camera was born with a meningomyelocele and a dislocated hip. She enjoys playing with Mary, age 2½. Compare physical development.

The practical nurse caring for the retarded child in the hospital needs to know his stage of maturation and his abilities. Communicating with the patient may be difficult. It is important to follow his home routines as closely as possible. Progress which he has made should not be allowed to slip during hospitalization. The habit and care sheet should be completed. Additional helpful details should be entered. Good communications between parents and nurse will help to make the transition from home to hospital as smooth as possible for the child.

The Eye

STRABISMUS (CROSS EYE)

Description. Strabismus, also known as *squint,* is a condition in which the child is not able to direct both eyes toward the same object. There is a lack of coordination between the eye muscles which direct movement of the eye.

There are several kinds of strabismus. In *monocular* squint (*mono*-one + *oculus* eye), one eye is used continuously for vision, and the other is turned inward or outward. In *alternating* squint either eye may be used for sight, while the alternate eye becomes crossed. Strabismus may be present at birth or acquired following a disease.

Treatment. When the condition is seen during early infancy, the doctor may recommend that the unaffected eye be covered by a patch until the baby is old enough to wear glasses. The affected eye may improve through use and often becomes normal. Eye exercises and glasses are effective ways of treating the condition medically. If this does not help, surgery should be considered. It is generally performed when the child is three or four; the condition should be corrected before the child starts school, to prevent him from becoming the subject of ridicule. Early correction also prevents the affected eye from suffering from lack of use. If this condition is left untreated, blindness may result, since the brain tends to obliterate the confusing double image.

Prevention of Eyestrain. The practical nurse should stress the importance of proper care of the eyes in her work and daily life. Little children who are beginning to read need books with large type in which the letters are spaced far apart. The lighting provided must be adequate and without glare. The child's chair and desk must be of the proper height.

Symptoms that may indicate eyestrain include inflamed, aching, or smarting eyes, frequent headaches, difficulties with school work, or inability to see the blackboards. They may occur suddenly. The child between 6 and 10 often becomes nearsighted, and has to hold his books very close to his eyes to read. An eye examination and in some cases a complete physical examination are indicated.

Nursing Care. The child undergoing surgery for strabismus is hospitalized for only a brief period. Some doctors prefer not to have the child restrained following surgery, since it is frightening and the child's struggles may increase. The surgery involves structures outside of the eyeball; therefore, the child is allowed up and about following. Eye dressings are kept at a minimum and elbow restraints may be all that is needed to keep the child from touching the dressings.

If the doctor feels that it is necessary to cover the eyes and restrain the patient's movement following surgery, the patient is told this before surgery and assured that the bandages and restraints will be removed as soon as possible. Since this is frightening for the patient, it is best that the parents remain with him and he be reassured that the bandages and restraints will be removed as soon as possible. Since he cannot move or see, diversions such as stories and records are necessary. When nausea has ceased, the child is placed on a regular diet. Tell the patient what he is about to eat when you are feeding him. Speak to the child before you touch him so that he will not be startled.

Communicable Diseases

The practical nurse student may experience her first contact with communicable diseases on the children's ward. Even if she has previously cared for the adult patient in isolation, she will find caring for the child unique. The basic principles of medical aseptic technique are the same, but the ability of the patient to adjust to the situation is markedly different.

Isolation is taxing psychologically on the child, because it accentuates the fact that he is separated from his parents. It is hardest on the infant over six months and the toddler, who especially need the security of their mothers. The toddler, in particular, needs company because his interest span is short. When confined to a crib, he becomes anxious and cries. He cannot amuse himself in play because he is afraid. He may cling or demand attention, or simply refrain from contact with anyone. These and other displays of anxiety must not be mistaken for "spoiled" behavior.

The school child can cope better with isolation for he can amuse himself somewhat. Nevertheless, life soon becomes dreary without visitors. Radio and television are no substitute for friends and play. When the illness is prolonged, the child will fall behind his classmates unless special arrangements are made.

Before the discovery of antibiotics, patients remained infectious for long periods of time, and hospitals maintained rigid rules to lessen the danger of cross-contamination. The number of patients and the detailed ritual involved in care kept the staff so busy that little attention was given to the individual child and his need for emotional support. With advances in medical knowledge, this approach has changed greatly. The majority of the common communicable diseases are cared for at home (e.g., mumps, chickenpox). The child is admitted to the hospital only if complications arise. As soon as the child's condition improves, and the dangers of cross-infection are over, the child is removed from isolation. Parents are encouraged to visit the patient. They should be provided with written instructions regarding the regulations of the individual hospital. These can be taken home and reviewed by them when they are more relaxed.

Review of Terms. A *communicable disease* is one that can be transmitted, directly or indirectly, from one person to another (see Tables 12-5 and 12-6). *Immunity* is natural or acquired resistance to infection.

In *natural immunity* (also called congenital), resistance is inborn. Some races apparently have a greater natural immunity to certain diseases than others. It also varies from person to person. If two people are exposed to the same disease, one may become very ill and the other may have no indications of the disease. However, a person who is immune to one disease is not necessarily immune to another.

Acquired immunity is not due to inherited factors, but is naturally acquired as a result of having had the disease or is *artificially* acquired through the use of vaccines and immune serums. Vaccines are not strong enough to cause the disease, but stimulate the body to develop an

Text continued on page 262.

Table 12-4. *Recommended Schedule for Active Immunization and Tuberculin Testing of Normal Infants and Children[1, 3]*

2 months..	DTP, trivalent OPV
3 months..	DTP
4 months..	DTP, trivalent OPV
6 months..	Trivalent OPV
12 months..	Tuberculin test[2]
	Live measles vaccine
15-18 months..	DTP, trivalent OPV, smallpox vaccine
4-6 years	DTP, trivalent OPV, smallpox vaccine
12-14 years..	Td, smallpox vaccine, mumps vaccine[3]
Thereafter	Td every 10 years
	Smallpox vaccine every 3-10 years
	Rubella vaccine[3]

[1]Reprinted by permission of American Academy of Pediatrics, from its *Report of the Committee on the Control of Infectious Diseases*, 16th Edition, 1969 (Red Book).

Abbreviations:

DTP is diphtheria and tetanus toxoids combined with pertussis vaccine.

Td is combined diphtheria and tetanus toxoids (adult-type).

OPV is trivalent oral poliovaccine. Trivalent OPV is recommended, but monovalent OPV may be substituted; the order of monovalent virus type fed is type 1 followed by type 3 and then type 2.

[2]Frequency of repeated tuberculin tests depends on the risk of exposure of children under care and the prevalence of tuberculosis in the population group.

[3]See text of 1969 Red Book for additional information.

Note: Mumps Vaccine (Mumpsvax), although most useful for susceptibles in pre-adolescents and older ages, is included by many among routine immunization and may be administered any time after the first year. At least one month should elapse between elective immunizations. The length of immunity is uncertain at this time. It is contraindicated during pregnancy. (See product package information, Merck, Sharp and Dohme, Division of Merck & Co., Inc., West Point, Pa. 19486.)

Rubella vaccine (Meruvax) is indicated for boys and girls from age one to puberty. Children in kindergarten and the first grades of elementary school are currently being given priority because they are often the major source of dissemination in the community. It is contraindicated in post-pubertal individuals and during pregnancy. At least one month should elapse between elective immunizations. (See product package information, Merck, Sharp and Dohme, Division of Merck and Co., Inc., West Point, Pa. 19486.)

Table 12-5. Common Communicable Diseases*

Disease	First Signs	Incubation Period	Prevention	How Long Contagious	What You Can Do
Chickenpox	Mild fever followed in 36 hours by small raised pimples which become filled with clear fluid. Scabs form later. Successive crops of pox appear.	2-3 weeks. Usually 14-16 days.	None. Immune after one attack.	6 days after appearance of rash.	Usually not serious. Trim fingernails to prevent scratching. Diluted alcohol or a solution of baking soda and water may ease itching.
German measles (3-day measles)	Mild fever, sore throat or cold symptoms may precede fine rose-colored rash. Enlarged glands at back of neck and behind ears.	2-3½ weeks. Usually 18 days.	Vaccine now available. Simple blood test determines whether individual has had rubella.	Until rash fades. About 5 days.	Not a serious disease, complications rare; give general good care and keep baby quiet. Avoid exposing any woman who is, or might be, in the early months of pregnancy unless she is sure she has had the disease.
Measles	Mounting fever; dry cough; running nose and red eyes for 3 or 4 days before rash which starts at hair line and spreads down in blotches. Small red spots with white centers in mouth (Koplik's spots) may occasionally be seen before rash.	1-2 weeks. Usually 10 or 11 days.	Vaccine can be given to provide immunity. A baby not vaccinated if exposed can be given gamma globulin to lighten or prevent measles.	Until 5 days after the rash has appeared	May be mild or severe with complications of a serious nature; follow doctor's advice in caring for a child with measles, as it is a most treacherous disease. If other children who have not had the disease are exposed, ask the doctor about protective inoculations for them.
Mumps	Fever; headache; vomiting; glands near ear and toward chin at jawline ache and these develop painful swelling. Other parts of body may be affected also.	14-28 days. Usually around 18 days.	Vaccine now available. (It is apt to be milder in childhood than in later years.)	Until all swelling disappears.	Keep child in bed until fever subsides; indoors unless weather is warm.
Roseola	High fever for 2 or 3 days which then falls to normal before appearance of a fine rash or large pink blotches on back and stomach or sometimes the whole body. Child may not seem very ill despite high fever (103-105) but he may convulse.	Not fully known.	None. Usually affects children from 6 months to 3 years of age.	Until the child seems well.	No special measures except rest and quiet. Force fluids during fever.
Strep throat (septic sore throat) and scarlet fever (scarlatina)	Sometimes vomiting and fever before sudden and severe sore throat. If followed by fine rash on body and limbs, it is called scarlet fever.	1-7 days. Usually 2-5	Antibiotics may prevent or lighten an attack if doctor feels it wise.	7-10 days. When all abnormal discharge from nose, eyes, throat has ceased.	Frequently less severe than formerly; responds to antibiotics which should be continued for full course to prevent serious complications.
Whooping cough	At first seems like a cold with low fever and cough which changes at end of second week to spells of coughing accompanied by a noisy gasp for air which creates the "whoop."	5-21 days. Usually around 10 days.	Give injections of vaccine to all children in infancy; if an unvaccinated child has been exposed, the doctor may want to give a protective serum promptly.	At least 4 weeks.	Child needs careful supervision of doctor throughout this taxing illness.

Table 12-6.   *Less Common Infectious Diseases**

Disease	First Signs	Incubation Period	Prevention	How Long Contagious	What You Can Do
Infectious hepatitis (catarrhal jaundice)	May be mild with few symptoms or accompanied by fever, headache, abdominal pain, nausea, diarrhea, general weariness. Later, yellow skin and white of eyes (jaundice), urine dark and bowel movements chalklike.	2-6 weeks. Commonly 25 days.	Injection of gamma globulin gives temporary immunity if child is exposed.	May last 2 months or more.	May be mild or may require hospital care. Requires special disinfection of needles. Stool precautions.
Infectious mononucleosis (glandular fever)	Sore throat, swollen glands of neck and elsewhere, sometimes a rash over whole body and jaundiced appearance, low persistent fever.	Probably 4-14 days or longer.	None	Probably 2-4 weeks but mode of transmission is not clear.	Keep in bed while feverish, restrict activity thereafter.
Meningitis	May be preceded by a cold; headache, stiff neck, vomiting, high temperature with convulsions or drowsy stupor; fine rash with tiny hemorrhages into the skin.	2-10 days	None	Until recovery. Only meningococcal meningitis is contagious.	Immediate treatment is necessary. Hospital care. Continued treatment with antibiotics as long as doctor advises.
Polio (infantile paralysis or poliomyelitis)	Slight fever, general discomfort, headache, stiff neck, stiff back.	1-4 weeks. Commonly 1-2 weeks	Give all children Salk or Sabin series.	1 week from onset of as long as fever persists.	Hospitalization.
Rocky Mountain spotted fever	Muscle pains, nosebleed occasionally, headache, rash on 3rd or 4th day.	About a week after bite of infected tick.	Injections can be given to a child who lives in a heavily infested area.	Spread only by infected ticks.	New drugs have improved treatment.
Smallpox	Sudden fever, chills, head and back ache. Rash which becomes raised and hard, later blisters and scabs.	6-18 days. Commonly 12 days.	Vaccination practically perfect protection. Vaccinate during first year and again before school.	Until all scabs disappear.	Doctor's care necessary.

*Adapted from United States Department of Health, Education, and Welfare: Your Child from One to Six, 1962, pp. 84-85.

immune reaction. Live or dead organisms may be used for this purpose. The Salk poliomyelitis vaccine is an example of the type in which dead viruses are used. In contrast, the Sabin oral polio vaccine is made with live, attenuated viruses. (See the immunization record, p. 259.)

If a person needs immediate protection from a disease, antibodies are obtained in immune serums from other sources; most are from animals, but some are from humans. For example, tetanus serum used to prevent lockjaw is procured from the horse, but *gamma globulin* is obtained from human blood. Gamma globulin is rich in antibodies and is particularly effective against measles. This type of immunity, passive immunity, though immediate in reaction, does not last as long as that which is actively produced by the body.

A *carrier* is a person who is capable of spreading a disease, but does not show evidence of it himself. Typhoid is an example of a disease spread by a carrier. The *incubation period* is defined as the usual amount of time that elapses between exposure to the disease and the onset of symptoms.

Tests are available to determine whether an individual is *susceptible* to a particular disease. Examples are the *Schick test* for diphtheria, the *Dick test* for scarlet fever, and the *tuberculin test* for tuberculosis. The practical nurse may commonly see the latter done by the Tine or intradermal skin test methods.

MEDICAL ASEPSIS

The purpose of medical aseptic technique is to prevent the spread of infection from one child to another, or from the child to the practical nurse. A person or object is considered *contaminated* if it has touched the infected patient or equipment which has come in contact with him. People or articles that have not had any contact with the patient are considered *clean.*

Articles that have come in direct contact with the patient must be *disinfected* before they can be used by others. When something is disinfected, microorganisms in or on it are killed by physical or chemical means. The autoclave which uses steam under pressure is considered very effective in killing most germs, when the article is adequately exposed and sterilized for the proper length of time. However, some materials, for example, the clinical thermometer, would be destroyed if autoclaved. A chemical disinfectant must be used instead. Before soaking an article in a disinfectant, the practical nurse must assure that it has been properly washed in soap and water and rinsed. The strength of the disinfecting solution is generally determined by the hospital pharmacist and dispensed to the wards in suitable containers. Seventy per cent alcohol is an example of one type used. The article must be totally submerged and remain in the solution for a *suitable length of time.* It is extremely important that articles in chemical solutions or in the autoclave be marked with the time in which they are to be removed. If the practical nurse fails to do this, an unsuspecting person may assume that what is in the autoclave or soaking are clean and may remove them before they are properly sterilized.

Throughout this text, emphasis has been placed on the role of the practical nurse in preparing a safe environment for the child and his parents. Of all dangers in our surroundings none is more serious than that of disease-bearing organisms. The nurse must understand the importance of protecting herself and others from the isolated patient. This is accomplished by specific procedures such as cleaning and disinfecting dishes, clothing, bedding, excreta, and hospital equipment. While doing this, the nurse must not, however, forget that the patient is her primary concern. As the student's confidence increases with repetition of the details of isolation, her approach to the patient and his problems will also be more effective.

Since isolation procedures vary from hospital to hospital and from hospital to home, a minimum of specific procedures are presented here. An attempt is made to better acquaint the student with the underlying principles of medical aseptic technique so that she may better judge the reliability of certain procedures, which may or may not be carried out. In general, measures of control are stricter for patients who have dangerous conditions than for those who have highly communicable but mild diseases. For example, the common cold is highly contagious, but patients are seldom isolated because of it. In contrast, meningococcal meningitis is now believed to be transmitted only by close contact with the infected person; nevertheless, most institutions carry out strict isolation procedures because of its seriousness. This practice is not necessarily ideal, but is a reality.

Preventing the Transmission of Infection

Respiratory Infections. These include most common childhood diseases. Precautions must be taken against discharges from the eyes, nose, throat, and ears. Paper tissues must be destroyed by burning or by placing them in the hospital sewerage system. Attendants wear gown and mask. Floors are damp mopped to control dust.

Wound Infections. Germs leave through the wound and may enter the body of the nurse through breaks in her skin, particularly those of the hands. Germs may also become airborne when a wound is dressed. An infected wound is kept covered. If the nurse must handle the dressing, she wears rubber gloves. The contaminated dressings and gloves are disinfected immediately after the completion of the procedure. In some hospitals the dressing and all articles used for the dressing are placed in special bags and autoclaved. In the home, the dressing should be burned immediately. Instruments used are boiled for 20 minutes. Articles of clothing and bed linen that some in contact with the wound are treated as precaution linen. The nurse wears a gown and mask for dressing changes. Linens in the home are boiled and aired in sunlight. Floors are damp mopped to control dust.

Skin Infections. If the lesions cannot be covered, the patient is isolated, and bedding, clothes, and dishes are disinfected. The nurse wears a gown.

Digestive Infections. Precautionary measures are taken against all discharges from the mouth, stomach, and intestinal tract. Dishes, toilet articles, bedding, and clothing are considered contaminated. Stools may require added disinfection in some diseases. The gown technique is employed.

Genital Infections. The danger of this type of infection lies in the discharge coming in contact with mucous membranes of the well person. The conjunctiva of the eye is particularly susceptible to infections from the same germs that invade the genitals. Discharges are burned or disposed of in the hospital sewerage system. Precautions include clothing, bedding, dishes, and toilet facilities. The gown technique is used.

Specific Techniques

Handwashing. Proper handwashing is essential to every procedure that the practical nurse performs, but it is doubly important when she is working with patients in isolation.* (See p. 52.)

Mask Technique. A mask is used once and discarded. It should never be allowed to hang about the neck and then be placed back over the face. It should cover the nose and mouth, and be changed at least once every hour. Do not touch a mask once it is in place. Remove it after the gown when leaving the unit, and do not touch the part that comes in contact with the face. Authorities disagree as to the effectiveness of the use of masks, so the practical nurse follows the procedures of the particular hospital in which she is employed.

Gown Technique. The practical nurse wears a gown to protect her clothing from contamination when she is giving direct care to the isolated child. If this were not done, disease germs would be carried on her uniform, and she would endanger the health of other patients as well as her own. The nurse must be particularly conscientious about proper gown technique on the children's ward, since small children need to be

---

*When foot pedals are not available for turning on water, faucets are handled with paper towels.

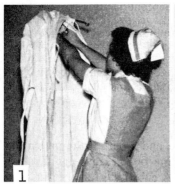
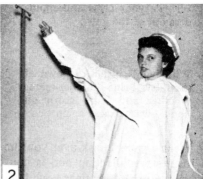
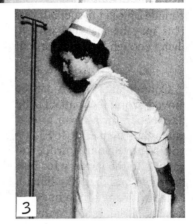

Figure 118. 1. Removing the gown from the hook. Grasp the gown at the inside of the neckband. 2. Keep one hand inside one sleeve while adjusting the other. 3. Draw the back edges of the gown together and away from the body before folding the back over and fastening the ties. (From Thompson, E., and LeBaron, M.: Simplified Nursing. 7th Ed. J. B. Lippincott Co., 1960.)

held for feedings and comforting and the nurse's relationship with the child is very direct. The gown must be long enough to lap over in the back. It is to be worn in the unit only, except for practices of group technique isolation of a specific disease.

The inside of the gown is considered clean, as is one inch around the neck. If either of these areas is contaminated accidentally, the gown is discarded and replaced. Generally the gown is hung in the unit with the contaminated surface on the outside. If the gown is to be *hung outside* the patient's room, the contaminated surface must be on the inside. More hospitals today are turning to the excellent practice of discarding the isolation gown after each use. Nevertheless, it is still not practical for some institutions because of the need for numerous gowns and additional laundering facilities. In such cases the practice of using the same gown for a 24 hour period is then used (see Fig. 118).

*Putting on the Gown**

1. Slip your hands inside shoulders of gown and lift it from hook.

Your clean hands touch only the clean inside of gown—hold gown away from uniform.

2. Slip your arms into the sleeves—then fasten gown at neck.

Be careful not to touch the front of the gown before you fasten the neck—keep sleeves from touching your hair.

3. Bring edges of gown together in back at waistline—draw away from your body and fold over—tie belt.

This part of the gown is contaminated so your hands are no longer clean.

Removing the Gown

1. Untie strings at waist.

The strings and hands are both contaminated.

2. Wash your hands—unfasten the strings at the neck.

The hands and the neck are clean.

3. Wiggle your arms and shoulders out of the gown.

When one hand is covered inside the sleeve, you can pull the other sleeve down by handling it with the protected hand.

4. With hands inside of gown at shoulders, bring shoulder seams together and hang gown on hook—wash hands again.

Hands are contaminated by touching outside of gown.

---

*From Thompson and LeBaron, Simplified Nursing, 1960.

Toys. Toys must be washable, and may be kept in a special cloth bag tied to the patient's crib so that they will not drop to the floor. The string of the bag is kept short, to avoid a situation in which it might become twisted about the child's neck. Since there is no satisfactory method of disinfecting books, reading should be limited to magazines or materials that are not highly prized by the owner. In highly communicable diseases, reading material is burned during terminal disinfection of the unit.

Visitors. Visitors are usually restricted to members of the immediate family. They should wear a gown and possibly a mask while in the patient's room. Articles brought to the patient must be washable or disposable. After the visitor's gown has been removed and deposited in the laundry hamper, he must wash his hands. Do not allow visitors to take articles from the room.

Isolation of the Child at Home

The child who is suspected of having a communicable disease should be kept away from other members of the family. Early symptoms may include fever, cold, runny nose, vomiting, headache, and abdominal pain. A doctor is consulted, because even some of the minor diseases can develop serious complications if left untreated. Once the diagnosis has been established, proper immunizations for other members of the family may be indicated.

The patient's room must be away from the center of family activities and near the bathroom. Most of the furnishings in a child's room are washable, so cleaning does not present much of a problem. Extra toys that the child will not be using should be removed for the convenience of the person caring for him. They may be placed in a large carton so that they will not become lost.

Equipment that is necessary for the patient's care may be placed on newspapers in his closet. It should be kept out of sight, and covered with a clean cloth. The doctor's orders are carried out in the patient's room unless there is a private bathroom. The patient's bath water and other fluid wastes are emptied into the toilet. Thick paper towels are used to lift the toilet cover to prevent contamination. The toilet seat is washed with hot soap and water after the toilet has been flushed to prevent possible contamination. When the patient is allowed bathroom privileges, the toilet seat is washed and disinfected after each use.

Since the majority of bedrooms do not have running water, the nurse must provide a pitcher of hot water and a basin. The pitcher is considered clean and is handled by the use of paper towels. The water is poured into the basin, and the hands are washed for two to three minutes with soap and water. The nurse grasps the handle of the pitcher with a paper towel to rinse one hand. This is repeated to rinse the other hand. Paper towels are burned once or twice a day as needed.

The practical nurse wears a gown while attending the patient. Contaminated linen may be collected in a large, covered kettle filled with cold water and soap. The contents are brought to a boil. After boiling 5 to 10 minutes, the linen is safe to handle.

The child's dishes must be kept separate from those of the rest of the family. They may be placed in a wash basin and boiled before being washed. Paper plates are convenient (see Fig. 119).

The practical nurse obtains information from the child's physician as to the advisability of visits from family members and friends, and any specific precautions which he may desire them to take.

The nursing care of the ill child in the home is basically the same as in the hospital. The doctor's orders are carried out, the patient is kept comfortable, and records of medications and treatments are maintained. Medications are the responsibility of the nurse and must be kept in a safe place. The person who administers the medication when she is off duty must be thoroughly instructed as to the name, time, and amount which the child is to receive. The nurse should confirm the administration of the medication when she returns the next day.

Diversions should be suitable to the age of the child. Children love stories, and the local librarian and parents can aid in choosing those that

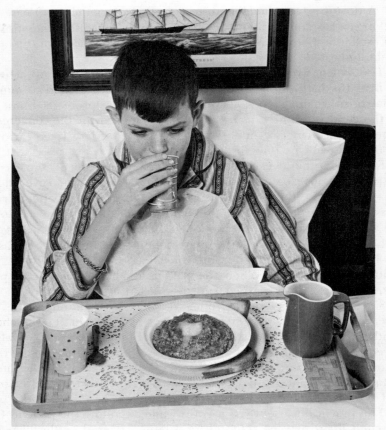

Figure 119. The use of paper plates in isolation. (Courtesy of Field Research Division, Paper Cup and Container Institute, Inc., New York City.)

appeal to the child of a certain age. Older children enjoy card games or those in which two can participate.

The practical nurse who establishes a good relationship with the child soon wins the confidence of the entire family. She should explain, in simple terms, procedures that are necessary, and she should let the child assist when possible.

STUDY QUESTIONS

1. Review the composition of the blood. What is the normal number of red blood cells? White blood cells? Platelets? What are the functions of each?
2. List several problems faced by the preschool child who is hospitalized.
3. Define the following: communicable disease, immunity, serum, gamma globulin, incubation period.

4. Discuss the postoperative care of the child who has had his tonsils and adenoids removed.
5. Billy, age four, has alternating strabismus. What is the cause of this condition? The treatment? The nursing care?
6. Why is it sometimes necessary to administer blood transfusions to the child with leukemia? What observations are necessary when a transfusion is running?
7. What is the cause of the bleeding from mucous membranes which is seen in leukemia?
8. How can diphtheria be prevented?
9. Rita, age five, has been in isolation for meningitis about a week. She is making satisfactory progress. How does her care differ from the care given to children who are not in isolation? List several diversions that appeal to the five year old.
10. Ken, age three, is recovering from the chickenpox. He is at home, and you are caring for him. What measures would you take to try to establish a good relationship with the child? His parents? What are the responsibilities of the practical nurse in this situation?
11. List the symptoms of the following diseases: mumps, chickenpox, measles, German measles, roseola.
12. Define acute glomerulonephritis. What nursing measures are specific to the condition?
13. What factors might conceivably precipitate an attack of asthma?

BIBLIOGRAPHY

Benz, G. S.: Pediatric Nursing. St. Louis, C. V. Mosby Co., 1964.
Bette, M. A.: Summer Work with the Retarded. Amer. J. Nurs. 67:1228-1229, 1967.
Blake, F., and Wright, F. H.: Essentials of Pediatric Nursing. 7th Ed. Philadelphia, J. B. Lippincott Co., 1963.
Broadribb, V.: Foundations of Pediatric Nursing. Philadelphia, J. B. Lippincott Co., 1967.
Culver, V. M., and Brownell, K. O.: The Practical Nurse. 6th Ed. Philadelphia, W. B. Saunders Co., 1964.
Flory, M. C.: Helping Parents Train a Retarded Child. Nurs. Outlook. 5:426, 1957.
Hammar, S. L., and Eddy, J.: Nursing Care of the Adolescent. New York, Springer Publishing Co., Inc., 1966.
Harmer, B., and Henderson, V.: Textbook of the Principles and Practice of Nursing. 5th Ed. New York, The Macmillan Co., 1957.
Hazel, S.: Lesson in Love for Retarded Pre-Schoolers. Amer. J. Nurs. 67:327, 1967.
Latham, H., and Heckel, R.: Pediatric Nursing. St. Louis, C. V. Mosby Co., 1967.
Marlow, D.: Textbook of Pediatric Nursing. 3rd Ed. Philadelphia, W. B. Saunders Co., 1969.
Memmler, R.: The Human Body in Health and Disease. Philadelphia, J. B. Lippincott Co., 1962.
Nelson, W. (Editor): Textbook of Pediatrics. 9th Ed. Philadelphia, W. B. Saunders Co., 1969.
Price, A.: The Art, Science and Spirit of Nursing. 3rd Ed. Philadelphia, W. B. Saunders Co., 1965.
Thompson, E., and LeBaron, M.: Simplified Nursing. 7th Ed. Philadelphia, J. B. Lippincott Co., 1960.
United States Department of Health, Education, and Welfare: Your Child from One to Six. Children's Bureau Publication No. 30, 1962.
United Sates Department of Health, Education, and Welfare: Infant Care. Children's Bureau Publication No. 8, 1963.

Chapter 13

THE SCHOOL AGE CHILD

VOCABULARY

Associate	*Embarrass*
Companion	*Exposed*
Concentrate	*Preoccupied*
Conflict	*Receptive*
Criticism	*Restless*

GENERAL CHARACTERISTICS

The school age child, from 6 to 12, differs from the preschool child in that he is more engrossed in fact that in fantasy. He has an ardent thirst for knowledge, and admires his teachers and adult companions, whom he considers wise. He uses the skill and knowledge he obtains to attempt to master the activities he enjoys, be it music, sports, and so forth. The child in school learns that he must cooperate with others. Participation in group activities heightens; gangs appear. Romantic love for the parent of the opposite sex diminishes, and the child identifies himself with the parent of the same sex. The type of acceptance he receives at home and at school will affect the attitude which he develops about himself and his role in life.

The child of this age is aware that his parents are human and make mistakes. Conflicts may appear, particularly if what the child learns in school is different from that which is practiced at home. Between six and twelve, children prefer friends of their own sex, and usually would rather be in the company of their friends than their brothers and sisters. Outward displays of affection of adults are embarrassing to them.

Growth is slow until the spurt directly before puberty. Weight gains are more rapid than gains in height. Muscular coordination is improved, and the lymphatic tissues become highly developed. The sinuses are frequently sites for infection. The six year molars, the first permanent teeth, erupt. The vital signs of the child of school age are near those of the adult. Temperature is 98.6; pulse, 85 to 100; respirations, 18 to 20. The systolic blood pressure ranges from 90 to 108 mm. Hg and the diastolic from 60 to 68 mm. Hg. Physical changes indicating puberty may appear. The average age of onset is 13 for girls and 14 to 15 for boys. This will vary about two years, plus or minus.

270

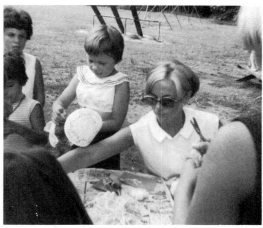

Figure 120.   The child of school age is creative and can cooperate with others. Well-planned summer programs appeal to children.

PHYSICAL, SOCIAL, AND MENTAL DEVELOPMENT

Six Years

The child of six bursts with energy and is on the go constantly. He soon becomes overtired, and it is necessary to set limits to his activities. He likes to start tasks, but does not always finish them, for his attention span is fairly brief. He tends to be bossy and sometimes rude, but is very sensitive to criticism. Sex investigations may still persist. The child's conscience is active and he finds it difficult to make decisions.

One of his most obvious physical changes at this age is the loss of the temporary teeth. The important six year molars erupt. The child can jump a rope, throw and catch a ball, and tie his shoe laces. He also performs numerous other feats that require muscle coordination. His language differs from that of the preschool child; he uses it for a purpose rather than for the pure joy of talking. He requires 11 to 13 hours of sleep a night.

Boys and girls play together at this age, although there is the beginning preference to associate with children of the same sex. Certain activities are common to both sexes. The boy in imaginative play is the soldier or trainman; the girl is the mother or nurse. Both sexes enjoy collecting objects that catch their fancy, e.g., leaves, stones, shells. Play at this time usually reflects events that occur in the immediate environment.

The child of six needs time and support to help him to adjust to school. If he has had nursery school or kindergarten experience, the

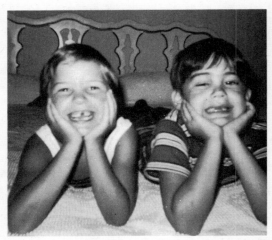

Figure 121. One of the most obvious physical changes of the six year old is the loss of the temporary teeth.

transition may be more comfortable. Most children go to school expecting the same reception that they are accustomed to in the home. If the parents are critical or overprotective, the child will assume that the teacher will be too. When this differs markedly from their expectations they begun to feel insecure and may even react hostile to the teacher. A trip to the school and a visit with the teacher if possible will give the child a better idea of what to expect. Children who are especially anxious benefit from having mother remain nearly for a few days. Not all children are ready for school merely because they have reached the proper age. Even those who are need time and support from parents and teachers before they can settle down to the job at hand. The child entering school is exposed to infection more frequently than he was at home. Preschool immunizations and a physical examination are indicated.

Seven Years

The child at seven is generally less of a problem than he was at six. It is a quieter age, and the child does not go looking for trouble. Some educators have noted that the second grader is the easiest to teach. He sets high standards for himself and for his family, has a good sense of humor, tends to be somewhat of a tease (e.g., wiggles his loose teeth to annoy adults), and is a little more modest than he was at an earlier age. He enjoys being active, but can also appreciate periods of rest. The second grader may acquire a "crush" on a friend of the opposite sex.

The child knows the months and seasons of the year and begins to tell time. He has a beginning concept of arithmetic, can count by two's and five's, and knows that money is valuable. His hands are steadier. Interest in God and heaven is heightened.

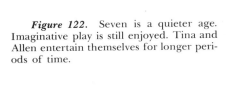
Figure 122. Seven is a quieter age. Imaginative play is still enjoyed. Tina and Allen entertain themselves for longer periods of time.

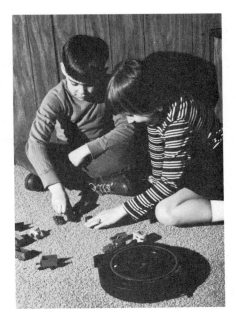

Active play is still important to both sexes. The boys are more apt to tease the girls rather than to participate in such games as jump rope or tag. Both sexes enjoy bike riding and table games. Realistic toys appeal to the seven year old, e.g., dolls that can be bathed and fed, trains that back up and whistle. Comic books are also popular. Becoming increasingly independent, the child imagines himself accomplishing feats more adventuresome than those of his parents, and cannot understand how they ever chose to lead such dull lives.

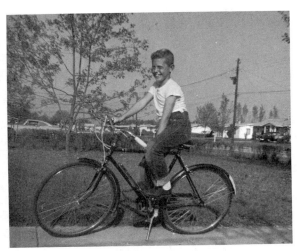
Figure 123. A bicycle opens new horizons for the child of school age.

One problem that may arise about this age is that of stealing. In many cases the child steals only to distribute his loot to neighborhood friends. This may in actuality be an attempt to buy friendship. His independence has separated him to a degree from his parents; if he cannot establish good relationships with his friends he may feel left out. When a child steals something, parents should tell him that they are aware of the fact, and insist on some form of restitution. They should not humiliate the child, but make it clear that such actions cannot be permitted. As always, accept the child but not the deed, and then try to understand the circumstances that are causing such behavior.

Eight Years

The eight year old wants to do everything, and can play alone for longer periods of time than the child of seven. Work is usually creative. Group activities such as the cub scouts are enjoyed, and companions of the same sex are preferred. Group fads begin to be seen. The eight year old likes to be considered important, particularly by adults. He behaves better for company than for the family. Hero worship is evident.

The arms and hands of the eight year old seem to grow faster than the rest of his body. The large and small muscles are better developed and movements are smoother and more graceful. The child can write rather than print, and he understands the number of days which must pass before special events (e.g., Christmas, birthdays, discharge from the hospital).

Competitive sports are enjoyed, but the child is generally a poor loser. Long involved arguments occur over decisions made by referees. Wrestling is frequent, and dramatic play is popular. Most children like to be the hero or heroine of their favorite programs. Neighborhood secret clubs are organized, and all members must pay strict attention to the rules.

Nine Years

The nine year old is dependable and not as restless as the child of eight. More interest is shown in family activities, more responsibility is assumed for personal belongings and for younger brothers and sisters, and tasks are more likely to be completed. The child resists adult authority if it does not coincide with the opinions or ideals of his group. He is, however, more able to accept criticism for his actions. Individual differences are very pronounced.

Worries and mild compulsions are common. Children avoid cracks in the pavement: "Step on a crack, break your mother's back." They realize that these actions are senseless, but still feel obliged to repeat them. Nervous habits, sometimes referred to as "tics," may also appear, and vary widely. Eye-blinking, facial grimacing, and shoulder shrugging

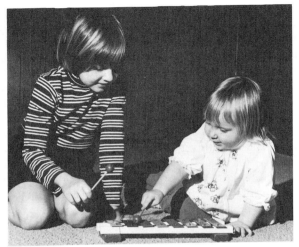

Figure 124. The child of school age entertains younger members of the family.

are but a few. The child cannot help such actions and should not be scolded for them because they are due mainly to tension; they usually disappear when home and social life become more relaxed.

Hand and eye coordination are well developed, and manual activities are managed with skill. The child works and plays hard, and becomes overtired. About 10 hours of sleep are needed a night. The permanent teeth are still erupting.

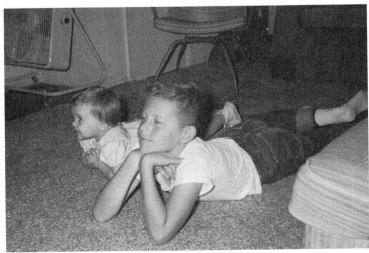

Figure 125. Children of all ages enjoy television. Parents should supervise the amount and types of programs viewed by children.

Competitive sports are still popular, as are reading, listening to the radio, and watching television and movies. Girls play for long periods of time with dolls. An interest in music is shown, and the child may desire to take lessons. The child knows the date, can repeat months of the year in order, and can multiply and do simple division. He takes care of his bodily needs, and by now his table manners are considerably improved.

10 Years

This marks the beginning of the preadolescent years. Girls are more physically mature than boys. The child begins to show self-direction, is courteous to adults, and thinks quite clearly about social problems and prejudices. He wants to be independent and resents being told what to do, but is receptive to suggestion. The ideas of the group are more important than individual ideas. Interest in sex and sex investigations continue to exist.

Girls in general are more poised than boys. Both sexes are fairly reliable about household duties. Slang terms are used. The 10 year old can write for a relatively long period of time, and maintains good speed. He uses fractions, and knows numbers over 100. Boys and girls begin to identify themselves with skills that pertain to their particular sex role. There is an intolerance of the opposite sex. The play enjoyed by the 10 year old is similar to that of the nine year old. The child takes more interest in his appearance.

10 to 12 Years (Preadolescent)

Adjectives that describe this age group include: intense, observant, all-knowing, energetic, meddlesome, and argumentative. This two year period before the onset of puberty is one of complete disorganization on the part of the child. Its beginning comes earlier in some children; the onset and rate of physical maturity varies greatly. Before the end of this period, the hormones of the body begin to influence physical growth. Posture is poor. There are 24 to 26 permanent teeth.

The child has an overabundance of energy, and is on the go every minute. Girls become "tom-boyish" in their actions. Table manners are a thing of the past, and the refrigerator is constantly emptied. The child is less concerned with his appearance. He seems to be preoccupied a great deal of the time, and this along with his physical activities and numerous anxieties account for some of the decline seen in school grades. Ability to concentrate decreases and the child never "hears anything his parents want him to." When asked to do a new task, he moans and groans.

Gangs are still important. The child is not ready to stand on his own feet, but cannot bear the thought of depending on his parents. He must overcome the problems that confront him without their help. His attitude implies, "Can't you see that I'm not a child anymore?"

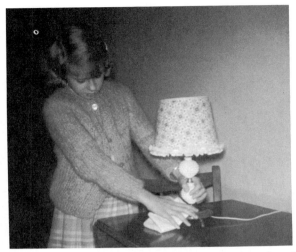

Figure 126. Becky, age 11, helps with the dusting to earn her allowance.

During prepuberty, the child is very much interested in his body, and watches for signs of growing up. Girls look forward to menstruation and to obtaining their first brassiere. Boys and girls tend to ignore the opposite sex, but in reality they are much aware of them. Their descriptions of each other are far from complimentary: "stupid, crazy, horrible," and so forth. Both sexes enjoy earning money by obtaining odd jobs. Boys usually deliver papers; girls mind younger brothers and sisters or help with housework. The preadolescent often seeks an adult friend of the same sex to idolize and to obtain emotional support.

Guiding the preadolescent is not easy. He needs freedom within limits and recognition that he is no longer a baby. He should know why parents make a decision, and not be expected to follow household rules blindly. The child's conscience enables him to understand reasonable punishment and he accepts it. Constant verbal nagging merely falls upon deaf ears. He should be provided with constructive opportunities to aid him in getting rid of pent-up emotions and energies. His irritating behavior is more easily accepted when one realizes that much of it indeed is "just a phase."

PHYSICAL CARE

The child of school age is gradually able to accept more responsibility for personal hygiene. He needs reminders, and in some instances, demonstrations as to how to do the task correctly. He is able to dress himself, brush his teeth, comb his hair, and wash his face and hands. (Most children of this age tend to forget that they have ears and a neck.)

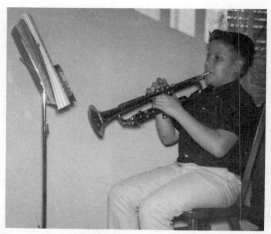

Figure 127. John, age 12, practices his trumpet lessons. Outlets such as this help the child to express his feelings in a constructive way.

He must be taught how to care for fingernails and toenails. Girls usually are more concerned with personal appearance than are boys.

Clothing need not be expensive, but simple in design and durable. Children must be taught the proper way to care for their clothes, but parents should anticipate temporary regressions in this area. Most mothers prefer that their children change into play clothes upon return from school. Play is rough and the school child is hard on wearing apparel. Shoes must be sturdy and of the proper size. Boots and rain-coats are necessary to protect the child from inclement weather. When heavy ski pants must be worn to school, lightweight slacks are worn beneath them, otherwise the child will have to wear the heavy outer pants during school, and will be too warm and uncomfortable. Stockings should fit properly to prevent irritation of the feet. All coats, sweaters, hats, boots, and so forth worn to school should be labeled.

The child of this age is so active during the day both physically and mentally that he soon becomes exhausted. His sleep is restless. The child from 6 to 8 years should have 11 to 13 hours of sleep a night. As he grows older, a little less is required. The 9 to 12 year old needs about 10 hours per night. Parents can judge the amount of sleep each of their children require. If the child is eating and playing well and keeping up with school work, chances are he is getting enough sleep.

The yearly preschool physical examination is given in the spring preceding admission. This allows time for correction of any problems that may be found. Booster shots should be given as required. The child also needs to have his teeth examined and any necessary dental work completed. School health programs aimed at maintaining and promot-ing health in the school systems are provided by most institutions. The nurses and other professional persons who participate in such programs play an important role in counseling parents. They also help in meeting the needs of handicapped children enrolled in their school.

The eating habits of the child of this age are basically good, and should not pose much of a problem when nutritious foods are offered. A good breakfast is important. The chief foods necessary are fruit, cereal, and milk. Eggs also add variety. Menus centered around these are more substantial than these consisting of toast or sweet rolls and coffee.

GUIDANCE

The child in school is in need of continuous understanding from persons concerned with his care. The types of relationships he has had previously are reflected in his behavior. He must known that he is wanted and loved, and that his parents are proud of his accomplishments, both in and out of school. He needs approval for tasks well done, and a minimum of criticism. At this age, the child is quite critical of himself, and needs help in self-acceptance. He is capable of good judgment, and should be allowed to make decisions and to take part in planning family activities. When he makes mistakes, he should be corrected and given explanations as to where his errors lie. Parents and nurses who show empathy toward school children can better understand their views.

The child wants to be accepted by his group; he imitates their speech, manner of dress, and actions. Interest in organizations is at its

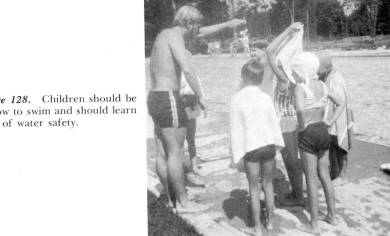

Figure 128. Children should be taught how to swim and should learn the rules of water safety.

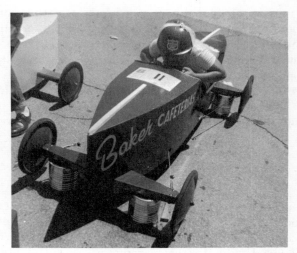

Figure 129.   The child of school age enjoys competitive sports.

peak. Children enjoy scouts and young people's groups affiliated with their church. Parents should encourage such group activities since they are both physically and morally strengthening.

The child needs time and a place to study. He should have a desk in his own room or at least in a private area of the house where he is able to concentrate. Furniture should be of the proper size; lighting should be adequate. He must learn to take responsibility for his assignments and school supplies, and to keep his room orderly. Parents can encourage him by showing interest in what he is learning, by joining parent-teacher organizations, and by visiting his teacher periodically. They must also vote on civic matters that will benefit the school system in their community.

At this age, an allowance or at least a means of earning money provides the child with opportunities to learn its value. It will take time and encouragement before he will learn to spend it wisely. Such experiences aid in making the school child a more responsible person.

Girls and boys need information and reassurance in advance about the changes that will take place in their bodies at puberty. This information is discussed in Chapter 15.

STUDY QUESTIONS

1. What are the average vital signs for the school child?
2. Describe the play of a six year old child. How does it differ from that of the child of nine?
3. What measures can be taken to help prepare a child for the first grade?

4. Johnny, age seven and one-half, came into the kitchen while you were serving diets. You notice that he helped himself to another piece of cake, and returned to his room. Discuss how you would deal with this situation.
5. Define the following: tic, puberty, hormone, sinus, compulsion.
6. You are working the evening shift. Visiting hours are over. When you enter the boy's ward, you find Fredie, age 10, and Don, age 12, engaged in a pillow fight. From your knowledge of this age group, would you consider this unreasonable behavior? How would you deal with this situation?
7. Discuss activities enjoyed by the child of eight. What diversion would you suggest for the long-term patient of this age?
8. Plan a day's menu for the school child. What foods should this menu be centered around?
9. What effect does the group have on the child from 10 to 12?
10. What hazards are most prevalent between the ages of 6 and 12? How can accidents resulting from such hazards be prevented?
11. You are playing checkers with Joan, age eight. You have just "jumped her king," when she bursts into tears. What is your reaction to this situation? How would you cope with it?
12. What factors should parents consider when selecting clothes for the school child?

BIBLIOGRAPHY

Blake, F.: The Child, His Parents and the Nurse. Philadelphia, J. B. Lippincott Co., 1954.
Blake, F., and Wright, F. H.: Essentials of Pediatric Nursing. 7th Ed. Philadelphia, J. B. Lippincott Co., 1963.
Breckenridge, M., and Murphy, M.: Growth and Development of the Young Child. 8th Ed. Philadelphia, W. B. Saunders Co., 1969.
Culver, V. M., and Brownell, K. O.: The practical Nurse, 6th Ed. Philadelphia. W. B. Saunders Co., 1964.
Hurlock, E.: Child Development. 3rd Ed. New York, McGraw-Hill Book Co., Inc. 1956.
Marlow, D.: Textbook of Pediatric Nursing. 3rd Ed. Philadelphia, W. B. Saunders Co., 1969.
Nelson, W. (Editor): Textbook of Pediatrics. 9th Ed. Philadelphia, W. B. Saunders Co. 1969.
New Hampshire State Department of Health. Child Development Chart. Maternal and Child Health.
Smith, C.: Maternal-Child Nursing. Philadelphia, W. B. Saunders Co., 1963.
Spock, B.: Baby and Child Care. Rev. Ed. New York, Duell, Sloan, and Pearce, Inc., 1968.

Chapter 14

DISORDERS OF THE
SCHOOL AGE CHILD

VOCABULARY

Alert	*Nodule*
Dietitian	*Shock*
Dressing	*Stenosis*
Forceps	*Sterile*
Graft	*Superficial*
Murmur	*Valve*

The child of school age is able to accept hospitalization more readily than the preschool child. He can endure separation from his parents if it is not prolonged. Children who have been cherished from birth can tolerate brief interruptions in their lives more easily than those who are denied a secure environment. If the practical nurse is to help the child, she should find out as much about him as possible. When you know a great deal about a patient, your interest in him is keener. This is evidenced by the concern one has for children of friends or relatives who are hospitalized.

The nurse will come in contact with many school age children who are handicapped and are long-term patients. Unfortunately many of them come from broken homes or because of their illness or poor family relationships have been unable to proceed along the lines of healthy emotional development. These children may be the ward problems. They need your help. Anyone can care for the cute, cooperative, well-adjusted patient. It takes an *exceptional* nurse to establish good relations with a sulky, unruly, unhappy child.

At this age the child is trying to establish an image for himself. He likes to talk with adults and to feel that his opinions are respected and he is important. Children seldom respond to direct questions from strangers. The new nurse can establish contact by engaging the patient in a competitive table game. As both patient and nurse become engrossed in the activity, the relationship becomes more relaxed and conversation flows more easily.

When the practical nurse first enters a noisy ward and sees that the children are bursting with pent-up energies, she feels inadequate and

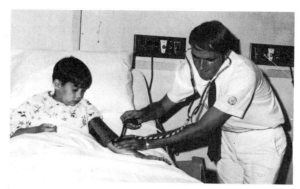

Figure 130. The practical nursing student explains what he is about to do so that the child's fears are lessened. (Courtesy of St. Barnabas Medical Center, School of Practical Nursing, Livingston, N.J.)

does not know how to cope with this new experience. Her first impulse is to "lay down the law" with a long list of "don'ts," but this is fruitless even if it brings about a certain amount of order. Instead, she should develop in children the ability to direct themselves through intelligent guidance. The pediatric ward is, after all, for children, and the nurse should not lose sight of this fact. Sometimes the nurse can enlist the help of an older child. If he knows that she needs his assistance, he will develop a feeling of responsibility. If the nurse has discovered the ring leader of the group, she is ahead of the game. Positive direction and consistency are tools of particular importance to the pediatric nurse.

The education of the school age child must continue throughout his infirmity. This gives him a sense of continuity with the outside world, provides him with periods of socialization, and may reinforce his weak academic areas. It involves the parents who may act as liaisons between the regular school and the hospital school. The teacher needs to be informed of his physical and emotional health if she is to deal effectively with the patient. The nurse provides the child with opportunities to study undisturbed so that he will be prepared for his classes.

School children are frequently brave during situations in which they are really quite upset. The nurse's presence is comforting to them in unfamiliar circumstances. She should not undermine this factor, even though the patient has not directly asked her to stay.

Circulatory System

RHEUMATIC FEVER

Description. Rheumatic fever belongs to a group of disorders known as *collagen* diseases. Their common feature is the destruction of connective tissue. Rheumatic fever, a systemic disease, is particularly detrimental to the heart. It is rare in the first three years of life, but reaches its peak of incidence between 5 and 15. The first attacks occur most often between 6 and 8 years of age. It has a high family incidence, and is more common in the lower income groups and when over-crowded conditions exist. It is more prevalent in winter and spring, and carrier rates among school children are believed to be increased during these seasons.

Rheumatic fever is considered to be a complication of streptococcal infection of the throat, i.e., group A beta hemolytic streptococci. The body becomes sensitized to the organism after repeated attacks, and develops an allergic response to it.

Symptoms. The symptoms range from mild to severe. The classic ones are *wandering joint pains* (polyarthritis), *skin eruptions, chorea* (a ner-vous disorder), and *inflammation of the heart.* Subcutaneous nodules may appear beneath the skin, but are not as common in children. Abdominal pain, often mistaken for appendicitis, may also occur. Fever varies from low grade to high elevations. Pallor, fatigue, anorexia, and unexplained nose bleeds may be seen. Rheumatic fever has a tendency to *recur*, and each attack carries the threat of further damage to the heart. The re-currences are greatest during the first five years following the initial attack, and decline rapidly thereafter.

POLYARTHRITIS (*poly-* many + *arthr-* joint + *-itis* inflammation of). The arthritis seen in rheumatic fever is distinctive in that it does not result in permanent deformity to the joint. It involves mainly the larger joints: the knees, elbows, ankles, wrists, and shoulders. The joints become painful and tender, and are difficult to move. This lasts for a few days, disappears without treatment, and frequently returns in another joint; this may continue over a period of weeks. The symptoms tend to be more severe in older children. The joint may be visibly swollen and inflamed. Relief is obtained by the administration of salicylates.

SKIN ERUPTIONS. The rash seen in rheumatic fever consists of small, red circles and wavy lines appearing on the trunk and abdomen. They appear and disappear rapidly and are of significance in diagnosing the disease.

CHOREA (St. Vitus' Dance). This is a disorder of the central ner-vous system characterized by involuntary, purposeless movements of the muscles. It may occur as an acute rheumatic involvement of the brain. It is seen primarily in children between the ages of 6 and 15. Recurrences may appear, but eventually the disease disappears spontaneously and recovery is complete.

Attacks of chorea, which begin slowly, are characterized by in-creased tension. The child may stumble and spill things, and may have difficulty buttoning his clothes and writing. When the face muscles are involved, grimaces appear. The child may laugh and cry inappropriate-ly, and show evidence of emotional strain. It severe cases, the child may become completely incapacitated. Fortunately, most cases are mild. The treatment is directed toward the relief of symptoms by physical and mental rest.

RHEUMATIC CARDITIS.   Inflammation of the heart, a manifestation of rheumatic fever, can be fatal. It occurs more often in the young child. The tissues that cover the heart and the heart valves are affected. The heart muscle, the myocardium, may be involved as well as the pericardium and endocardium. The *mitral valve*, between the left atrium and left ventricle, is frequently involved. Vegetations form which interfere with the proper closing of the valve and disturb its normal function. When this valve becomes narrowed, the condition is called *mitral stenosis*. The burden on the heart is great because it has to pump harder to circulate the blood. As a result, it may become enlarged. Symptoms of poor circulation and heart failure may occur.

The patient has an irregular low grade fever, is pale and listless, and has a poor appetite. Moderate anemia and weight loss are apparent. The child may experience dyspnea upon exertion. The rate of the pulse and respirations are out of proportion to the body temperature. The doctor may detect a soft murmur over the apex of the heart.

Diagnosis.   The diagnosis of rheumatic fever is difficult to make and is based on the entire clinical picture. A careful physical examination is done and a complete history of the patient is taken. Certain blood tests are helpful. The *sedimentation rate** and the white blood cell count are elevated. These indicate infection or an excessive breakdown of body

---

*An expression of the extent and velocity of the sedimentation of red blood cells in fresh citrated blood.

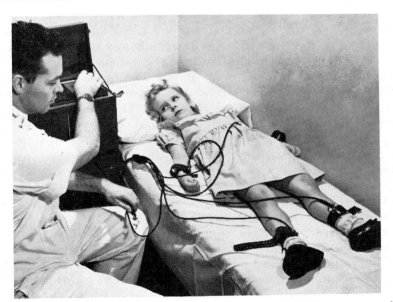

Figure 131.   The electrocardiogram is a graphic report of electric currents produced by activity of the heart muscle. (Presbyterian Hospital, Chicago, Illinois.)

tissues. Abnormal proteins, e.g., C-reactive protein, may also be evidenced in the serum. Additional studies may include x-rays of the chest and lung tests. The *electrocardiogram,* a graphic record of the electrical changes caused by the beating of the heart, is very useful. These tests are repeated throughout the course of the disease so that the doctor may determine when the active stage has subsided.

Prognosis. Prognosis of rheumatic fever is improving. In the United States its incidence has declined in the past 20 years. The immediate outlook for recovery without residual heart damage during the acute stage is good. Death from uncomplicated rheumatic fever is unusual. Recurrent infections may cause further damage to the heart, however, and result in chronic defects. The damaged heart may lead to early death in adulthood or invalidism. Research is now being conducted in an attempt to develop a vaccine which will prevent streptococcal infections in children.

Treatment and Nursing Care.   The doctor directs his treatment toward complete physical and mental rest, relief of pain and fever, and management of cardiac failure if it occurs.

Medications include the *salicylates,* usually aspirin, and *steroids* such as cortisone, ACTH, or prednisone, which relieve fever and pain, and make the patient more comfortable. They have undesirable side effects which the nurse should be aware of and watch for. High dosages of aspirin can result in gastric upset, ringing in the ears, and headaches. Cortisone, prednisone, and ACTH may cause acne, moonface, edema, hypertension, and excessive hairiness.

Morphine is given to control chest pain. Children are more sensitive to this drug than adults, and a relatively smaller amount is prescribed. The signs of excessive dosage are the same in children as adults. However, the child may react more rapidly and more violently. Early toxic symptoms of morphine are slow respirations (below 12 per minute), deep sleep, and constricted pupils. The nurse always counts the patient's *respirations* before she administers morphine. *Digitalis* may be given to slow and strengthen the heart. The *pulse* rate is counted carefully before giving this drug. If it is markedly lower or has changed in quality, the doctor is contacted before giving the dose. Since the pulse and respiration rates of children vary with age, the nurse consults the patient's chart to see what the previous readings have been before she administers such drugs. *Phenobarbital* may be given as a sedative. The doctor may order the use of *oxygen.* Small daily dosages of *penicillin* or *sulfadiazine* are given to protect the child from further streptococcal infection. Many physicians recommend that it be given for five years or longer following the first attack.

The patient is placed on strict bed rest during the intial attack, i.e., he is to remain in bed at all times. He does not have bathroom privileges and must be bathed, fed, moved in bed, and so forth. The amount of work the heart has to do must be limited by resting the entire body. In

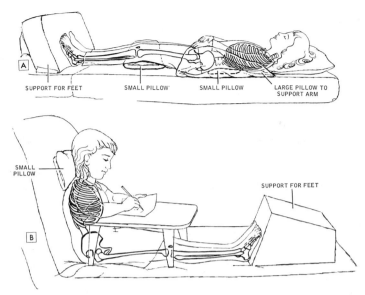

Figure 132. Methods of positioning a child for good body alignment. *A*, flat in bed. *B*, in a sitting position. (From Marlow, D.: Textbook of Pediatric Nursing, 1969.)

this way the body requires slower blood circulation and the heart does not have to work as fast or as hard as it does when a person is active. The nurse should explain this to her patient since he will cooperate better if he understands the reasons for his confinement. She also reassures him that this restriction is only temporary.

Nursing procedures are carried out quickly and skillfully so that they will not be painful or tiring to the patient. They should be organized so as to assure as few interruptions as possible. A bed cradle is used to prevent the weight of the bedclothes upon the painful extremities. The practical nurse should support the joints with her hands when moving the patient.

Care includes special attention to the skin, especially that over bony prominences, light back care (a brisk rub would tire the cardiac patient), good oral hygiene, and small, frequent feedings of nourishing foods. The intake and output of fluids is recorded. Regular bowel habits should be established. Vital signs are taken at designated intervals. The pulse is counted for a *full* minute. The doctor may also order sleeping pulses which are taken without disturbing the patient. The nurse tries to anticipate the needs of the child. She tells him what she is about to do, and explains the reasons for it. If she has a respiratory infection, she does not care for the rheumatic fever patient. All attempts must be made to shield him from persons who harbor infections.

In severe cases, the child looks acutely ill. His temperature is higher. The face is flushed and cyanosis may be evident. It may be necessary for the child to sit up in order to breathe. The child remains in bed and may complain of pain about the heart, stomach, and abdomen. The white blood cell count becomes greatly increased. An electrocardiogram provides valuable information in detection and follow-up of carditis.

School Work.   Provisions must be made for the child to carry out his school work as his condition permits. It is the nurse's responsibility to prepare him for his sessions with the teacher. If the patient does not feel well that day, the practical nurse notifies the nurse in charge. The room is adequately ventilated and lighted. The patient rests for at least a half hour before instruction begins and then is offered the bedpan. His face and hands are washed and some form of nourishment is given. He is dressed unless this is contraindicated. The back rest is elevated, and the over-bed table is cleared and placed at a convenient level. The footrest is properly positioned. A chair is provided for the teacher. The nurse should place a sign on the door so that no one will interrupt.

Since a period of convalescence is needed upon discharge, a tutor will be required unless closed circuit television or a school-to-home telephone is available.

Emotional Support.   All efforts are made to give emotional support to the child and his family during this long illness. When a person is ill, he tends to intensify feelings of failure which everyone experiences from time to time. The patient may brood and becomes obstinate. The child is prohibited from participating in many of the natural rag-tag activities of childhood; therefore, his return to the community may find him poorly coordinated and self-conscious. To prevent intensive problems from arising, the child needs to be kept occupied within his capacity. He also needs the companionship of his friends via mail, telephone, and, when possible, visits. This and a close relationship with the rest of his family will keep the child from feeling left out. The spiritual needs of the patient should not be neglected.

Suggested passive diversions include: an aquarium, a mirror hung so that he may see the activities in the corridor, plants of various types, a canary or other similar housebird (this may not be permitted in the hospital, but is acceptable in the home), stories, and quiet music. As his condition improves, part of his time may be taken up by doing simple tasks for himself. Hobbies such as soap carving and stamp collecting are interesting and fun to start. Boys can be encouraged to follow certain baseball activities or similar sports on television. This may help them to communicate with their peers.

Close medical supervision and follow-up care is essential. Today physicians try to instill positive attitudes in the child. They emphasize what he can do rather than what he cannot. Persons caring for the long-term patient must try to instill confidence, rather than make the child overdependent. It is wise not to continually stress the fact that he has a heart condition. If the home environment is not suitable for the type of care the child needs, he may be placed in a convalescent home for

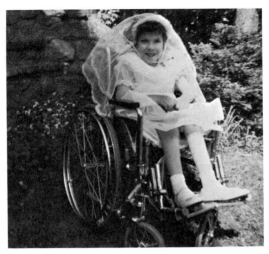

Figure 133. Suzanne has her very special day. The spiritual needs of all long-term patients should not be neglected. (Courtesy of Crotched Mountain Foundation. Greenfield, New Hampshire.)

chronically ill children until he is in good health. This further isolation can be extremely taxing on the physical and psychological development of the child and calls for ingenuity on the part of all concerned with his care.

Digestive System

APPENDICITIS

Description. Appendicitis occurs when the opening of the appendix into the cecum becomes obstructed. (This may be due to a number of reasons, e.g., blockage by fecal matter, infection, allergy.) It is rare under the age of one, uncommon under five and does not occur as often in children as in adults.

Symptoms. The symptoms in older children, similar to those in adults, are nausea, vomiting, abdominal tenderness, fever, constipation, and an increase in the number of white blood cells. The symptoms of appendicitis in the small child are more obscure. The patient has to be observed carefully over a period of hours to determine the diagnosis. The child cries and is restless. He runs a low grade fever. Pain is more generalized and harder to pinpoint. Nausea and vomiting may occur. Since these symptoms are indicative of many childhood upsets, the diagnosis is more difficult to establish.

Treatment.   This condition is treated by surgical operation called an *appendectomy*. The child may be hospitalized prior to surgery for a brief time during which he is kept on bed rest and his vital signs are taken periodically. The doctor may order the nurse to place an ice bag on the involved area to relieve pain and to decrease peristalsis. Fluids and feedings are withheld pending surgery.

Penicillin, streptomycin, or the sulfonamides may be given to prevent and minimize the danger of infection. If the appendix ruptures, the infected contents spill into the abdominal cavity and a generalized infection called *peritonitis* results. Cathartics are withheld when a patient has abdominal pain, to prevent precipitation of this, which of course is to be avoided, but today it is not considered as dangerous to the life of the child as it was before the discovery of the so-called "miracle drugs." The prognosis of uncomplicated appendicitis is good.

Nursing Care.   This discussion is limited to the care of the child upon his return from the recovery room. The immediate postoperative care is similar to that discussed on page 127 for the patient with a herniorrhaphy.

A recovery bed is prepared to receive the child upon his return to the ward. The furniture is arranged so that the stretcher can be wheeled easily to the bedside. The bed should be equipped with side rails. An emesis basin and tissues are placed on the bedside table, and an intravenous pole is brought into the room. The patient is transferred gently from the stretcher to the bed. Temperature, pulse, respiration, and blood pressure are taken upon his arrival, and the dressing is observed for drainage. If an intravenous is running, the kind, amount, and rate are observed. The nurse records her observations and the time the patient arrived on the ward, his state of consciousness (e.g., alert, groggy, nausea or vomiting), and any drainages. The practical nurse reports to her team leader or head nurse to review the postoperative orders left by the physician.

During the course of the day the following nursing measures are carried out: The patient's position is changed frequently. He is taught to take deep breaths and to cough. His hands and face are washed, and a clean hospital gown is applied. An accurate record of intake and output is kept. The practical nurse reports the first voiding to the head nurse. If the patient has not voided during her shift, this should also be brought to the head nurse's attention. Small sips of water are given by mouth as nausea ceases. As soon as the child is able to take water and other fluids by mouth, intravenous feedings are discontinued. Vital signs are taken as ordered. The patient is encouraged to move about in bed. Evidences of pain are reported. Pediatric patients recuperate quickly from uncomplicated surgery. Ambulation is generally not a problem.

Sterile Dressings.   The practical nurse is frequently shown how to change simple sterile dressings, such as those on the patient following an appendectomy. She is observed by the registered nurse while changing the dressing until she feels secure in doing the procedure by herself.

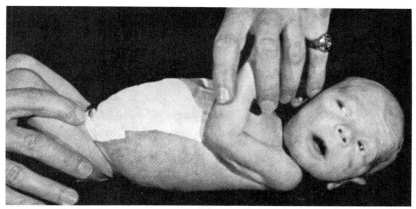

Figure 134. A surgical dressing helps to prevent contamination of a wound. This premature baby had undergone surgery for intestinal obstruction. (From Gross, R. E.: Surgery of Infancy and Childhood, 1964.)

Surgical dressings are used to protect the wound, to absorb drainage, to prevent the wound from becoming contaminated, to apply pressure, to keep the wound edges close together to promote healing, and to apply medications locally. All surgical dressings are done using *aseptic technique.*

Sterile supplies and equipment are kept on a dressing cart. When it is necessary to change a dressing, the child is brought to the treatment room, unless it is contraindicated, so that other children in the ward are not upset. If the dressing is changed at the bedside, the patient is screened. The windows and doors of the room are shut to prevent the movement of air in the room. This lessens the chances of contaminating the wound by airborne germs. When personnel are sufficient, another person assists with the dressing change. One person remains contaminated and pours solutions, obtains extra supplies, and so forth. The nurse should provide adequate lighting. She explains what she is going to do to the child, and drapes him. She prepares the unsterile equipment first: a newspaper is placed at the foot of the bed to receive soiled dressings and adhesive tape is cut into needed lengths.

SPECIAL CONSIDERATIONS. The transfer forceps found on the dressing cart are used only to transfer sterile supplies from the cart to a sterile field, *never* to apply a dressing to the patient. They are held with their tips *down* to prevent the disinfecting solution from running back onto the contaminated handles and then flowing back onto the sterile tips when the forceps are inverted. Transfer forceps are held above the waist at all times. The practical nurse must be very careful not to hit the forceps against unsterile objects in the environment.

Covers of sterile containers are carefully removed to prevent contaminating the insides, and are placed upside down. A sterile towel is · spread open in a convenient area. Usually the over-bed table or bedside stand is safer than the bed on the children's ward. The stand is positioned so that the nurse does not have to turn her back on the sterile field. The child is instructed not to touch the towel or wound. An attempt should be made to distract the child by conversation.

The sterile articles needed for the dressing change are dropped onto the sterile field. The transfer forceps should not come in direct contact with the towel. If the wound needs to be bathed or requires similar treatment, wear sterile gloves. When handling sterile instruments without gloves, touch only the handles. These unsterile handles must be kept off the sterile surgical field. For practical purposes, consider that one inch of the outer edge of the sterile towel is contaminated. *Never reach across the sterile field.* Do not handle sterile supplies unnecessarily. If you do not have assistance and find it necessary to return to the dressing cart for further supplies, always wash your hands first.

After the dressing has been completed, the patient is made comfortable. The nurse observes the type and amount of drainage on the soiled dressing before she discards it. Instruments used are washed, rinsed, and sterilized. The dressing cart is replenished. The practical nurse should chart the time of the dressing, the area to which it was applied, the color and amount of drainage (scant, moderate, excessive), the odor, any unusual findings, medication if applied, and how the patient tolerated the procedure.

ASSISTING THE DOCTOR WITH A DRESSING CHANGE. The doctor will appreciate the nurse's assistance when he changes a dressing. If the practical nurse has never helped with the particular dressing before, she should mention this fact to him, but also show her willingness to be of assistance. The dressing cart contains most of the necessary articles and supplies. The nurse checks that it has been properly restocked. The doctor prepares the sterile field. When he needs more sterile sponges, the practical nurse drops them on the sterile field by using the transfer forceps. Cleanse the lips of solution bottles by pouring a small amount from them before pouring the liquid upon the sterile sponge. *The lip should not come in direct contact with the sterile article.* Provide a waste receptable to be used by the doctor. The nurse cares for the equipment and soiled dressings following the procedure. She makes the patient comfortable. Charting includes the time and area of the dressing change, by whom, the type and amount of drainage, how the patient tolerated the procedure, and any other pertinent information, e.g. removal of stitches.

The Skin

BURNS

Description. Burns occur frequently during childhood. The prevalence is higher among boys than girls because of their natural aggressiveness. These burns may be caused by many factors, such as stoves, heaters, vaporizers, radiators, irons, fireplaces, bath water, coffee, defective wiring, unguarded outlets, and strong acids and alkalis such as lye or ammonia.* A burn affects the entire body, not merely the specific area. If one-third to one-half the skin surface is burned, the chances for recovery are not good. Death usually occurs within 48 hours in the majority of severe burns. The prognosis depends on the depth of the burn as well as the extent. There are three degrees of burns:

FIRST DEGREE. The skin becomes reddened, but the burn is superficial. First aid: Apply white petrolatum U.S.P. or other suitable sterile ointment or immerse in ice water.

SECOND DEGREE. Blisters appear. First aid: If the injured area is small, treat as for first degree burns, otherwise cover with a sterile dressing or the cleanest cloth available. (This keeps the air out, and decreases pain.) Avoid breaking the blisters. Call the doctor.

THIRD DEGREE. The skin is charred and the underlying tissues are injured. First aid: Cover with a sterile dressing. If extensive, wrap the child in a clean sheet. Do not attempt to remove clothing that sticks to the area. Keep the child warm through the use of blankets, and take him to the emergency room of the nearest hospital. Do not apply ointment or any other substance.

Second and third degree burns must be thought of as open wounds with the added danger of infection. Do not apply greasy ointment such as lard or butter, which may infect the wound and will have to be removed for adequate treatment. Absorbent cotton is never used, since it will stick to the injured area.

The chief cause of death from burns is shock and the toxic condition that arises from it. This is due to the sudden loss of large amounts of *plasma,* the fluid portion of the blood. The fluid passes from the blood vessels into the tissues. There is a decrease in blood *volume* and a change in the composition of the blood. Circulation becomes sluggish. This affects the normal function of vital organs. They suffer from lack of oxygen and nutrients. Waste products accumulate in the blood. Without proper treatment, death will result. The practical nurse should learn well the early symptoms of shock. These are:

Increase in pulse and respirations.
Decrease in blood pressure.
Decrease in temperature.
Pallor.
Cold, clammy skin.
Prostration.
Dilated pupils.

*Blake and Wright, p. 479.

Treatment. The immediate treatment of shock in cases of severe burns is handled by the doctor and the registered nurse in the hospital emergency and in some instances the operating room. Specimens of blood and urine are obtained. A pain reliever such as morphine or codeine is administered. Intravenous fluids or plasma are begun, and oxygen is given when necessary. Dyspnea, sternal retractions, and stridor may indicate a tracheotomy. Tetanus antitoxin is given if the patient has not had tetanus toxoid. A booster dose of tetanus toxoid may be given if the child has had prior inoculations, as well as an antitoxin against gas gangrene. A urinary catheter may be inserted.

Local treatment of the wound varies. The most widely used methods are the *open technique* or the *pressure bandage (closed) technique*. In the open technique no dressing is applied. The doctor may clean the wound but no covering is placed over it. A protective crust (*eschar*) will form in several days and prevent the further loss of fluids. The patient is placed on *sterile* sheets. Personnel caring for him wear *sterile* gowns and masks obtained from the operating room or central supply. Thorough hand-washing is essential. Special burn tents of plastic with portholes through which the nurse cares for the patient are now available. These provide increased protection from infection, like the Isolette protects the premature. In the closed bandage method the wound is tightly bandaged to prevent fluid loss. The bandages are not removed for two to three weeks. Some surgeons use a light plaster of paris cast instead of a bandage. Protective antibiotics are usually administered.

Newer methods of treating burns through the use of various solutions are gaining popularity. Wet soaks of 0.5 per cent silver nitrate solution changed several times daily have helped to reduce infection and odor. Skin grafting can sometimes be commenced earlier and its need may be lessened by the use of this method. *Debridement* or removal of dried crusts is done in all methods, when needed to clean the wound and prepare the new *granulation* tissue for grafting. When a graft is done, skin is transplanted from one individual to another or from one part of the body to another to cover the burned area. The latter called an autograft (*auto* self + graft) is the only kind of skin graft accepted permanently by the tissues except for the skin which comes from an identical twin. The site from which the skin is removed is referred to as the *donor* area. Both sites are covered with sterile dressings following the procedure.

Role of the Practical Nurse. Children who have suffered extensive burns and survive the early dangers face a long period of hospitalization and require specialized care. The practical nurse is often called upon to care for the child who is convalescing. The various aspects of nursing care vary with the age of the patient, the area of the burn, and the type of treatment instigated.

Preventing Infection. Every effort must be made to prevent the injured area from becoming infected. With a young child, arm restraints may be necessary to keep him from touching the area with his fingers.

The nurse must wash her hands carefully before caring for the patient and assisting with dressing changes. All articles that come in contact with the wound must be sterile. When enemas are given, waterproof materials must be used to prevent contamination of the dressing. The nurse should report signs of infection immediately. These are: elevation of temperature, pulse, and respiration; restlessness; pain; and a foul odor to the dressing. All infection must be cleared before skin can be grafted.

Fluids and Nourishment.   The physician plans the amount of fluids to be given by the results of tests made on the patient's blood. The loss of plasma in the blood results in an increase in the concentration of red blood cells. A simple hemoglobin count or a hematocrit (which indicates the proportion of red blood cells to a specific amount of blood) provides the necessary information.* Typing and crossmatching for transfusions are also done. Parenteral therapy is given to replace fluids and electrolytes. Oral fluids, though restricted initially to prevent nausea and vomiting, are necessary during the convalescent stages to aid the body in getting rid of poisons, to prevent kidney damage, and to maintain body fluid requirements. The nurse must use her ingenuity to persuade the child to take sufficient amounts of fluids. *An accurate record of intake and output is kept.* Poor appetite is frequently encountered in these patients. Frequent feedings of foods high in calories, protein, and iron are necessary. A high protein diet is a normal diet with added amounts of meat, milk, eggs, cheese, fish, or poultry.† Iron therapy may be instigated when anemia begins to develop. Eggnogs are nourishing between-meal drinks for such patients. Offer small amounts frequently. Vitamins B and C are given to hasten healing and to stimulate the appetite. Gavage feedings may be necessary.

Position.   The foot of the crib is raised. The doctor will designate the later positions of the child. If the doctor applies a dressing to an extremity, he places it in correct alignment before applying the bandage. He may also use a splint to maintain it in correct position. The practical nurse should bear in mind that the other parts of the body that are not affected need exercise and proper positioning to prevent painful contractures. The child's position is changed every two to four hours unless contraindicated. A footboard is used to prevent footdrop. Support should be given by means of pillows, sandbags, and rolled towels as necessary. The physical therapist may be asked to visit the child regularly to carry out exercises to keep the joints limber and healthy. The nurse is gentle when positioning her patient to prevent injury to the delicate skin which is healing beneath the bandage.

Skin Care.   The unaffected parts of the patient's body must be kept

---

*Mason, Basic Medical-Surgical Nursing, 1967.
†Mowry, Basic Nutrition and Diet Therapy for Nurses, 1966.

clean and dry. Special attention is given to the skin around the injury. It should be kept free of exudate by gentle cleansing. Petrolatum may be applied for protection. The buttocks and perineal area are given special care, particularly if the dressing borders these areas. Crib sheets are pulled taut, and kept dry, clean, and free from crumbs. A Bradford frame is often used to facilitate nursing care (see p. 180). Pressure areas may develop, particularly when immobilization is necessary. The nurse observes the child's skin closely when giving the daily bath.

Comfort Measures. The child with severe burns requires medication to relieve pain during the early stages of his illness. Pain contributes to shock and must be controlled for this purpose as well as for the well-being of the patient. Morphine may be given to relieve the immediate distress. The doctor may also order a sedative such as phenobarbital to be given periodically. As the child recuperates, the need for such drugs is generally diminished. The doctor may request that the child be given a pain reliever such as *Demerol* before dressing changes.

The room should be kept well ventilated to prevent offensive odors. A deodorizer is used when necessary. The patient's unit is kept neat, clean, and adequately lighted.

The use of a bed cradle prevents the weight of the covers from touching the affected areas. The urinal is emptied p.r.n. and the amount is recorded. The child's hair is combed and arranged neatly. Back rubs are given, and good oral hygiene is maintained.

The practical nurse observes the patient for discomfort or signs of bleeding from the gastrointestinal tract which could indicate a stress or *Curling's ulcer,* sometimes seen in patients with burns.

Emotional Support. This type of injury is taxing to the child and his parents. It requires long periods of hospitalization and frequent readmissions. The accident itself is terrifying for the child but it is made even worse if it was caused by his disobedience. The practical nurse encourages the child to express his feelings. She should not be upset if he screams during dressing changes or takes out his frustrations on her. She must maintain a calm but firm manner and assure him that she understands how he feels. She should keep from showing her reaction to the wound, since children are quick to recognize an expression of alarm or disgust, and may take it personally.

The long-term patient requires diversions of various types. Toys are kept within easy reach to prevent excessive movement. The crib is placed near the door so that the child may observe the activities outside. As his condition improves, he should enjoy the companionship of other children. Older patients enjoy helping with routine ward functions, which gives them a feeling of accomplishment.

The practical nurse gives constant support to the parents, who usually feel guilty in cases of accidents. She should indicate by her manner that she does not blame them for what has happened.

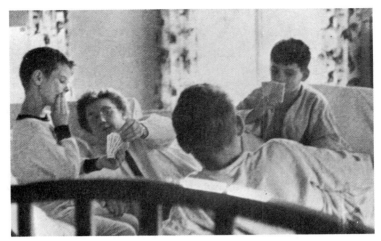

Figure 135. Planned and supervised competitive games for the same age group in the hospital setting will compensate for restricted activity. (From Tender Loving Care. The Journal of the American Medical Association. *157*:25, 1955.)

The importance of prevention of burns cannot be overemphasized (see p. 171).

PEDICULUS CAPITIS

Description. This disease, known as *head lice*, affects the scalp and hair. The eggs, called nits, attach to the hair, become numerous, and hatch within three or four days. Head lice is more common in girls than boys because of their long hair. It is easily transferred from one child to another and is seen most frequently in the school age child.

Symptoms. The child suffers from severe itching of the scalp. He scratches his head frequently and often causes further irritation. The hair becomes matted. Pustules and excoriations may be seen about the face.

Treatment and Nursing Care. The treatment is directed toward killing the lice, getting rid of the nits, and treating any infections of the face and scalp. Several preparations are available. One containing DDT powder is often used, as well as Kwell (benzene hexachloride). Pesticides should be used under the physician's direction since they can be irritating to the skin and mucous membranes. Nits are removed by combing the hair with a fine tooth comb dipped in hot vinegar. The hair is washed following. In some cases, recovery is hastened by cutting the hair. Clothing and bedding are boiled to prevent reinfection. Wool clothing requires dry cleaning. Children should be cautioned against swapping headgear. Proper cleansing of the hair and scalp as well as periodic examinations are preventive measures.

Endocrine System

DIABETES MELLITUS

Description. Diabetes is a condition in which the body is not able to utilize carbohydrates properly owing to a deficiency of *insulin,* an internal secretion of the pancreas. The cause and cure of this disease are unknown. It is inherited as a recessive gene characteristic. Diabetes is uncommon but more severe in children. Those who develop it are not overweight, as is characteristic of adults. The peak years of onset are three, six, and twelve.* Acute infections are believed to be responsible at times for activating dormant diabetes.

Symptoms. The symptoms of this disease appear more rapidly in children. The patient complains of excessive thirst (polydipsia), is constantly hungry (polyphagia), and excretes large amounts of urine frequently (polyuria). The child who is bladder trained may begin wetting the bed or begin to have frequent "accidents" in his pants during play periods. He loses weight and is irritable. The skin becomes dry, and boils may develop. These symptoms may go unrecognized until an infection becomes apparent or until coma results. Laboratory findings indicate *glycosuria,* sugar in the urine. Excessive amounts of sugar appear in the blood (*hyperglycemia* [*hyper-* above + *glyc-* sugar + *-emia* blood]). One test performed to determine the amount of sugar in the blood is called the *glucose tolerance* test. The diagnosis is based on the results of the laboratory findings, the past history of the patient, and the symptoms presented.

Diabetic acidosis. Diabetic acidosis is also referred to as diabetic coma, although a person may have diabetic acidosis with or without coma. It may result if a diabetic patient contracts a secondary infection and does not take care of himself or, as occurs fairly often in diabetic children, the disease proceeds unrecognized until coma occurs. Even minor infections such as a cold increase the severity of diabetes. The symptoms range from mild to severe. They occur *slowly* and the patient looks sick. The skin is dry and the face flushed. The patient appears dehydrated. He is thirsty but may vomit if fluids are offered. He perspires and is restless. There may be generalized pain in the abdomen and throughout the body. A characteristic *fruity odor* of the breath is apparent. As the condition becomes worse, the patient becomes weak and drowsy. His breathing patterns are peculiar in that there is no normal period of rest between inspiration and expiration. This is termed *Kussmaul* breathing. The patient becomes unconscious. Death will result

---

*Martin, p. 107.

unless insulin, fluids, and salt are administered. Response to treatment is *gradual* over a period of hours.

Treatment.   The aims of treatment in juvenile diabetes are those of assuring normal growth and development, providing the child with a happy active childhood, and preventing complications. This involves four areas basically: diet, insulin, exercise, and proper education of the child and his parents.

DIET.   The diabetic diet prescribed for children has gradually changed over the years. Today doctors and dietitians attempt to provide a diet that is as close to that of the normal child as possible. The eating patterns of the entire family are taken into consideration, as well as their financial situation. The principal differences seem to be whether the diet is to be *free* or *measured.* The general considerations of management are the same, but there is a vast difference in the exactness of correction desired.

Advocates of the free diet feel that the patient does not require a specific diet as long as his weight remains normal, he is not excreting acetone in the urine, and no complications of diabetes are present. The mother is instructed in the requirements of a good diet. An exact intake is not prescribed, but regular and consistent meals are stressed. Excessive carbohydrate intake and between-meal snacks are discouraged, but not forbidden. Food intake is appraised periodically by the doctor and the dietitian to assure that the essential amounts of calories, protein, minerals, and vitamins are obtained. Adjustments in the diet are made when indicated. If acetone appears in the urine, the doctor is consulted. Those who suggest free diet management feel that children rebel less often to this type of program and the majority of patients can adjust to it without becoming too careless about the disease.

Other doctors prescribe a measured diet in diabetes. It is usually begun in the hospital. The doctor specifies the total number of calories and the proportions of the three basic types of food (carbohydrates, proteins, and fat) that the patient is to receive daily. The patient's age, size, sex, and activity are taken into consideration. The dietitian calculates the diet after she receives the prescription. She determines the type and amounts of food which the child will receive each day, and consults frequently with the child and his parents during hospitalization to determine the food patterns and preferences of the family. Follow-up consultations are held after discharge. Once the disease is brought under control with insulin, the diabetic child has the same nutritional requirements as a normal child except that he must follow a pattern and eat the same amounts of food each meal every day. Exchange lists compiled by a joint committee of the American Dietetic Association, the American Diabetes Association, and the United States Public Health Service provide for variety in the diet. For instance, crackers may be substituted for bread when soup is served as long as the specified amounts are adhered to. Mothers can gain valuable information in meal planning by subscribing to the ADA Forecast.* School children should bring their lunch to school rather than eat in the cafeteria. This keeps them from being tempted by foods that are not on their diet, and gives the mother a more accurate idea of the amount of carbohydrates consumed.

The practical nurse has a number of responsibilities as a member of the nursing team concerned with the patient and his diet management. This begins by preparing the child for his meals. He is offered the bedpan about a half hour before he is to eat. The nurse tests the specimen of urine for sugar and acetone if ordered. The child's face and hands are washed, and distracting toys are removed for the time being. The child is served his tray in his crib on a bed table or at a regular table suited to his size. Small children require bibs. The tray is served *on time*. Patients who receive regular insulin before meals may have an insulin reaction if food is not taken within 20 minutes. If the nurse is scheduled for lunch when diets are served, she should notify her team leader and not presume that others will feed the child.

Be sure that the tray is served to the *right patient*. A mistake can occur, particularly if several children are on special diets. It can happen more easily on the pediatric ward where patients roam about freely. Food should be cut into small pieces. Toast or muffins are buttered, and eggs are removed from their shells. A child who is able to feed himself is encouraged to do so. The nurse uses her powers of observation to determine when help is needed. She notices the foods that he especially enjoys.

When the child has finished, the tray is removed. The nurse observes the types and amounts of foods that the patient did not eat. She charts them in the nurses' notes, and also informs the nurse in charge. These are brought to the attention of the dietitian, who determines the number of calories the patient did not receive, and orders a between-meal snack such as orange juice to make up the differences. The nurse washes the child's hands and face, straightens his crib, and returns his toys to him.

INSULIN. Insulin is used principally as a specific drug for the control of diabetes mellitus. It is a specially prepared extract obtained from the pancreas of cattle or pigs. When injected into the diabetic patient, it enables the body to burn and store sugar. In adults, certain mild cases of this disease may be controlled by diet alone. All diabetic children, however, require insulin.

Tolbutamide (Orinase)†, a sulfonylurea compound given orally, has not proved satisfactory in the treatment of children. It is sometimes erroneously referred to as "oral insulin." Although it does lower the

---

*American Diabetes Association. 1 East 45 St., New York, New York 10017.
†Product of the Upjohn Company.

blood sugar, it is completely different from insulin in origin and method of action.

The dosage of insulin is measured in units, and special syringes are used in its administration. The scale of each type of syringe corresponds in color to the type of insulin used. (A syringe for U-40 insulin is scaled in red enamel, the color of the label and carton of all types of U-40 insulin. The scale for U-80 syringes is green.) Syringes are available in both short and long forms. Double scaled syringes containing a U-40 scale on one side and a U-80 scale on the other are also used in hospitals. A single scaled syringe is safer, and should be obtained for the diabetic at home.

The two most commonly used strengths of insulin are U-40 (red label and cap) and U-80 (green label and cap). U-40 insulin is used when the dosage is small. U-80 insulin is stronger than U-40 and enables the patient to take a larger dose in a smaller amount of solution.

Insulin is administered *subcutaneously*. Parents and children must be taught the reasons why it is necessary to take the hormone, and how to administer it by injection. A child from 7 to 10 can generally be taught to give his own injections. The earlier he learns, the better. Proper instruction of the patient is one of the most important aspects of the treatment of diabetes. The doctor prescribes the type and amount of insulin and specifies the time. In the hospital the nurse may be requested to notify the physician after each urine test. The site of the injection is rotated to prevent poor absorption and injury to the tissues. (See Fig. 136.) Unused insulin is refrigerated. It should not be stored in the freezer compartment.

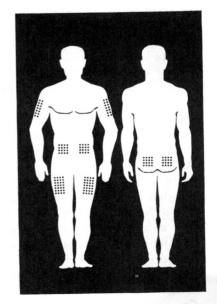

Figure 136. Sites of injection of insulin. The site of injection should be changed daily to prevent poor absorption and injury to tissues. (Courtesy of Eli Lilly and Company, Indianapolis, Indiana.)

The various types of insulin and their action are listed in Table 14-1. The main difference is in the amount of time required for effect and the length of protection given. Regular and crystalline insulin have had nothing added to them. Crystalline insulin is a purified form of regular insulin and is less likely to cause allergic reactions. Both NPH, an intermediate type, and PZI, a long-lasting insulin, have had small amounts of chemicals added to prolong their action and to make them more stable, and offer protection over a period of hours, which enables the patient to do without repeated injections of unmodified insulin. They are cloudy and require mixing before being withdrawn from the vials. This is done by rolling the bottle gently between the palms of the hands. Insulin is not used if it is discolored.

Frequently the doctor will order a combination of a short-acting insulin and a longer-acting one, e.g., give 10 units of NPH insulin and 5 units of regular insulin at 7:30 A.M. This offers the patient immediate and long-lasting protection. NPH or lente insulins may be given in the same syringe as regular or crystalline insulins. PZI insulin should not be given in the same syringe as the regular or crystalline types because a chemical reaction occurs which produces more PZI insulin. Two injections are required in such cases unless ordered otherwise.

EXERCISE.   Exercise is important for the patient with diabetes because it causes the body to use sugar and promotes good circulation. It lowers the blood sugar, and in this respect acts like more insulin. The diabetic patient who has planned vigorous exercise should carry extra sugar with him to avoid insulin reactions. The blood sugar level is high directly after meals so that active sports can be participated in at such times. Less active games should be enjoyed directly before meals. The diabetic child is able to participate in almost all active sports. Poorly planned exercise, however, can lead to difficulties. The diabetic child should not be allowed to swim unsupervised.

EDUCATION OF THE CHILD AND HIS PARENTS.   The child and his family must be taught how to live with diabetes. This is ideally begun when the diagnosis has been confirmed. Many hospitals hold special group clinics for diabetic patients. These sessions are conducted by the physician, dietitian, and registered nurse. Patients who have had the disease over a period of years provide encouragement for the new patient. Topics for discussion include: dietary management, urine testing, administration of insulin, the importance of exercise, and proper skin care. The patient is taught to recognize the symptoms of insulin shock and diabetic coma, and what to do when they occur. He should wear an identification medal or bracelet designating his condition. Regular health habits to prevent secondary infection are also stressed.

The practical nurse, although not directly responsible for the immediate instruction of the patient, can contribute much to instill confidence in him and the members of his family. She should listen to the parents to determine some of their apprehensions. Many simple questions asked by

Table 14-1.   Insulin Activity*

Name	Time and Route of Administration	Onset	Peak	Duration of Action	Most Likely Time for Insulin Reaction	Most Likely Time for Sugar in the Urine
Fast action						
Regular	15–20 minutes before meals, S.C. (I.V. in emergency)	Rapid, within 1 hour	2–4 hrs.	5–8 hrs.	10 A.M. to lunch	During night
Crystalline	Same	Same	Same	Same	Same	Same
Semilente	½–¾ hr. before breakfast, deep S.C. (never I.V.)	Same	6–10 hrs.	12–16 hrs.	Before lunch	Same
Intermediate action						
Globin	½–1 hr. before breakfast. S.C.	Within 2–4 hrs. (rapidity increases with dose)	6–10 hrs.	18–24 hrs.	3 P.M. to dinner	Before breakfast and lunch
NPH	1 hr. before breakfast. S.C.	Within 2–4 hrs.	8–12 hrs.	28–30 hrs.	Same	Before lunch
Lente	Same	Same	Same	Same	Same	Same
Slow action						
Protamine Zinc	Same	Within 4–6 hrs.	16–24 hrs.	24–36 hrs. plus	2 A.M. to breakfast	Before lunch and bedtime
(PZI) Ultralente	1 hr. before breakfast, deep S.C. (never I.V.)	Very slow–8 hrs.	Same	36 hrs. plus	During night and early morning	

*Adapted from Bergersen and Krug, p. 627.

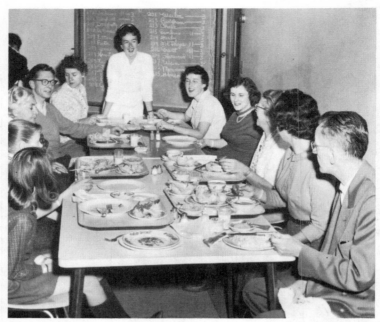

Figure 137. Diabetic patients in the cafeteria of a teaching center. Education of the patient is a key factor in the treatment of this disease. (Courtesy of Hospital Teaching Unit of New England Deaconess Hospital, Boston, Mass.)

children themselves may be answered. She must have a positive attitude toward the disease. It can be controlled, is not deforming, and the child who is under correct supervision is able to lead a normal life. A child should not be permitted to use his disease as a crutch against accepting his normal responsibilities.

The nurse should stress the following care pertinent to the child with diabetes:

Shoes.   Inexpensive ones that can be replaced often as the child grows.

Skin.   Breaks in the skin require immediate attention. The child should bathe at least every other day.

Infections.   Sensible clothing. This becomes a problem, particularly during preadolescence and adolescence. Obtain proper immunizations against communicable disease.

Exercise.   Moderate and regular each day in home and hospital.

Records.   Keep a daily record of insulin dose, diet, and urine tests until illness is under control and patient understands it clearly.

Diet.   Adherence to diet. Your understanding that it is difficult at times.

Urine Specimens.   Stress the importance of regular urine tests (sugar and acetone). Respect the privacy of the child who collects his own specimens.

Tests for Sugar in the Urine

CLINITEST

Equipment. Clinitest tablets, test tube, urine specimen, water, dropper.

1. Place 5 drops of urine in a test tube.
2. Add 10 drops of water.
3. Add 1 Clinitest tablet.
4. Read after bubbling has ceased. Compare to color guide.
5. Record results.

BENEDICT'S TEST

Equipment. Test tube, dropper, Benedict's solution, small pan with handle, test tube holder (or spring type clothespin in the home), urine specimen.

1. Place 5 cc. of Benedict's solution into test tube.
2. Add 8 drops of freshly voided urine.
3. Heat test tube in pan of boiling water for 5 minutes.
4. Remove. Allow to cool.
5. Read, and compare to color guide.
6. Record results.

Test for Ketone Bodies in the Urine

ACETONE TEST

Equipment. Reagent (Acetest* tablet or powder), urine specimen, dropper, paper towel.

1. Place reagent on white background. A folded paper towel may be used.
2. Add 1 or 2 drops of urine to tablet or powder, according to specific directions.
3. Compare to color guide. A prompt appearance of lavender or a color denotes acetone. There must be a *definite* color change for the test to be positive. False positives are the most common type of error made in this procedure.
4. Record results.

Reagent strips, specially impregnated paper, are a new and quick means of detecting ketone bodies in the urine. The test end of the reagent strip is dipped into the urine specimen. Color changes are

---

*Ames Company.

compared to a color guide. Some reagent strips may be used for a variety of urine tests.

Acknowledgment of the Disease.   Teachers and other persons caring for the child should be told that he is a diabetic so that they are prepared to help him in an emergency.

Psychological Aspects.   The child is interested in his illness when he is encouraged to care for himself rather than constantly coddled by his parents. Summer camps for diabetic children promote socialization and try to instill confidence in the child. Rebellion against routines is natural, particularly during adolescence. This is usually temporary and requires patience and understanding by adults caring for the youngster. Adolescent girls need to understand that motherhood is not out of the question for them. Although babies of diabetic mothers run a greater risk of survival, modern medical practice has done much to improve their chances. Close medical supervision for mother and baby are of great importance.

Insulin Shock.   Insulin shock, also known as *hypoglycemia* (*hypo-* below + *glyc-* sugar + *-emia* blood) occurs when the blood sugar level becomes abnormally low. This condition is caused by too much insulin. Factors that may account for this imbalance include poorly planned exercise, reduction of diet, improvement of the condition so that the patient requires less insulin, and errors made through improper knowledge of insulin and the insulin syringe.

Children are *more prone* to insulin reactions than adults because the condition itself is more unstable in young people, and because their activities are more irregular. *Poorly planned exercise* is frequently the cause of insulin shock during childhood.

The symptoms of an insulin reaction, which range from mild to severe, are generally noticed and treated in the early stages. They appear *suddenly* in the *otherwise well* person. Examinations of the blood would reveal a lowered blood sugar level. Urine tests indicate an absence of sugar and acetone. The child becomes irritable and may behave poorly. He looks pale, and may complain of feeling hungry and weak. Sweating occurs. Symptoms related to disorders of the nervous system arise, since glucose is vital to the proper functioning of nerves. The child may become mentally confused, and his muscular coordination is affected. If left untreated, coma and convulsions can occur.

The immediate treatment consists of administering sugar in some form such as orange juice, Coca-Cola, ginger ale, ice cream, or candy. If it cannot be distinguished whether the patient is having an insulin reaction or is suffering from diabetic acidosis, and the patient is fully conscious, give sugar. It will bring about an immediate recovery if the patient is in insulin shock, and will not make much difference if he is in acidosis. If the patient does not respond rapidly, contact his physician. When the patient is unconscious, keep him warm by covering him with a blanket. Do not give anything by mouth; get medical attention immediately.

THE CHILD WITH AN EMOTIONAL
DISTURBANCE

Growing up can be painful even under the best circumstances. It is difficult for the child in the early school years to live up to so many rapidly developing standards. Guilt and anxiety feelings develop. Finger sucking, nail biting, excessive fears, stuttering, and conduct problems are reflections of nervous tension. Disorders which may or may not be traced to emotional problems include constipation, diarrhea, stomach aches, dermitis, obesity, frequent urination, enuresis, and the common cold. The term *psychosomatic* has come to refer to the bodily dysfunctions which seem to have an emotional as well as an organic basis.* Each person has a different potential for coping with life. Truancy, lying, stealing, failure in school, or a crisis, such as the death or divorce of parents, are but a few of the difficulties which may require the services of the child guidance clinic.

The first psychiatric clinic for children in the United States was established in Chicago in 1909 to serve delinquents. The basic staff of the child guidance clinic is composed of a psychiatrist, a psychologist, and a social worker; frequently, a pediatrician is also a member of the staff. Usually the child guidance clinic provides both diagnostic and treatment services. It may be part of a hospital, a school, a court, a public health or welfare service, or it may be an independent agency.†

The various psychiatric specialties may be confused by the average person. A *psychiatrist* is a medical doctor who has specialized in mental disorders. The *psychoanalyst* is usually a psychiatrist, but may be a psychologist (lay analyst). All psychoanalysts have advanced training in psychoanalytic theory and practice. The *clinical psychologist* should have a doctorate of philosophy in clinical psychology from a recognized university. Many work in the school systems with children, teachers, and families in an attempt to prevent or resolve problems.

There are also emotionally disturbed children who require the type of care provided in residential treatment centers. Their home situations may be such that they can only respond to therapy by a complete change of environment. In both areas the total situation to which the child reacts needs to be treated rather than just the individual patient.

The Role of the Practical Nurse.   In order for the practical nurse to work effectively with the disturbed child, she must first understand the types of behavior considered within a normal range as the two are so intimately related. She is a valuable member of the medical team in that

---

*L. Dennis, Psychology of Human Behavior for Nurses (Philadelphia: W. B. Saunders Co., 1967) p. 223.

†H. Wallace, Health Services for Mothers and Children (Philadelphia: W. B. Saunders Co., 1962) p. 247.

she works closely with the hospitalized child and the long term patient in particular. She keeps a careful record of his behavior and notes his relationship with members of his family. Such notations are meaningful to the physician who is as concerned with preventing problems from arising as he is with treating them. Is four year old Janice wetting the bed? What about Bobby who continually bangs his head against the crib during naptime? What does Allan do in the playroom? Is he sitting alone in a corner? Does he hit the other children? Is he constantly in motion? Does Eric act indifferent to your attempt to establish rapport with him? Is there a physical cause for his behavior? Each action in itself might be considered well within the normal limits of behavior, but when carried to extremes, such actions may interfere with reality and should be investigated further. The nurse should bear in mind that behavior which one might typify as "bratty" may be interpreted very differently by persons skilled in understanding deeper levels of personality. She should feel free to discuss the conduct problems of her patients with other members of the staff and not consider these problems a threat to her own abilities.

One might ask where else does the practical nurse see such children? Wherever children are — in the home, in nursery school, in residential institutions, in child health conferences, in special clinics, in the doctor's office. Perhaps they may even belong to her. Every day, everywhere, children are trying to cope with stress. Many succeed and grow stronger. Many do not.

When parents request assistance from the nurse she should encourage them to seek help from their family physician or pediatrician, or from a community mental health center. If the child is in school, the services of the school psychologist may prove valuable. The nurse should support organizations concerned with mental health, vote on issues which are pertinent to the welfare of children in her community, and volunteer her services when they are needed.

STUDY QUESTIONS

1. What other diseases do you know of besides rheumatic fever that are considered "collagen" diseases?
2. List the symptoms of rheumatic fever.
3. Mrs. Rogers, your neighbor, is upset because the doctor wants to do further tests on her son John to rule out rheumatic fever. She is hysterical and says that her boy will die or be crippled for life. From your knowledge of this disease, how would you manage this situation?
4. Differentiate between first, second, and third degree burns.
5. What are the symptoms and first aid for shock?
6. Discuss the nursing care of a patient convalescing from third degree burns of both legs.

7. What is meant by "sterile technique"? What does the practical nurse need to know about the use of transfer forceps?
8. Observe one of your classmates setting up a sample sterile field. How could she have done this more effectively? Did you notice any faults in her sterile technique?
9. How do you sterilize a syringe in the home?
10. How does the treatment and nursing care of diabetes differ in the child?
11. List several mannerisms that may indicate nervous tension in the child.
12. What importance does body position play in the treatment of the long-term patient?
13. Discuss the postoperative care of Jim, an eight year old patient recovering from an appendectomy.

BIBLIOGRAPHY

Bergersen, B., and Krug, E.: Pharmacology in Nursing. 11th Ed. St. Louis, The C. V. Mosby Co., 1969.
Blake, F., and Wright, H.: Essentials of Pediatric Nursing. 7th Ed. Philadelphia, J. B. Lippincott Co., 1963.
Dennis, L.: Psychology of Human Behavior for Nurses. Philadelphia, W. B. Saunders Co., 1967.
Harmer, B., and Henderson, V.: Textbook of the Principles and Practice of Nursing. 5th Ed. New York, The Macmillan Co., 1957.
Marlow, D.: Textbook of Pediatric Nursing. 3rd Ed. Philadelphia, W. B. Saunders Co., 1969.
Martin, M.: Diabetes Mellitus. Philadelphia, W. B. Saunders Co., 1960.
Mason, M.: Basic Medical-Surgical Nursing. New York, The Macmillan Co., 1967.
Mowry, L.: Basic Nutrition and Diet Therapy for Nurses. St. Louis, The C. V. Mosby Co., 1966.
Nelson, W. (Ed.): Textbook of Pediatrics. 9th Ed. Philadelphia, W. B. Saunders Co., 1969.
Price, A.: The Art, Science and Spirit of Nursing. 3rd Ed. Philadelphia, W. B. Saunders Co., 1965.
Rapier, D., Koch, M., Moran, L., Geronsin, J., Cady, E., and Jensen, D.: Practical Nursing. St. Louis, The C. V. Mosby Co., 1966.
Sadler, S.: Rheumatic Fever. Nursing Care in Pictures. Philadelphia, J. B. Lippincott Co., 1949.
Shearman, C.: Diets Are for People. New York, Appleton-Century-Crofts, 1963.
Wallace, H.: Health Services for Mothers and Children. Philadelphia, W. B. Saunders, 1962.

Chapter 15

THE ADOLESCENT

VOCABULARY

Adjustment	*Menstruation*
Authority	*Peer*
Curriculum	*Puberty*
Function	*Reassure*
Mature	*Recognition*
Menarche	*Responsible*

GENERAL CHARACTERISTICS

Adolescence is defined as the period of life beginning with the appearance of secondary sex characteristics and ending with cessation of growth. Perhaps one of its most certain characteristics is its uncertainty. It is a period of life that lasts a comparatively long time in our culture, and involves a great number of adjustments on the part of the child.

Life is never dull when there are adolescents in the family. The adolescent's surge toward independence becomes pronounced. This desire makes it practically impossible for him to get along with his parents, who represent authority. When he submits to their wishes, he feels humiliated and loses confidence in himself. If he revolts, conflicts arise within the family. Parents and teenagers have to weather the storm together, and try to come up with solutions that are relatively satisfactory to all. Numerous other factors also account for the restlessness of youth. Their bodies are rapidly changing, and they experience intense sexual drives. They desire to be accepted by society, but are not sure how to go about it. Adolescents question life, and search to find themselves. "Who am I?" "What do I want?" In late adolescence they must think about choosing a career and finding a suitable mate.

These facts sound complicated in themselves, but they are intensified by a world that is constantly changing. Even parents are confused by the rapid pace of living and the many advances in technology. The constant threat of a totally destructive war also adds to their insecurities. The adjectives commonly and not surprisingly used to describe the teenager are irritable, aggressive, unstable, and seemingly ignorant to the needs of others.

There is no perfect way to guide adolescents. Their reactions to such pressures are individual. A great deal depends on the experiences they have already encountered in early life. Amazingly enough, the majority of children come through with flying colors and relatively few residual scars, perhaps because youth learns to live with the insecurities of this era, having never known any other.

PHYSICAL DEVELOPMENT

Preadolescence is a short period immediately preceding adolescence. In girls, it is between 11 and 13 years of age, and is marked by rapid changes in the structure and function of various parts of the body. It is

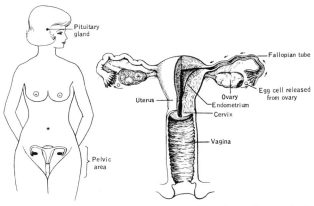

Figure 138. *Menstruation.* (Courtesy of Personal Products Corportion).

The *pituitary gland* is a small gland at the base of the brain. It sends out chemical messengers through the blood to various parts of the body. These messengers, or hormones, are responsible for many steps of growth and change as we grow up. When a girl reaches the age of puberty, the pituitary sends out a new hormone that affects the functions of a group of organs concerned with menstruation.

The *pelvic area* is located in the lower part of the body in the region of the hips. It is here that the organs associated with menstruation are located.

The *ovaries* are two small female organs that manufacture human egg cells. When a girl reaches the age of puberty, these little cells wake up and begin to grow. Each month a cell escapes from an ovary and starts to travel along a passageway—one of the fallopian tubes. This movement of the egg cell is called ovulation. If one of these cells becomes fertilized by a male cell, it can develop into a baby.

The *fallopian tubes*, into which the egg cells pass, lead toward the uterus.

The *uterus* is often called the womb. This is where the egg cell develops, if it has been fertilized. Each month a soft, thick lining (endometrium) of tissue and blood vessels forms inside the uterus.

The *endometrium*, or uterus lining, serves as a warm nest to shelter and nourish the unborn child until it has grown enough to be ready to come into the world as a baby. But unless an egg cell has been fertilized and a baby started on its way toward birth, there is no need for the cell, or for the blood and tissues of the endometrium. And so they are passed from the body.

The *cervix* is the lower part of the uterus, connecting it with the vagina.

The *vagina*, a passageway leading to the outside of the lower part of the body, carries away these materials in a slight flow of blood. This is called menstrual flow. When it occurs, it lasts for several days each month, and is known as menstruation.

distinguished by *puberty*, the age at which the reproductive organs become functional and secondary sex characteristics develop. Hormonal changes affect both physical and emotional development. The age at which this phenomenon takes place varies, and is about two years earlier in girls than in boys. It is preceded by spurts in height and weight in both sexes. General appearance tends to be awkward, i.e., long-legged, gangling. The sweat glands are very active, and greasy skin and acne are common.

Puberty is easily recognized in girls due to the onset of *menstruation*. The first menstrual period is called the menarche. It frequently occurs about the age of 13, but this varies. It may occur as early as 10 or as late as 15 years of age. Certain bodily changes take place prior to the menarche. Fat is deposited in the hips, thighs, and breasts, causing them to enlarge. Growth of the external genitals also takes place. Hair develops in the pubic area and underarms. In short, girls take on a definite female look. The body reaches its final measurements about three years from the onset of puberty. At this time the ends of the long bones knit securely to their shafts, and further growth can no longer take place.

In boys, there is no clearcut event that marks puberty. The depth of the shoulders increases and the pectoral muscles enlarge. Voice changes are also noticeable. Hair begins to grow on the face, chest, axillae, and pubic areas. The genitals enlarge. Erections and nocturnal emissions take place. The production of sperm occurs about the age of 15.

This period is reached with some uncertainties by the child. He needs to be told what bodily changes to expect and the purpose for these changes. Two years too soon is better than one day too late. Parents who have answered their child's questions truthfully throughout childhood offer him a secure and natural foundation to build upon. Even though most children anticipate puberty, the actual occurrence may be alarming to them. They need to be reassured that such body discharges are normal, and that they need not be alarmed or embarrassed about them.

Adults working with teenagers should try to create an atmosphere of understanding. The adolescent needs to known that his parents and the nurse realize that his new feelings are sometimes difficult to handle. The adolescent needs help in redirecting his sexual energies to more socially acceptable behavior such as sports, hobbies, wholesome social experiences, and studies.

Children may experience certain problems peculiar to puberty. The girl who begins to experience physical changes at about the age of nine may feel self-conscious, for she towers over her friends or has to wear a brassiere. She may be the subject of ridicule because she is different. On the other end of the scale are the late comers who begin to feel abnormal. Their friends look more feminine, and they feel unattractive.

Such situations are not limited to girls. Of particular concern is the boy who is on a slow time schedule of development. Still a "shrimp" at

15, he is unable to compete for placement on school teams because of his size. He sees his male friends being admired for their height and strength, and this presents a threat to him. Fears such as these are natural and usually can be alleviated by reassurance from adults. Their time will come as surely as the day begins and ends.

Adolescents are very self-conscious, and skin blemishes are always a problem. They observe their faces carefully in the mirror, and squeeze and pick at pimples, which makes the situation worse, for the pus that escapes can infect the surrounding skin. Germs on the child's hands also lead to reinfection as he touches other areas of his face. Permanent scarring can result. When acne is severe, a doctor should be consulted. He may be able to improve the child's appearance and prevent permanent disfigurement. This will boost the youth's morale, for he will feel that someone really is concerned with his problem.

Difficulties in school social life appear during puberty. Many girls are more mature than the boys in their own class. Not only are their interests different, but the size of the girls in comparison with the boys presents certain difficulties, particularly at dances. This can be a touchy situation because both sexes are oversensitive. As a result, social functions that include diverse age groups are enjoyed more than those limited to classmates.

MENTAL AND SOCIAL DEVELOPMENT

Need for Independence. The teenager's desire for freedom is intense. He can generally think up some issue to debate if he works at it enough. The usual disagreements revolve around dating, the use of the family car, money, chores at home, school grades, and choice of friends. He can also go into long discourse about trivial matters. This gives him practice in asserting his own opinions. He would be disappointed if everyone continually agreed with him.

The adolescent is too old to accept the direction of his parents without question yet is too young to accept adult responsibilities. He joins a gang, dresses differentialy, and adopts slang language in an attempt to find a niche for himself. He values the opinions of his *peers* (a group made up of his equals), and shares his thoughts and inspirations with them. He needs to *belong.* Parents will accomplish more by welcoming the group than by antagonizing them. It is better to have them underfoot, than in less desirable places than the home.

Need for Knowing His Role in Life. Parents must constantly bear in mind the fact that most children will someday be husbands and wives. They should attempt to give them an understanding of the male and female roles in society. Children gain their deepest impressions about such roles from their parents. A mother who is unhappy and dwells on the dark aspects of motherhood will convey her feelings to her daughter. On the other hand, if she enjoys being a mother she can create favorable

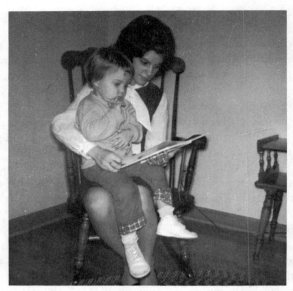

Figure 139. During adolescence a girl's interest in child care is at its peak.

feelings that cannot truly be measured. The nurse dealing with adolescents in the hospital has many excellent opportunities to demonstrate through her work the qualities that are becoming to womanhood.

Boys too are confused about being able to fit into their expected patterns. The more secure a boy is in his relationship with his father, the easier it is for him to accept the responsibilities of manhood. Parents who make no secret of their love for one another help to prepare young men and women for comfortable supportive relations in married life.

Need for Recognition. The adolescent needs to be recognized as an important member of the family. Sometimes parents become so used to dictating that they fail to listen to their children. Teenagers need to be able to express their points of view, and in cases where they show wisdom, their ideas can be incorporated into use. Instead of making a long list of rules for the teenager to follow, his help should be enlisted in determining activities that he is ready to accept. Parents should give him reasons for their requests, and be liberal with praise. Praise can be given directly for a good job done, or it may be recognized through money or by allowing him more responsibility because of his good judgment. His good features should be concentrated on rather than his bad. This does not mean being totally unrealistic, but the teenager needs confidence in himself, and it can be so easily instilled or destroyed. The teenager should not be compared with others of his age. He should be judged by his own capabilities.

Need for Responsibility. Young people look forward to challenges. Parents must watch for ways that they may free their children to take on

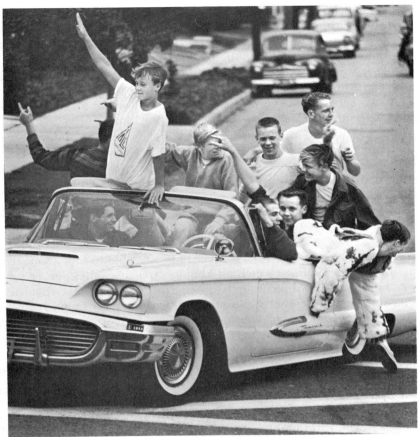

Figure 140. Feats of daring and unique activities with his peers are part of the teenager's search for independence. (Reprinted by permission of The Saturday Evening Post, 1961, The Curtis Publishing Company and Mr. William Bridges.)

new responsibilities. Perhaps some of the reasons teenagers appear so lazy is because the tasks which we ask them to do are rather uninteresting (e.g., take out the garbage, wipe dishes, dust). Even these routine jobs can be made more inspiring if youth are taught to see them in relation to their overall objective. (In this case, making the home a more pleasing place in which to live.) Astronauts have a certain amount of dull routine to their jobs; so do doctors, nurses, and scientists. They are able to accept routine tasks because they contribute to the effectiveness of the entire project. The more kinds of work youth can learn to enjoy, the better they are able to accept dull routines. To be able to work and to take pride in accomplishments is one of the greatest satisfactions of man.

Children must also be taught the value of money. An allowance is helpful because the child learns to budget his money. If it is simply handed out when needed, the adolescent does not develop a sense of responsibility concerning it. Allowances should be increased from time to time to comply with the age and needs of the child. If it is impossible to give an allowance one week, the parents should simply say so. This is a valuable lesson in itself. Parents generally find that they save money by planned distribution, since it comes and goes so quickly otherwise.

As the child grows more capable, he learns to save for items that he desires. He should be allowed to shop a bit for himself. If a boy buys an old car, he will soon discover it takes money to run and repair it. Experiences such as this provide valuable lessons in finance. Today people marry younger than ever. Nothing is more detrimental to a family than heavy debts. It is better for youth to make their financial mistakes early rather than later when they cause real trouble. Girls as well as boys need to understand how to spend wisely. Today many wives handle the budgets because husbands must be away from home more often.

Worries.   Teenagers worry a lot. They are able to talk about fears that are not too imtimate, such as school exams or clothes. Other problems, however, are difficult to express. Johnny may feel that he is disliked or left out. Jane thinks she is ugly, and stays home from the school dance. Adolescents who have to live with deep anxieties such as alcoholism or mental illness need support. Of course the ability to bear trouble varies widely. When youth has reached the end of his emotional rope, he manifests it by calling attention to himself, sometimes in rather wild ways.

Daydreams.   Adolescents spend a lot of time daydreaming. This can be done in the solitude of one's room or during a biology lecture. Most of this is normal and natural for this age group. Daydreaming is usually

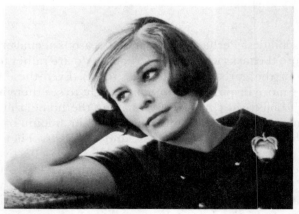

Figure 141.   Adolescents spend a good deal of time daydreaming. Most of this is normal and natural for this age group.

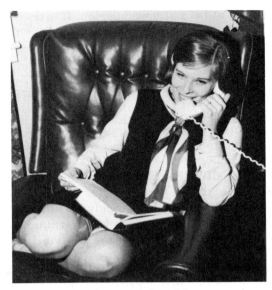

Figure 142.   The telephone and the adolescent are inseparable.

considered harmless, if the child continues his usual active pursuits. It also serves several purposes. Adolescence is a lonely, in-between age; daydreaming helps to fill the void. Acting out imaginatively what will be said or done in various situations prepares the girl or boy in dealing with the opposite sex, so that when confronted with the real situation he is better able to cope with it. Daydreams are also a valuable safety valve for the expressions of strong feeling.

It is also common for teenagers to swoon over their favorite singers, movie stars, and others. They form fan clubs, and direct their attention to a real person. All such manifestations are natural and useful to the child in his search for self-discovery.

Dating.   Adolescents need to meet and become acquainted with members of the opposite sex, so that they can learn to be comfortable with them. This usually begins by admiration from afar, and is accompanied by daydreams as the boy or girl attempts to think of ways to attract the attention of the object of his affection. Boys in particular need to test their powers of conquest. Competition and rivalry are keen. A good deal of the conversation heard in youth revolves around the stolen girl or boy friend. Girls need to feel attractive and desired by the opposite sex. When the boy or girl has satisfied himself that he is popular, he advances to the next stage where tenderness and love become more prominent features.

The practice of "going steady" is currently popular with youth. This insures them of a date for school functions and gives them a chance to evaluate the qualities of the particular person. It is detrimental in that it limits the number of persons the boy or girl dates. This is particularly significant since the current generation is marrying so much younger than in previous years.

CHOOSING A CAREER

Some adolescents graduate from high school with a definite idea of what they would like to do. Many, however, are unsure of what they want. In order to choose a career that he is best suited for, the youth must first know himself. What particularly interests him? What is he good at? What are his shortcomings?

By this time the boy or girl has already taken some rather definite steps toward a goal. Choice of high school curriculum and grades determine eligibility for college entrance or preparation for a specific vocation.

Parents should observe the interests of their children and encourage them to take advantage of their particular talents. Whenever possible, they should investigate various fields by direct inspection. Valuable information can also be obtained through pamphlets. The school guidance counselor administers aptitude tests as a further guide, and can work with the child so that he is exposed to as wide a selection of careers as possible. The final decision must be made by the adolescent. If a person is to be happy in his work, he must choose it of his own free will, and not merely because his parents expect him to follow in their footsteps.

Both white and blue collar jobs have their respective importance. The salaries today tend to be relatively equal. If a person is happy and satisfied with is work, and is contributing to the particular field by his skill or knowledge, he has chosen wisely. Many girls select marriage and motherhood as a career shortly after graduating from high school. They need to be well prepared through home, church, and school for this extremely important role.

PROBLEMS OF PARENTS

It is difficult at times for parents to cope with adolescents. The shift from the rigid rules of discipline, to permissiveness, to the current middle-of-the-road position leads to confusion. Some parents are unsure of their own opinions, and may hesitate to exert authority. Others refuse to change any of their theories to accommodate youth. The child who is the subject of heavy concentrations can become over-anxious. Mothers have a particular problem because they have to find substitute satisfactions for the loss of a dependent child. As the adolescent matures, he becomes more secure, and is able to develop a new and more satisfactory relationship with his parents.

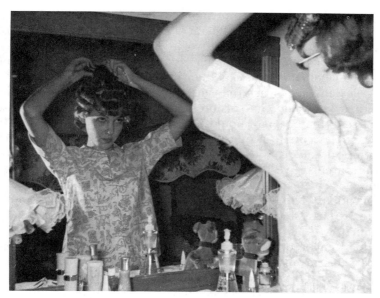

Figure 143. The adolescent is particular about appearance.

CARE AND GUIDANCE

Grooming. The adolescent is self-sufficient in respect to personal hygiene. Grooming improves and he begins to care about his appearance. He follows the group's standard of dress. (In some circles today, the "in" thing is to be disheveled, as is brought to mind by the term "hippie.") Now that he is able to earn money he can buy some of his own clothes. He is particular about the way they are pressed. He spends hours combing his hair. Girls tend to be equally concerned with the details of grooming. Teenagers become more conscious of the appearance of other members of their family. This is particularly true when they are entertaining at home. Most of the emphasis placed on clothes and looks is a welcome relief to parents who have up to now been constantly prodding their children to improve their personal hygiene. Parents must, nevertheless, help to develop healthy attitudes in adolescents, so that they will keep clothing and looks in proper perspective.

Nutrition. Teenagers need three well balanced meals a day. Most of them have too many other things on their minds to bother about good nutrition. Not that they don't eat! The refrigerator becomes somewhat of a mania to them. Boys are larger and participate in more active sports, so they eat more than girls. Girls tend to watch their figures. Sometimes they go on crash diets and will eat very little for several days. Such valuable foods as milk, potatoes, and bread are omitted with the *mistaken* idea that they are in themselves fattening. They fail to realize that good looks and proper nutrition go hand in hand. The teenage girl who marries and becomes pregnant is faced with the completion of her own growth, *plus* the extra needs of the baby. If her nutritional background is poor, she runs a higher risk of facing complications such as premature labor and toxemias than if it were adequate.

Adolescents may learn the value of good nutrition, but getting them to put their knowledge into action is another matter. Dictating is useless. The nurse in the hospital should not expect miracles. Be patient. If you can get adolescents to acquire one or two good habits, credit yourself with some success. If you are working in the home, you might suggest that the parents give them practice in meal planning, marketing, and cooking. Listen to their ideas, and try to straighten out some of their misconceptions. The nurse or nutritionist has a more attentive audience than do parents, since teenagers look up to those whom they consider authorities.

Adolescents require foods that aid in the development of bones and muscles. This means sufficient amounts of protein, minerals (particularly calcium), and vitamins C and D. A moderately active pubertal girl requires 2200 to 2800 calories per day. A very athletic boy in a similar stage of growth may require 3000 to 4000 calories per day. Rate of physical growth, stage of sexual maturation, and the amount of activity pursued must be taken into consideration in determining requirements.

It is important to distribute protein-rich foods throughout the various meals. This begins by a substantial breakfast. For example, juice, a bowl of cereal, an egg, a glass of milk, and toast (see also p. 152). Realizing the importance of breakfast, the nurse should stress the necessity of allowing adequate time for it. This may mean getting the children to bed earlier at night, so that they can arise sooner. It also helps if everyone sits down together rather than eating in relays.

Good eating habits established in the home are fortified by schools that serve nutritionally desirable foods. Many adolescents take part of their lunch from home and supplement it at the cafeteria. Let the adolescent make his own sandwiches, and be sure that they include such protein foods as meat or fish, peanut butter, or eggs. Jam and jelly sandwiches are not as nourishing. Milk should be drunk at lunch. The eating habits that the teenager develops will be passed on to another generation. Let them be good ones.

Sleep. Eight or nine hours of sleep at night are generally indicated. Adolescents are very enthusiastic about projects and their interest span is wide. Some just do not known when to slow down, and become exhausted. This fatigue is felt later and they become tagged "lazy." The teenager needs a bed with a firm mattress, and preferably a room of his own. Sufficient rest and proper nutrition contribute to general wellbeing. Parents and nurses must stress their importance as a safeguard against disease and as fundamental necessities for good physical and mental health.

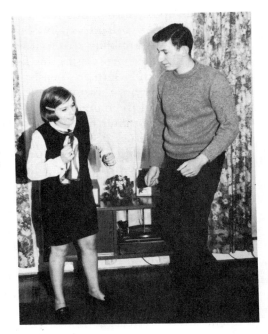

Figure 144.   Adolescents enjoy dancing. Mixed parties help them to better understand the opposite sex.

Safety.   The chief hazard to the adolescent is the automobile. It kills and cripples teenagers at alarming rates. Many schools today offer driver training courses as an integral part of the educational program. Students learn how to drive, and the responsibilities that accompany it. Preventing motor vehicle accidents is of utmost importance to every community. Adolescents who ride motorcycles, motor scooters, or motorbikes should know the rules of the road and should wear special safety equipment such as helmets for protection.

Other common causes of death in this age group are drowning and firearms, most of which are avoidable. Boys and girls should learn how to swim, and the safety measures that pertain to the sport. If a boy is interested in hunting or similar sports that require the use of a gun, he must be instructed in the proper care of it and the dangers involved.

Other Health Factors.   The medical profession is beginning to take a longer look at the problems of the adolescent. Clinics are being set up designed with him in mind. Prior to this time, the adolescent group was more or less left drifting between the area of pediatrics and adult study. Hospitals did not have facilities to accommodate them. They were either placed with adults or small children. Now many institutions have adolescent wings with personnel experienced in dealing with the problems of this particular age. This new branch of medicine dealing with adolescents is called *ephebiatrics* (ephēbos-puberty). Physicians trained in this area are called *ephebiatrists.*

The prevention of illness in this group as in all others is of primary importance. Booster immunizations against communicable disease, particularly smallpox and tetanus toxoid, should be administered periodically (see p. 259). Girls especially should receive the Shick test to determine their susceptibility to diphtheria. As mothers, their immunity will protect the newborn during his first months of life. Immunizations against mumps and German measles are now available. The German measles vaccine is not recommended for individuals who have reached puberty because of the danger of an unknown pregnancy or conception within a short time after inoculation. Even the weakened virus may be damaging to the fetus.

The adolescent should receive periodic medical and dental examinations. The 11 to 13 year old has all the permanent teeth except the four wisdom teeth which generally appear late in the teens or early twenties. Cavities during adolescence tend to increase because of the large consumption of sweets. Boys and girls are also prone to neglect brushing as often as they should, because they are so busy. The adolescent should begin to take responsibility for his six month dental check-ups so that he will carry through on this in adult life. He may also benefit from visiting his physician alone. The doctor may be able to gain his cooperation more easily than his parents, and the boy or girl will feel more free to discuss parental problems with the doctor.

The adverse effects of smoking should also be pointed out as many smokers are teenagers. Sound educational programs are now in effect which attempt to discourage youngsters from acquiring the habit.

The teenager needs to be informed of the consequences of certain social problems. Drinking, drug addiction, and premarital sex relations are not problems peculiar to this generation, but seem to be on the increase. Venereal diseases such as syphilis and gonorrhea caused by illicit sex relations still appear in somewhat alarming degrees. The underlying factors that precipitate such problems are unfortunately harder to diagnose and treat than the disease itself. The mere fact that adolescents turn to such extremes of behavior reflects serious problems. It is the duty of parents, the medical profession, and society in general to help adolescents to develop a sound philosophy of life. This cannot be accomplished by preaching, but by example. We cannot wait until children become adolescents to begin our work on moral standards. It begins in infancy, and is continuous. Adolescents have to learn what is morally right for them as individuals, not as compared to others. A great deal of adolescent behavior is a reflection of the amount of training he receives in the home, his religious instruction, and the circles in which he moves.

STUDY QUESTIONS

1. Define the following: preadolescence, adolescence, puberty, menstruation, menarche, peer.

2. List the signs of puberty in the male and female.
3. Do you feel that you were well prepared for the changes that took place at puberty? How might you have been helped to meet this adjustment more satisfactorily?
4. Alice, age 16, spends a great deal of her time daydreaming. Of what value is this to her? How can it be detrimental?
5. At what age do you feel boys and girls should begin to date? Discuss your answer with your classmates.
6. Mike, age 14, has a long, shaggy hair style. His parents want him to get a crew cut, but he refuses. Do you think this is typical of this age group? Why?
7. Plan a day's menu for a family with a 15 year old daughter and a 17 year old son. What foods in particular need to be stressed?
8. List several needs of the adolescent.
9. What hazards are peculiar to teenagers? How can they be prevented?
10. What are some of the social problems that appear during this age group?
11. Discuss various ways in which parents can help adolescents to develop a sense of responsibility.
12. What is meant by "preparing the teenager for his role in life"?

BIBLIOGRAPHY

Blake, F.: The Child, His Parents and the Nurse. Philadelphia, J. B. Lippincott Co., 1954.
Marlow, D.: Textbook of Pediatric Nursing. 3rd Ed. Philadelphia, W. B. Saunders Co., 1969.
Metropolitan Life Insurance Co.: Your Teen Years. New York, 1958.
Nelson, W. (Editor): Textbook of Pediatrics. 9th Ed. Philadelphia, W. B. Saunders Co., 1969.
Smith, C.: Maternal-Child Nursing. Philadelphia, W. B. Saunders Co., 1963.
Spock, B.: Baby and Child Care. Rev. Ed. New York, Duell, Sloan and Pearce, Inc., 1968.
United States Department of Health, Education, and Welfare: The Adolescent in Your Family. Children's Bureau Publication No. 347, 1955.

Chapter 16

DISORDERS OF THE ADOLESCENT

VOCABULARY

Chemotherapy	Lavage
Cramp	Malaise
Dysmenorrhea	Obese
Gynecology	Pasteurize
Intradermal	Toxic

Adolescence is a relatively healthy period. The girl or boy by now has become immune to the common infectious diseases. Deaths resulting from other types of illness are comparatively low. Accidents still pose a major threat and head the mortality rate list. The emotional upheaval seen during this stage of life is particularly significant. Minor physical complaints are magnified and it is difficult to establish a clear diagnosis. The adolescent who is handicapped faces numerous social problems at this time. The child who has had a prolonged illness since early childhood may find facing adolescence very difficult, especially if his basic needs have been neglected during early childhood. Separation from home is not generally a problem during this period. Most teenagers have had some experiences away from home. Minor homesickness may still be apparent.

The younger student practical nurse may feel inadequate when she cares for adolescents since she is barely out of that age group herself. Sometimes a problem results when the student becomes too friendly with the patient and confuses her role of authority. She may be unable to be objective about the patient and his problems.

Adolescents are very interested in their appearance. The nurse may be able to gain a girl's confidence by helping her to style her hair, care for her fingernails, and so on. Both boys and girls need to be made to feel important, especially in front of their peers. The same courtesy given to adults should be given to adolescents and their visitors. The nurse should always provide privacy for her patient during a procedure that might embarrass him.

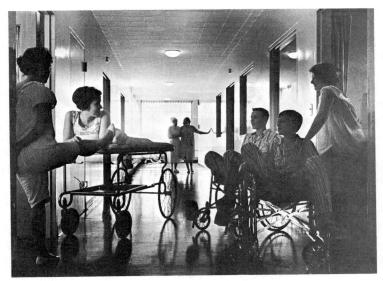

Figure 145. A hall in an adolescent unit. A nurse in these units must like teenagers, understand them, and be willing to work with their problems. (Courtesy of Joern Gerdts. Reprinted by permission of the Saturday Evening Post, 1961, and The Curtis Publishing Company.)

Respiratory System

TUBERCULOSIS

Description. Tuberculosis is an infectious disease caused by the *tubercle bacillus,* which is found throughout the world, especially in areas where poor living conditions exist. The fatality rate is higher during infancy and adolescence than in other childhood years. Tuberculosis is more prevalent in adolescent girls than boys. It is also more common in the Negro race.

There are two types of tuberculosis that affect people, *bovine* and *human.* The bovine strain, which can be transmitted through the milk of infected cows, usually attacks parts of the body other than the lungs, and is not common in the United States today, owing to pasteurization of milk and careful control of dairy herds. The human form is transferred from one person to another. It is commonly referred to as *pulmonary tuberculosis* because the lungs are the main site of infection. It is responsible for more than 90 per cent of all tuberculosis in this country today.

The *tubercle bacillus* deserves special consideration because of its rather unique properties. It is covered by a tough capsule and is capable of living outside of the body for weeks on dust, furniture, clothing, floors and so on. It also can remain dormant within the body tissues for long periods of time. When the body's resistance becomes lowered through disease, fatigue, or improper nutrition, it revives and produces further infection.

The organism gains entry to the body through the respiratory or digestive tract. It is transmitted to others by droplet infection and by direct contact. Children are often infected by adults through kissing, by eating utensils and environmental dust. Newborn infants must be separated from infected mothers for this reason. Grandparents may also be possible sources of infection, for the incidence of tuberculosis after the age of 50 is relatively high. The organism does not always cause the disease when it enters the body. Infection depends on the *number* of bacilli present, the *frequency* of exposure, and the child's age, nutrition, and general state of health.

Symptoms. The symptoms and severity of tuberculosis vary greatly in children. The disease may be well advanced with only a few manifestations. Once the organisms enter the body they attack the tissues of the lung, and may also invade the regional lymph nodes. In some cases they are killed or immobilized for longer periods of time. The practical nurse may hear this referred to as a *healed primary lesion.* The infection may, however, spread to other areas of the lung, and to the digestive tract through the swallowing of infected sputum. If the germs filter out into the blood stream, the infection can be carried to all parts of the body. Localized tuberculous infection can appear in the brain, liver, spleen, and kidneys. Widespread infection, called *miliary tuberculosis,* occurs mostly in infants and young children. The death rate from miliary tuberculosis has been reduced markedly through the use of modern drugs. Symptoms of a primary lesion may include malaise, fatigue, anorexia, weight loss, and irritability.

A *secondary* infection, a more destructive process than a primary infection, may occur during adolescence or early adult life. This may be due to reinfection or activation of a healed lesion. Extensive inflammation occurs and healing is accompanied by scarring. The apex of the lung is frequently the site for a secondary infection. The symptoms resemble more closely those in adult patients, e.g., cough, expectoration, fever in the late afternoon, weight loss, night sweats, and bloody sputum.

Diagnosis. Tuberculin tests are used to detect tuberculosis along with chest x-rays, examination of sputum, and examination of stomach contents. A positive tuberculin test in a young child is particularly significant because it means the child has recently been infected. A positive reaction in adults and older children may mean only that the person has a healed lesion, and is hypersensitive to the protein of the tubercle bacillus. Further examination is required to determine whether or not the lesion is active. A negative tuberculin test with a few exceptions rules out the possibility of tuberculosis.

Two types of tests currently used are the *intradermal (Mantoux) test*

A

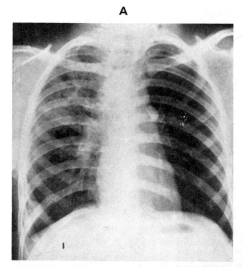

Figure 146. *A*, calcified node in left hilar area and tuberculous lesions in upper part of right lung in a Negro child 12 years of age. *B*, extensive tuberculous lesion in the chest of the mother, who disclaimed any knowledge of illness or history of tuberculosis in any member of the family. Sputum was positive for tubercle bacilli. Roentgenogram of the mother was taken as part of a survey of the family because of detection of tuberculosis in the child. (From Nelson, W. E., (Editor): Textbook of Pediatrics, 1969.)

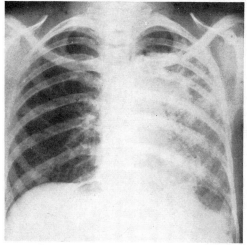

B

and the Heaf Multiple Puncture test, or its modification the Tine Test. The types of tuberculin available are Old Tuberculin (OT) and purified protein derivative (PPD). A tuberculin syringe is used for the Mantoux test. A very small amount of material is injected intradermally. The injection site is examined after 48 hours for redness or thickening which indicate a positive reaction.

Each tuberculin Tine Test consists of a stainless steel disk with four prongs or tines attached to a plastic handle (See Figure 148). The tines have been dip-dried with "old tuberculin." The entire unit has been sterilized and will remain sterile until it is removed from its individual

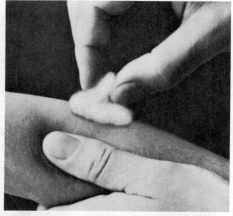

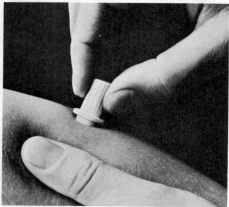

Figure 147. How to apply the tuberculin, Tine test. 1. Clean site with alcohol, acetone, ether, or soap and water. Allow arm to dry. The volar surface is the preferred site for accurate, standardized tuberculin testing. 2. Grasp patient's arm firmly since the sharp momentary stinging may cause the patient to jerk his arm, resulting in scratching. Stretch the skin of the forearm tightly, and apply the Tine test with the other hand. Hold for one second. Sufficient pressure should be exerted so that four puncture sites and a circular depression of the skin from the plastic base are visible. 3. Discard unit. The Tine test should never be reused. Local care of the skin site is not necessary. (Courtesy of Lederle Laboratories, division of American Cyanamid Company, Pearl River, New York, 1966.)

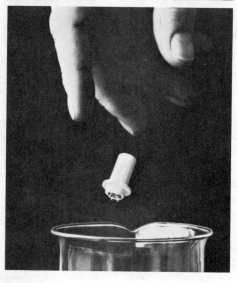

protective cap. Tests should be read in 48 to 72 hours. The test is considered positive if the induration around one or more of the puncture sites is 2 mm. or more in duration.*

Drugs. The drugs used against this disease act mainly to prevent the tubercle bacillus from multiplying. Once chemotherapy is begun, it should be continued faithfully until the doctor decides it is no longer required. The tubercle bacilli can become highly resistant to medication, particularly when therapy is interrupted. One of the responsibilities of the nurse is to help her patient understand the importance of taking medication, because it generally has to be taken for at least a year and sometimes longer, which is discouraging to the patient. Streptomycin, isoniazid (INH), and para-aminosalicylic acid (PAS) are most frequently used in various combinations.

Streptomycin, an antibiotic, is given by intramuscular injection. The dosage is carefully regulated to prevent toxicity. When the drug is used for prolonged periods of time, it may cause damage to the auditory nerve, which results in deafness.

Isoniazid (INH) is a synthetic substance that comes from isonicotinic acid. It can be given orally or intramuscularly and the side effects are relatively few. It is considered the most potent of the three. As with streptomycin, the tubercle bacilli may become resistant to it.

Para-aminosalicylic acid (PAS), a synthetic drug given orally, is not very effective when used alone. When combined with streptomycin or isoniazid, it delays the formation of resistant tubercle bacilli and increases the effectiveness of the drug with which it is combined. The isoniazid-PAS combination is convenient since both can be given by mouth. The toxic effects are usually related to gastric irritation, e.g., nausea, vomiting, anorexia, and sometimes diarrhea.

Prevention. One of the most effective ways of preventing tuberculosis is to keep young children and adolescents away from possible sources of infection. Since it is spread from one person to another, children should be shielded from those who have coughs of unknown origin and from those who are known to have the disease. Raw milk and food made from raw milk may also be a possible means of transmission. Parents who hire others to care for their children should check into the health background of the persons employed. Teenagers should be taught the value of good nutrition and sufficient rest.

An expectant mother should have a chest x-ray early in the prenatal period to rule out the possibility of tuberculosis. All babies need to be given some type of tuberculin tests during infancy. This should be repeated periodically throughout childhood. If a child is known to have been exposed, he should be examined by the doctor as soon as possible.

---

*Adapted from Lederle Laboratories: *Tuberculin, Tine Test.* Pearl River, New York, 1966.

Early diagnosis and treatment are essential. BCG vaccine (bacillus of Calmette and Guérin), given to prevent tuberculosis, is not used extensively in this country since its value is a subject of controversy. Mobile x-ray units are valuable in screening large numbers of people.

A person who is known to have this disease and is in a general hospital is placed on isolation precautions (see p. 263). His diet should be high in protein, calcium and vitamins. He requires both physical and mental rest. As the lesion heals the patient's activity can be increased. Channels of communication between home and school should be kept open. Diversions suitable to the age of the patient are necessary. All those who come in contact with a patient before the diagnosis of tuberculosis has been definitely established must be examined. Children who have the disease cannot attend school, so special provisions for education must be made. Once the child has been cured, he should still be examined periodically. Widespread education of the public is important. Yearly physical examinations which include chest x-ray and blood tests are a major step toward the prevention of this disease.

OBESITY

Description.   Obesity is the accumulation of excess body fat. It is distinguished from the term overweight by the degree. The problems involved in obesity are generally more complex than those of persons who are a few pounds overweight. Weight gain between the years of 7 to 12 is common. Most children stay plump during puberty and then return to their normal size.

Obesity becomes particularly significant during adolescence, when feelings of inadequacy are pronounced. Obese adolescents are concerned about their personal appearance but are unable to conform to the standards of the group. They are often the subject of cruel ridicule. Obese teenagers date less, and may feel rejected, unattractive, and unloved. Accompanying the mental anxieties are the more obvious physical handicaps. They may be unable to participate in sports or other school activities. They are more accident prone. Their choice of careers is more limited. Girls especially find it difficult to obtain youthful clothes.

The causes of obesity are numerous. Contrary to popular belief, obesity due to abnormal function of the glands is rare. Parents sometimes overfeed their children, falsely thinking that "a fat child is a healthy one." An unhappy teenager may seek satisfaction through food. There is also a general surge in the appetite of adolescents due to the rapid gains in growth which are taking place.

Treatment.   Dieting is difficult. When the problem begins in early childhood, a person is faced with a lifetime of fighting calories. This is complicated by the fact that food is readily available in this country, and advertisers bombard the public with tempting tasty treats. Parents must be keenly interested in helping their child to lose weight if the diet is to be successful. Sometimes it is necessary for the entire family to go without some of the richer dishes. Mother should refrain from buying cookies and cakes, and fresh fruits should be substituted as between-meal snacks. The nurse should emphasize the fact that diets should be carefully prescribed and controlled by a physician. Adolescents are apt to go on self diets that are dangerous to their health. Whenever such a major satisfaction as eating is denied, it must be replaced with something equally as satisfying and rewarding, such as new social activities, hobbies, friends, or sports.* The nurse should approach the obese adolescent in a non-threatening way. She should try to recognize his achievements and increase his self-esteem. The basic dignity of the individual should always be foremost in her mind.

The Skin

ACNE VULGARIS

Description. Acne, an inflammation of the skin commonly referred to as pimples, occurs frequently in adolescence owing to the changes which take place in the skin at puberty. There is also a familial tendency involved. The pores enlarge and secrete more oil. Dust or dirt may enter the pores, forming blackheads which cause further enlargement and thus germs can easily enter the pores. A small infection takes place and pimples form. When these pimples become filled with pus they are called *pustules.* Acne is usually seen on the chin, cheeks, and forehead. It can also develop on the back and shoulders.

Treatment. The treatment is aimed at improving the general health of the adolescent through proper nutrition, cleanliness of the skin, and adequate rest. Doctors and nurses must be concerned about the teenager as a person, and how the acne affects his impression of himself. It can be very distressing. When the patient becomes emotionally upset the condition may worsen. Vigorous exercise in the fresh air and direct sunshine helps to improve the complexion. The doctor may recommend that the patient avoid chocolates, peanuts, sea foods, cola drinks, and other food high in carbohydrate content. These are favorites of the teenager and are often eaten during periods of socialization. He may prescribe a local medication. Broad spectrum antibiotics may also be used. X-ray therapy may be indicated in severe cases. The

---

*Hammar and Eddy, p. 85.

teenager should assume responsibility for the physician's orders. He should receive emotional support from the adults in his life.

Reproductive System

DYSMENORRHEA

Description. Dysmenorrhea, or painful menstruation, is experienced by some adolescent girls. Few, however, find it so uncomfortable that it interferes with their normal activities. The problem is hard to evaluate clearly because of the adolescent's emotional tension, and because during this time preoccupation with bodily complaints is common. Parents should take an optimistic attitude when explaining menstruation to their daughters. They should emphasize the fact that it is a normal process.

Treatment.   Good personal hygiene, fresh air, and moderate exercise contribute to the well-being of the individual during menstruation. Girls should avoid becoming chilled. When necessary, local heat may be applied to the abdomen for the relief of cramps. A mild sedative might also be indicated. The practical nurse should be considerate of the teenager and listen to her feelings about menstruation and about her

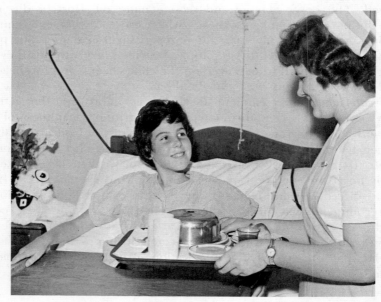

Figure 148.   Good nutrition means good health for both patient and practical nurse student. (Courtesy of Hanover School of Practical Nursing, Hanover, N.H.)

role in life. This added support is time well spent. Continued, severe dysmenorrhea requires further investigation by a gynecologist, a doctor who specializes in the diseases of women.

Drug Abuse

The use of marihuana (pot) in the United States has increased rapidly. Marihuana enters the bloodstream swiftly and acts on the brain and nervous system. Rapid pulse, decreased body temperature, reddening of the eyes, and incoordination of movement may be seen. There may be a distortion in the person's sense of distance, hearing, and time. In large doses, marihuana can cause visual hallucinations or illusions. Although it is at present classified as a drug on which dependence rather than true addiction develops, persons using it may proceed to other forms of abuse.

LSD (acid), also a "hallucinogen," affects the mind. Its continued use impedes concentration. "Trips" can be very frightening to youngsters and have been known to contribute to acts of murder or suicide. It can also lead to acute or chronic mental illness. The use of LSD is thought to produce changes in the chromosomes of the body which could cause malignancy in the patient or malformation of the offspring. It is against the law to illegally possess marihuana or LSD and the teenager using either of them is subject to punishment by law. This may mean a police record and interruption of his education. His personality may be further affected, since he is in a precarious stage of emotional growth and development.

Drugs such as Benzedrine, Dexedrine, and Methedrine from the amphetamine family are also subject to abuse. Normally used to control fatigue and appetite, they may disguise the normal warning signs of fatigue when used promiscuously. These drugs are known in slang terminology as "pep pills," "bennies," or "speed". The practical nurse should be aware that such abuses by teenagers do take place. She should report behavior which she considers bizarre. The nurse should also avail herself of community opportunities to learn about the prevention and treatment of such conditions.

STUDY QUESTIONS

1. Differentiate between the human and bovine types of tuberculosis.
2. Define the following: BCG vaccine, miliary tuberculosis, Mantoux test, PPD, Tine test.
3. Mrs. Wright, a practical nurse student, has just finished mopping the floor in the room of her patient who has tuberculosis. Discuss how she would safely care for the mop and water following this

procedure. From your knowledge of the tubercle bacillus, what is the potential danger of failure to carry out this procedure properly?

4. How do the symptoms of tuberculosis differ in the child?

5. Name three drugs currently used in the treatment of tuberculosis.

6. What practical everyday matters would be of greatest concern to you if you were told that you had to enter a sanatorium as soon as possible?

7. What is the role of the practical nurse in the prevention of tuberculosis?

8. What problems confront the obese adolescent?

9. What are the dangers of obesity?

10. Mrs. Harris, a practical nurse, states, "Weight reduction is merely a matter of will power." Do you agree with this statement? how will her dealings with obese patients be affected by this attitude?

11. Why is acne such a problem during adolescence?

12. What problems confront the teenager who uses drugs indiscriminately?

BIBLIOGRAPHY

Blake, F., and Wright, F. H.: Essentials of Pediatric Nursing. Philadelphia, J. B. Lippincott Co., 1963.

Hammar, S., and Eddy, J.: Nursing Care of the Adolescent. New York, Springer Publishing Co., Inc., 1966.

Lederle Laboratories: Tuberculin Tine Test. Pearl River, New York, 1966.

Marlow, D.: Textbook of Pediatric Nursing. 3rd Ed. Philadelphia, W. B. Saunders Co., 1969.

Mason, M.: Basic Medical-Surgical Nursing. New York, The Macmillan Co., 1967.

Nelson, W. (editor): Textbook of Pediatrics. 9th Ed. Philadelphia, W. B. Saunders Co., 1969.

Shearman, C.: Diets Are for People. New York, Appleton-Century-Crofts, 1963.

Spock, B.: Baby and Child Care. Rev. Ed. New York, Duell, Sloan and Pearce, Inc., 1968.

United States Department of Health, Education, and Welfare: Hung on LSD . . . Stuck in Glue? 1968.

GLOSSARY

Amniocentesis: A needle is placed into the uterus of an expectant mother to obtain a specimen of amniotic fluid for analysis. This is done to determine possible damage to the fetus by Rh incompatability.

Angioma: A tumor, usually benign, which is made up chiefly of blood and lymph vessels.

Ascariasis: Roundworm infestation.

Atelectasis: Incomplete expansion of the lungs at birth or a collapse after expansion due to mucus plug, tumor, pressure from organs and other causes.

Atresia: A congenital anomaly in which a normal opening is absent, e.g., atresia of the esophagus.

Bradford frame: A special oblong frame made of one inch pipe, covered with canvas strips, and supported by blocks to raise it from the mattress. The canvas strips are movable, thus the patient can urinate and defecate without moving the spine.

Bryant traction: A type of traction apparatus commonly used for toddlers suffering from a fractured femur. Vertical suspension is used.

Cardiac decompensation: Heart failure.

Celiac syndrome: An inability to absorb fats which results in malnutrition, vitamin deficiency, foul bulky stools, and a distended abdomen.

Cephalocaudal: The orderly development of muscular control which proceeds from head to foot and from the center of the body to the periphery.

Chronic ulcerative colitis: A serious chronic inflammatory disease of the large intestine.

Circumcision: The surgical removal of the foreskin of the penis.

Cleft lip and palate: Congenital anomalies due to failure of the embryonic structures of the face to unite. Characterized by an opening in the upper lip or palate.

Clubfoot: A congenital orthopedic anomaly, characterized by a foot which has been twisted inward or outward.

Coarctation of the aorta: A constriction of the aortic arch or of the descending aorta.

Congenital anomaly: A malformation present at birth.

Cretinism: A congenital defect in the secretion of the thyroid hormones, characterized by physical and mental retardation.

Cryptorchidism: Failure of the testicles to descend into the scrotum.

Cystic fibrosis: A generalized disorder of the exocrine glands, especially the mucous and sweat glands. The lungs and pancreas in particular are involved.

Cystic hygroma: A lymphangioma most frequently seen in the neck and the axillae.

Deciduous teeth: Baby teeth.

Denis Browne splint: Two separate footplates attached to a crossbar and fitted to a child's shoes, used in the correction of clubfeet.

DNA (Deoxyribonucleic acid): A complex protein believed to be the storehouse of hereditary information. It is present in the chromosomes of cell nuclei.

Down's syndrome: A form of mental retardation caused by chromosomal defects; formerly known as mongolism.

Ductus arteriosus, patent: A congenital anomaly in which the opening between the aorta and the pulmonary artery fails to close after birth.

Dyspnea: Difficult breathing.

Eczema: An inflammation of the skin, frequently associated with an allergy to food protein or environment.

Empyema: Pus, especially in the chest cavity.

Encephalitis: An inflammation of the brain.

Enuresis: Abnormal inability to control urine; may be due to organic or psychological problems.

Ephebiatrics: A specialty concerned with the problems of young people.

Epilepsy: A convulsive disease, characterized by seizures and loss of consciousness.

Erythroblastosis fetalis: Physiologic hemolytic anemia due to blood incompatability. Associated with babies born of Rh positive fathers and Rh negative mothers.

Fontanels: Openings at the point of union of skull bones, often referred to as "soft spots."

Gavage: Feeding the patient by means of a stomach tube or with a tube passed through the nose, pharynx, and esophagus into the stomach.

Genetics: The study of heredity.

Hemangioma: A benign tumor of the skin which consists of blood vessels.

Hemophilia: A hereditary disease, characterized by an abnormal tendency to bleed.

Hirschsprung's disease: Megacolon; enlargement of the colon without evidence of mechanical obstruction. There is a congenital absence of ganglionic cells in the distal segment of the colon.

Hyaline membrane disease: Respiratory distress often seen in prematures in which a membranous substance lines the alveoli of the lungs, preventing the exchange of gases.

Hydrocele: An abnormal collection of fluid surrounding the testicles, causing the scrotum to swell.

Hydrocephalus: A congenital anomaly, characterized by an increase of cerebrospinal fluid of the ventricles of the brain which results in an increase in the size of the head and in pressure changes in the brain.

Hyperbaric oxygen therapy: Oxygen administered under increased atmospheric pressure to increase the oxygen pressure within the blood. The patient is enclosed in a sealed chamber.

Hypospadias: A developmental anomaly in which the urethra opens on the lower surface of the penis.

Imperforate anus: A congenital anomaly in which there is no anal opening.

Impetigo: An infectious disease of the skin, caused by staphylococci or streptococci.

Infant mortality: The ratio between the number of deaths of infants less than one year of age during any given year and the number of live births occurring in the same year.

Infectious mononucleosis: A generalized disease causing enlargement of the lymph tissues throughout the body. There is an increase in the number of mononuclear leukocytes in the blood. It occurs mainly in older children and adolescents.

Interatrial septal defect: An abnormal opening between the right and left atria of the heart. Blood which contains oxygen is forced from the left to the right atrium.

Intertrigo: A chafe of the skin which occurs when two skin surfaces come together.

Interventricular septal defect: An opening between the right and left ventricle of the heart. Blood passes directly from the left to the right ventricle.

Kernicterus: A grave form of jaundice of the newborn, accompanied by brain damage.

Laryngotracheobronchitis: Inflammation of the larynx, trachea, and bronchi.

Lonalac: Low salt formula.

Meckel's diverticulum: A congenital blind pouch, sometimes seen in the lower part of the ileum. A cord may continue to the umbilicus or a fistula may open at the umbilicus. An intestinal obstruction may occur if the cord becomes strangulated. Corrected by surgery.

Meconium: The first stool of the newborn; a mixture of amniotic fluid and secretions of the intestinal glands.

Meconium ileus: A deficiency of pancreatic enzymes in the intestinal tract in which the meconium of the fetus becomes excessively sticky and adheres to the intestinal wall, causing obstruction. Occasionally seen in babies born with cystic fibrosis.

Megacolon: See *Hirschsprung's disease.*

Meningocele: A congenital anomaly, caused by a protrusion of the *meninges* or membranes through an opening in the spinal column.

Meningomyelocele: A congenital anomaly, characterized by a protrusion of the *membranes* and *spinal cord* through an opening in the spinal column.

Microcephaly: A congenital anomaly in which the head of the newborn is abnormally small.

Miliaria: Prickly heat; inflammation of the skin caused by sweating.

Mongolism: See *Down's syndrome.*

Moro reflex: When a newborn is jarred, he will draw his legs up and fold his arms across his chest in an embrace position.

Mucoviscidosis: See *Cystic fibrosis.*

Murmur: A sound heard when listening to the heart, caused by blood leaking through openings that have not closed.

Muscular dystrophy: Wasting away and atrophy of muscles. There are several forms, all having some common characteristics.

Nevus (pl. *nevi*): A congenital discoloration of an area of the skin, such as a strawberry mark, mole, and so forth.

Niemann-Pick disease: A hereditary disease in which there is a disturbance in the metabolism of lipoids (substances resembling fats), causing physical and mental retardation.

Omphalocele: A herniation of the abdominal contents at the umbilicus.

Ophthalmia neonatorum: Acute conjunctivitis of the newborn, caused by the gonococci of gonorrhea, a venereal disease.

Orthopnea: The patient has to sit up in order to breathe.

Osteogenesis imperfecta: A congenital bone disease in which the bones fracture easily.

Otitis media: Inflammation of the middle ear.

Paraphimosis: Impaired circulation of the uncircumcised penis due to improper retraction of the foreskin.

Patent ductus arteriosus: One of the most common cardiac anomalies, in which the ductus arteriosus fails to close. Blood continues to flow from the aorta into the pulmonary artery.

Phenylketonuria (P.K.U.): An inborn error of metabolism causing retardation; the body is unable to utilize phenylalanine, an amino acid.

Phimosis: A tightening of the prepuce of the uncircumcised penis.

Poliomyelitis: An acute infectious disease of the brain stem and spinal cord.

Pyloric stenosis: A congenital narrowing of the pylorus of the stomach due to an enlarged muscle.

Rapport: Harmonious relation.

Rectal prolapse: A dropping or protrusion of the mucosa of the rectum through the anus.

Retrolental fibroplasia: Blindness of a premature infant, caused by an over-exposure to oxygen. The blood vessels of the retina become damaged.

Rickets: A disease of the bones, caused by lack of calcium or vitamin D.

Rooting reflex: The infant turns his head toward anything which touches his cheek as a means of reaching food.

Rubella: German measles.

Rubeola: Measles.

Scoliosis: Lateral curvature of the spine.

Scurvy: A disease caused by the lack of vitamin C in the diet, and characterized by joint pains, bleeding gums, loose teeth, and lack of energy.

Shunt: A bypass.

Spina bifida: A congenital defect in which there is an imperfect closure of the spinal canal.

Talipes equinovarus: See *Clubfoot*.

Tay-Sachs disease: Infantile amaurotic family idiocy.

Tetralogy of Fallot: A congenital heart defect involving pulmonary stenosis, ventricular septal defect, dextroposition of the aorta, and hypertrophy of the right ventricle.

Thalassemia: A hereditary blood disorder in which the patient's body cannot produce sufficient hemoglobin.

Thrush: An infection of the mucous membranes of the mouth or throat caused by the fungus *Candida*.

Tinea: A contagious fungus infection; ringworm.

Torticollis: Wryneck; a condition in which the head inclines to one side because of a shortening of either sternocleidomastoid muscle.

Tracheoesophageal fistula: The esophagus, instead of being an open tube from the throat to the stomach, is closed at some point. A fistula between the trachea and the esophagus is common.

Truncus arteriosus: A single arterial trunk leaves the ventricular portion of the heart and supplies the pulmonary, coronary, and systemic circulations.

Turgor: Good elasticity of skin.

Varicella: Chickenpox.

Variola: Smallpox.

Ventriculography: X-ray examination of the ventricles of the brain following the injection of air into the ventricles.

Vernix caseosa: A cheese-like substance which covers the skin of a newborn.

Volvulus: A twisting of the loops of the small intestine, causing obstruction.

Wilms' tumor: A malignant tumor of the kidneys.

INDEX